T0261794

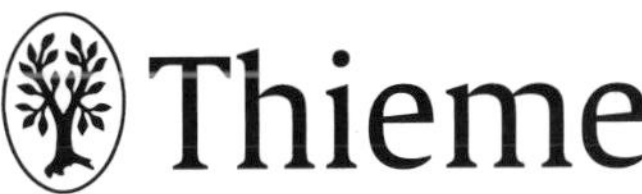
Thieme

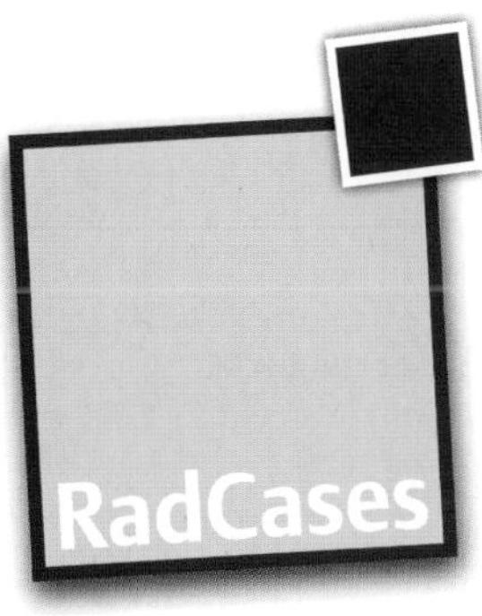

RadCases Ultrasound Imaging

Edited by

Nami Azar, MD
Associate Professor of Radiology
Director, Center for Interventional Radiology
Section Head, Ultrasound
Abdominal and Cross-Sectional Intervention Fellowship Director
Department of Radiology
University Hospitals Case Medical Center
Cleveland, Ohio

Carolyn Donaldson, MD
Clinical Assistant Professor
University of Chicago, Pritzker School of Medicine
Chicago, Illinois
NorthShore University HealthSystem
Evanston, Illinois

Series Editors

Jonathan Lorenz, MD
Associate Professor of Radiology
Department of Radiology
The University of Chicago
Chicago, Illinois

Hector Ferral, MD
Senior Clinical Educator
NorthShore University HealthSystem
Evanston, Illinois

Thieme
New York • Stuttgart • Delhi • Rio

Executive Editor: William Lamsback
Managing Editor: J. Owen Zurhellen IV
Editorial Assistant: Heather Allen
Senior Vice President, Editorial and Electronic Product Development: Cornelia Schulze
Production Editor: Teresa Exley, Maryland Composition
International Production Director: Andreas Schabert
International Marketing Director: Fiona Henderson
Director of Sales, North America: Mike Roseman
International Sales Director: Louisa Turrell
Senior Vice President and Chief Operating Officer: Sarah Vanderbilt
President: Brian D. Scanlan
Compositor: MPS Limited

Library of Congress Cataloging-in-Publication Data

RadCases ultrasound imaging/edited by Nami Azar, Carolyn Donaldson.
p. ; cm.–(RadCases)
Ultrasound imaging
ISBN 978-1-60406-322-6
I. Azar, Nami, editor. II. Donaldson, Carolyn (Diagnostic radiologist), editor. III. Title: Ultrasound imaging. IV. Series: RadCases.
[DNLM: 1. Ultrasonography–Case Reports. 2. Diagnosis, Differential–Case Reports. WN 208]
RC78.7.U4
616.07'543–dc23 2014025179

Important note: Medicine is an ever-changing science undergoing continual development. Research and clinical experience are continually expanding our knowledge, in particular our knowledge of proper treatment and drug therapy. Insofar as this book mentions any dosage or application, readers may rest assured that the authors, editors, and publishers have made every effort to ensure that such references are in accordance with the **state of knowledge at the time of production of the book**.

Nevertheless, this does not involve, imply, or express any guarantee or responsibility on the part of the publishers in respect to any dosage instructions and forms of applications stated in the book. **Every user is requested to examine carefully** the manufacturers' leaflets accompanying each drug and to check, if necessary in consultation with a physician or specialist, whether the dosage schedules mentioned therein or the contraindications stated by the manufacturers differ from the statements made in the present book. Such examination is particularly important with drugs that are either rarely used or have been newly released on the market. Every dosage schedule or every form of application used is entirely at the user's own risk and responsibility. The authors and publishers request every user to report to the publishers any discrepancies or inaccuracies noticed. If errors in this work are found after publication, errata will be posted at www.thieme.com on the product description page.

Some of the product names, patents, and registered designs referred to in this book are in fact registered trademarks or proprietary names even though specific reference to this fact is not always made in the text. Therefore, the appearance of a name without designation as proprietary is not to be construed as a representation by the publisher that it is in the public domain.

Thieme Publishers New York
333 Seventh Avenue
New York, NY 10001 USA
1-800-782-3488, customerservice@thieme.com

Thieme Publishers Stuttgart
Rüdigerstrasse 14 70469 Stuttgart, Germany
+49 [0]711 8931 421, customerservice@thieme.de

Thieme Publishers Delhi
A-12, Second Floor, Sector -2, NOIDA -201301
Uttar Pradesh, India
+91 120 45 566 00, customerservice@thieme.in

Thieme Publishers Rio, Thieme Publicações Ltda.
Argentina Building 16th floor, Ala A, 228 Praia do Botafogo
Rio de Janeiro 22250-040 Brazil
+55 21 3736-3631

Printed in China by Everbest Printing Ltd.

ISBN 978-1-60406-322-6

Also available as an e-book:
eISBN 978-1-60406-323-3

To our daughters, Marie and Julia, for their resilience and many sacrifices on behalf of my work. I hope that you too will be passionate about whatever it is you do in life. And to Jim, who has always been my rock.

Carolyn Donaldson, MD

I would like to dedicate this book to my wife, Dana, and my daughter, Nelly, for their endless support. Great thanks for my friends in the ultrasound department at University Hospitals of Cleveland for the amazing work, great cases, and continuous encouragement.

Nami Azar, MD

RadCases Series Preface

The ability to assimilate detailed information across the entire spectrum of radiology is the Holy Grail sought by those preparing for the American Board of Radiology examination. As enthusiastic partners in the Thieme RadCases Series who formerly took the examination, we understand the exhaustion and frustration shared by residents and the families of residents engaged in this quest. It has been our observation that despite ongoing efforts to improve Web-based interactive databases, residents still find themselves searching for material they can review while preparing for the radiology board examinations and remain frustrated by the fact that only a few printed guidebooks are available, which are limited in both format and image quality. Perhaps their greatest source of frustration is the inability to easily locate groups of cases across all subspecialties of radiology that are organized and tailored for their immediate study needs. Imagine being able to immediately access groups of high-quality cases to arrange study sessions, quickly extract and master information, and prepare for theme-based radiology conferences. Our goal in creating the RadCases Series was to combine the popularity and portability of printed books with the adaptability, exceptional quality, and interactive features of an electronic case-based format.

The intent of the printed book is to encourage repeated priming in the use of critical information by providing a portable group of exceptional core cases that the resident can master. The best way to determine the format for these cases was to ask residents from around the country to weigh in. Overwhelmingly, the residents said that they would prefer a concise, point-by-point presentation of the Essential Facts of each case in an easy-to-read, bulleted format. This approach is easy on exhausted eyes and provides a quick review of Pearls and Pitfalls as information is absorbed during repeated study sessions. We worked hard to choose cases that could be presented well in this format, recognizing the limitations inherent in reproducing high-quality images in print. Unlike the authors of other case-based radiology review books, we removed the guesswork by providing clear annotations and descriptions for all images. In our opinion, there is nothing worse than being unable to locate a subtle finding on a poorly reproduced image even after one knows the final diagnosis.

The electronic cases expand on the printed book and provide a comprehensive review of the entire subspecialty. Thousands of cases are strategically designed to increase the resident's knowledge by providing exposure to additional case examples—from basic to advanced—and by exploring "Aunt Minnie's," unusual diagnoses, and variability within a single diagnosis. The search engine gives the resident a fighting chance to find the Holy Grail by creating individualized, daily study lists that are not limited by factors such as radiology subsection. For example, tailor today's study list to cases involving tuberculosis and include cases in every subspecialty and every system of the body. Or study only thoracic cases, including those with links to cardiology, nuclear medicine, and pediatrics. Or study only musculoskeletal cases. The choice is yours.

As enthusiastic partners in this project, we started small and, with the encouragement, talent, and guidance of Tim Hiscock at Thieme, we have continued to raise the bar in our effort to assist residents in tackling the daunting task of assimilating massive amounts of information. We are passionate about continuing this journey, hoping to expand the cases in our electronic series, adapt cases based on direct feedback from residents, and increase the features intended for board review and self-assessment. As the American Board of Radiology converts its certifying examinations to an electronic format, our series will be the one best suited to meet the needs of the next generation of overworked and exhausted residents in radiology.

Jonathan Lorenz, MD
Hector Ferral, MD
Chicago, IL

Preface

This book of the RadCases series is a comprehensive review of all specialties from vascular ultrasound (US) to obstetrics. The advantage of this US review is that it includes video clips, which is how the boards are now conducted. Although the RadCases series typically presents pathology, some normal cases are included. It is important to be able to recognize the normal appearance of things such as the endometrium and the different carotid waveforms.

Unlike other imaging modalities, US is widely used in multiple medical specialties by many persons of varied levels of expertise. Many urologists and gynecologists have ultrasound machines in their offices. Currently, there is discussion about medical students being given a portable US machine at the same time as they receive their stethoscopes. Therefore, it is important as radiologists that we maintain a level of expertise in ultrasound.

Ultrasound is the least sexy imaging modality in radiology. It is labor intensive, operator dependent, and the random planes of section make it difficult for the radiologist to interpret. With the RVU pressure, radiologists shy away from scanning. However, because of the lack of radiation, need for contrast, and the relatively inexpensive cost, US will not be phased out by CT or MR. With the image optimization provided by harmonics, Doppler, and elastography, US continues to evolve, ensuring its staying power.

The history of US is relatively short. Sonar, the initial use of US, was developed by the U.S. Navy in the 1950s to direct submarines. US was first used in clinical medicine in the 1970s. US equipment continues to improve with imaging optimization, including harmonics, and the diagnostic abilities of ultrasound allow for its staying power.

All of the cases are real-life patients whose studies have been read in the last several years. We are confident they will prepare you for the boards. They will provide confidence in your diagnostic capabilities practicing radiology, especially US.

Best of luck on boards,

Carolyn Donaldson, MD
Nami Azar, MD

Acknowledgements

I would like to acknowledge Hector Ferral for inviting me to coauthor this ultrasound book of the RadCases series. To Marie, who launched me electronically on this project from the start. Julia, who spent hours studying with me at Starbucks. To the University of Chicago residents and fellows, who reviewed and edited my cases while rotating on the ultrasound service. And, lastly, to the sonographers whose talent and tireless attention to detail allow me to look like I know what I am doing.

Carolyn Donaldson, MD

Thank you to Dr. Noam Lazebnik for your contributions to the cases.

Nami Azar, MD

Case 1

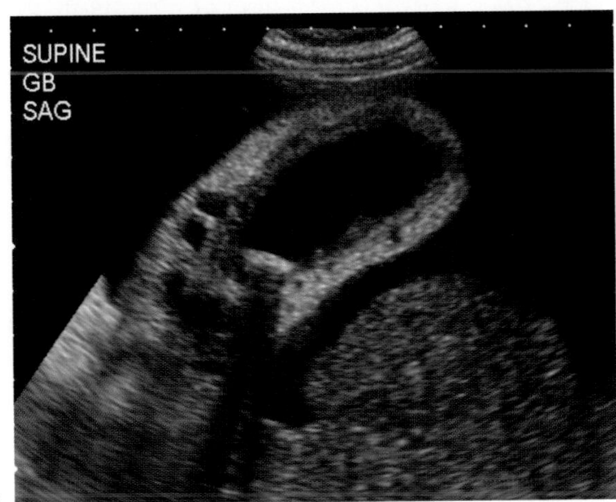

A

Clinical Presentation

A 49-year-old woman with history of hepatitis C presents for liver evaluation.

Further Work-up

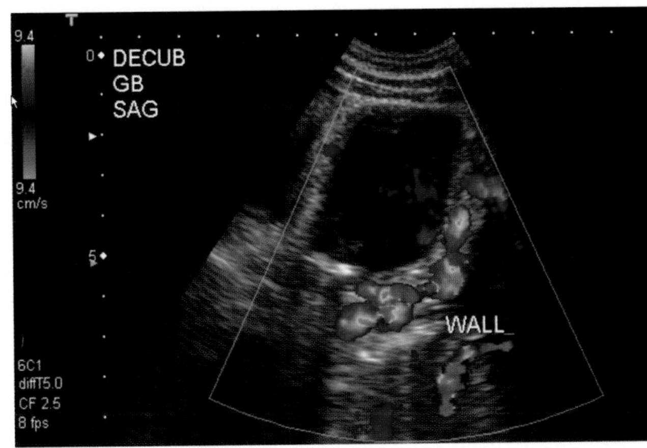

B

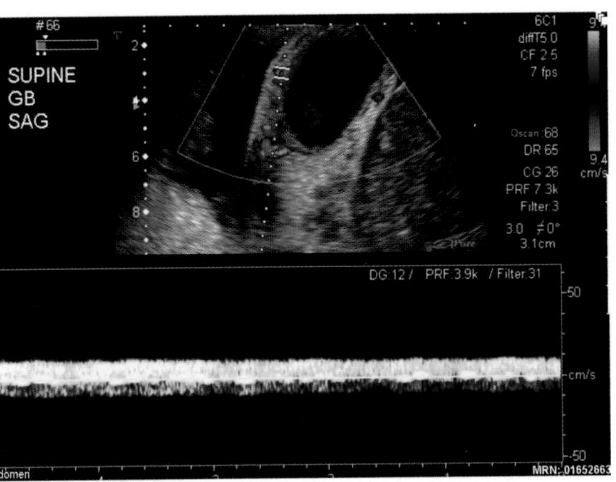

C

Imaging Findings

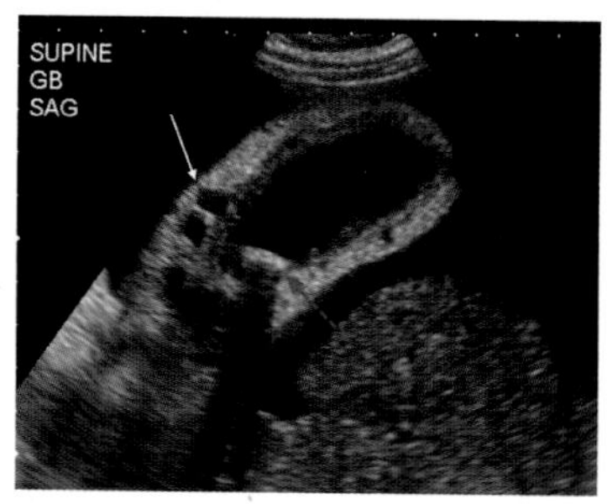

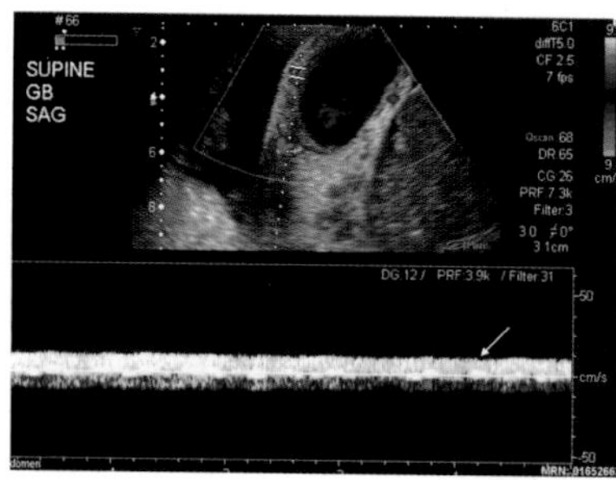

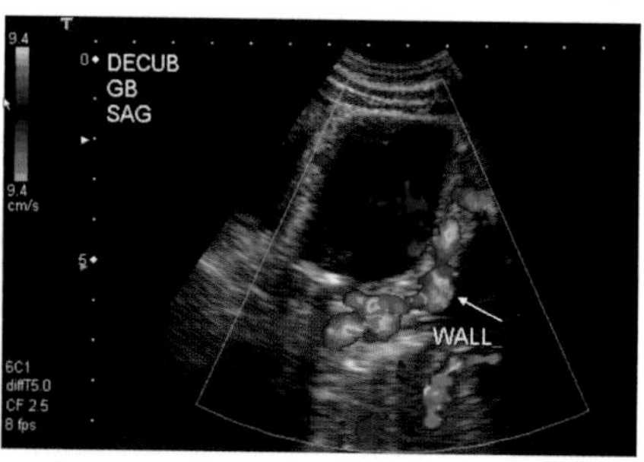

(A) Gray scale ultrasound image shows signs of liver cirrhosis and ascites. Cystic changes and wall thickening (*white arrow*) are noted in the gallbladder. Gallstone is also present (*red arrow*). **(B)** Color ultrasound demonstrates flow within the cystic lesion in the wall (*white arrow*). **(C)** Pulse Doppler tracing confirms the presence of flow, demonstrating monophasic (*arrow*), venous flow pattern (similar to the portal vein).

Differential Diagnosis

Vascular lesions of the gallbladder include wall varices, diffuse adenomyomatosis, and gallbladder cancer.

- ***Gallbladder varices:*** Usually seen as portosystemic collateral, a monophasic flow is usually present.
- *Diffuse adenomyomatosis:* The diffuse form is seen in 20% of patients with adenomyomatosis. The presence of twinkle artifact (noise on Doppler tracing) is suggestive of the diagnosis.
- *Gallbladder wall carcinoma:* Irregular wall thickening is seen. The presence of invasion and arterial flow raises the possibility of malignancy.

Essential Facts

- Likely associated with portal hypertension and or portal vein thrombosis. Rarely as a normal pathway.
- Portosystemic shunt linking the cystic vein branch of the portal vein to the anterior abdominal wall systemic collaterals.
- Could be formed as bypass around a focally thrombosed extrahepatic segment of the portal vein.
- Gallbladder varices may be related to dilated veins due to back pressure within the portal venous system in patients with chronic portal hypertension.

✓ Pearls & × Pitfalls

✓ The presence of portovenous flow in the gallbladder wall with cystic changes is characteristic of gallbladder varices.

× The presence of color in the gallbladder without characterizing the waveform/type of flow could be misleading with potential misdiagnosis.

Case 2

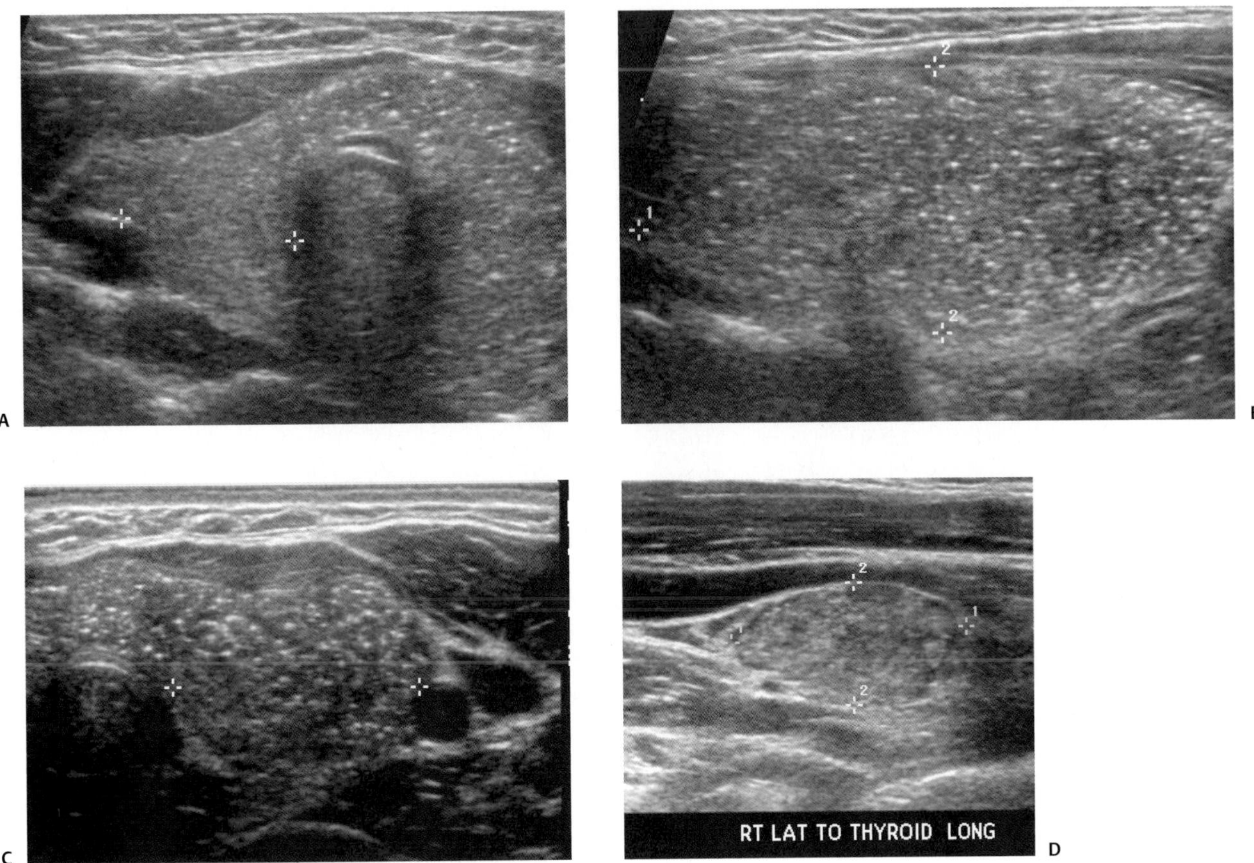

Clinical Presentation

A 15-year-old girl with enlarged left thyroid on exam.

Imaging Findings

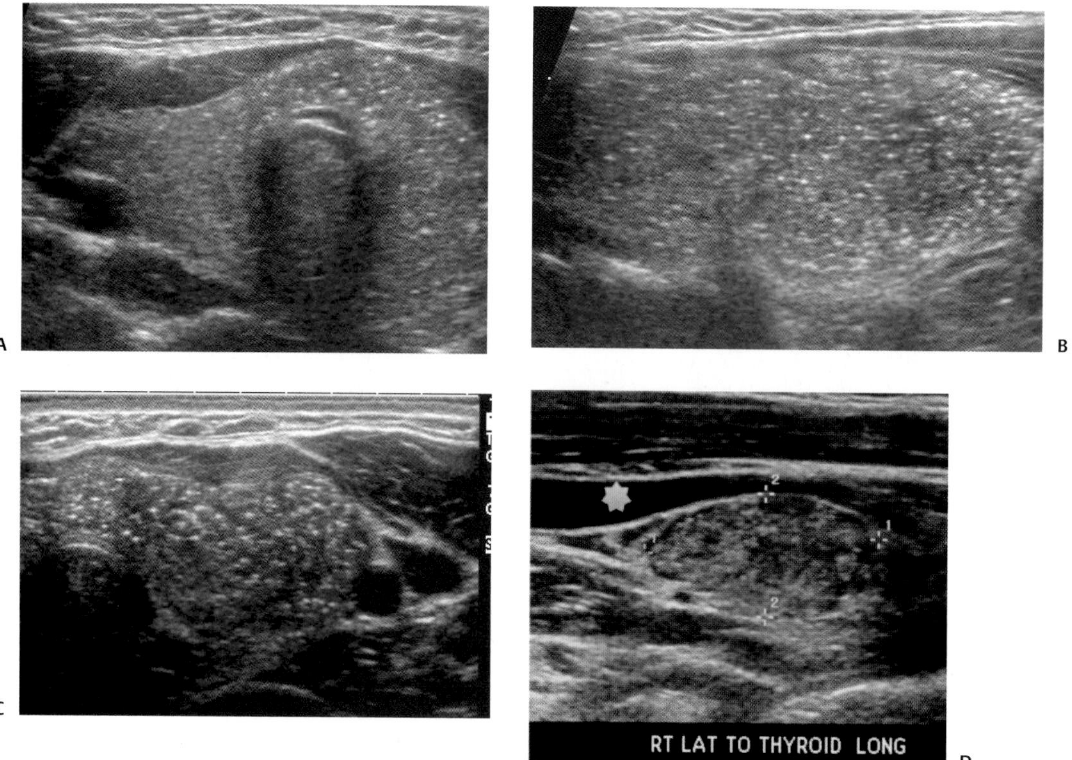

(A) Transverse image of the thyroid gland reveals an enlarged left lobe with distinctly different echotexture than the normal right lobe. Longitudinal **(B)** and transverse **(C)** images reveal a heterogeneous enlarged left lobe with innumerable echogenic foci throughout the gland. **(D)** An enlarged lymph node lateral to the thyroid is heterogeneous and contains microcalcifications. *Asterisk* denotes the jugular vein.

Differential Diagnosis

- ***Metastatic papillary thyroid cancer:*** Diffuse psammomatous calcifications or microcalcifications in the thyroid and a cervical lymph node is consistent with metastatic papillary thyroid cancer.
- *Diffuse thyroiditis:* The echotexture of the thyroid gland will be coarse or inhomogeneous in the setting of diffuse thyroiditis but punctate echogenic foci will not be present. It is usually symmetric bilaterally.
- *Chronic lymphocytic thyroiditis (also known as Hashimoto's thyroiditis):* A diffusely heterogeneous echotexture is seen with Hashimoto's thyroiditis. It is usually bilateral and fairly symmetric.

Essential Facts

- Microcalcifications even without an associated mass are highly suspicious for papillary thyroid cancer and warrant FNA.
- Psammoma bodies are laminated, basophilic, spherical concretions and are a characteristic finding of papillary thyroid carcinoma.
- Most microcalcifications seen with thyroid ultrasound represent psammoma bodies and are highly sensitive for malignancy.
- Diffuse microcalcifications from papillary thyroid cancer have a significant incidence of metastatic cervical nodes.
- Microcalcifications and cystic changes within a lymph node are suspicious for metastatic involvement.
- Loss of the normal fatty hilum and rounded shape of a lymph node are suspicious features of lymph nodes.

✓ Pearls & × Pitfalls

✓ Psammomatous calcifications are highly specific for papillary thyroid cancer (95% specific).

✓ Most psammomatous calcifications are seen in solid nodules.

✓ A cluster of microcalcifications in the thyroid gland is suspicious for malignancy even without an obvious mass lesion.

✓ Psammomatous calcifications can be seen in metastatic lymph nodes, including nonenlarged nodes.

✓ When areas of microcalcification are detected within the thyroid gland, evaluation of the cervical lymph nodes should be performed.

Case 3

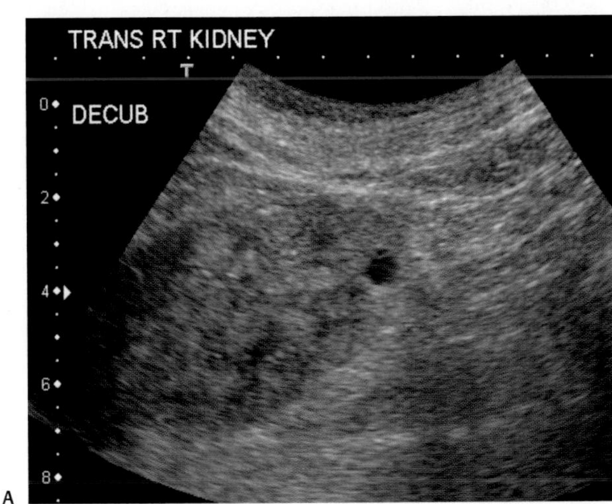

A

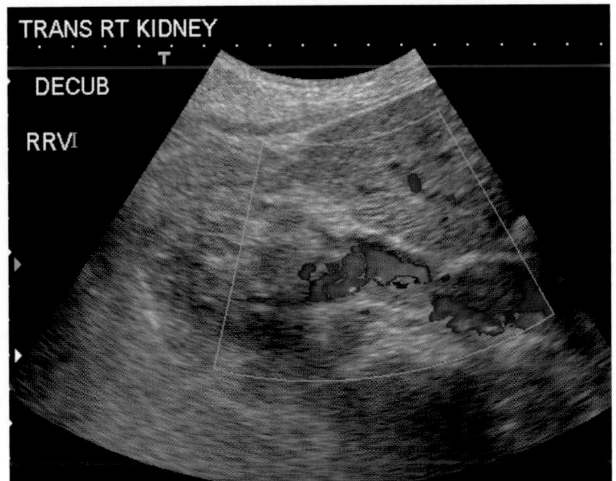

B

Clinical Presentation

A 82-year-old female presents with hematuria.

Further Work-up

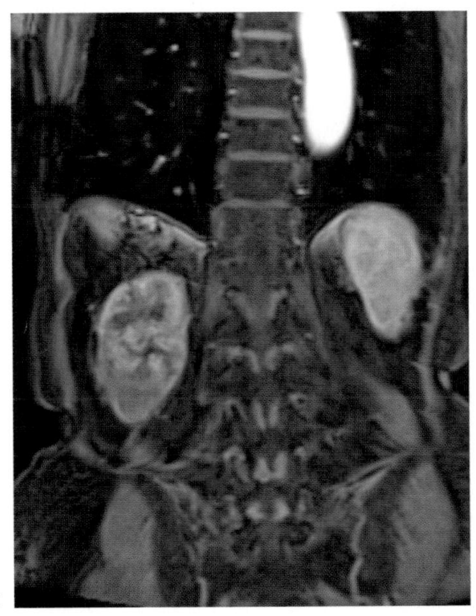

C

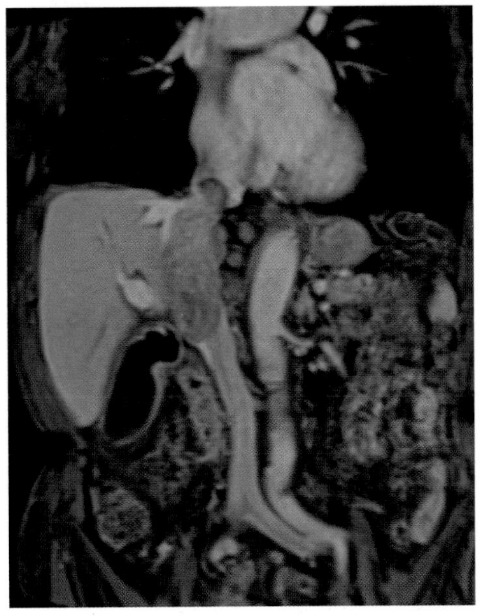

D

Imaging Findings

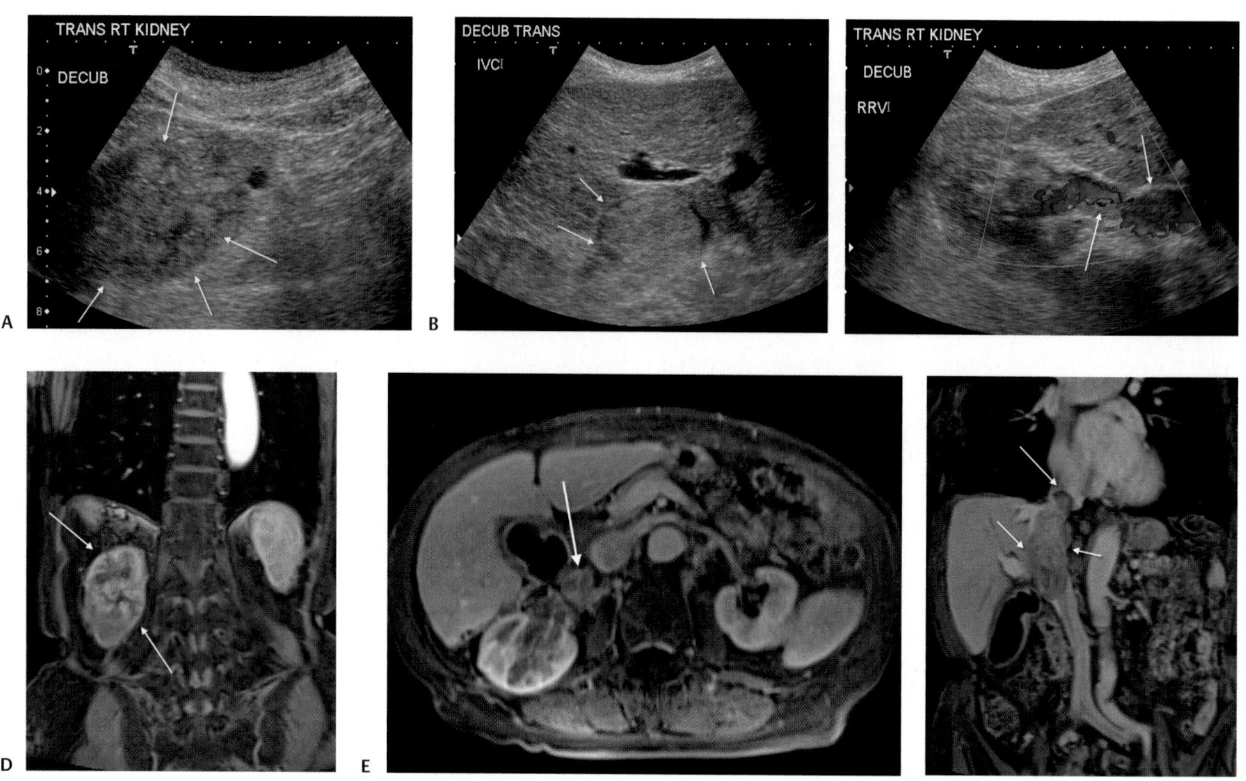

(A–F) Ultrasound images show a hypoechoic lesion in the posterior aspect of the right kidney (*arrows*, image **A**). Filling defect within the renal vein is noted extending into the IVC (*arrows*, image **B**). The invasion into the IVC is confirmed on color Doppler (*arrows*, image **C**). Contrast-enhanced MRI images of the kidneys show a hypervascular, enhancing mass in the posterior aspect of the right kidney (*arrows*, image **D**) with large filling defect in the renal vein (*arrow*, image **E**) with extension into the hepatic and thoracic segments of the IVC (*arrows*, image **F**).

Differential Diagnosis

- ***Renal cell carcinoma (RCC) with extension to the IVC:*** Appears as a hypoechoic, isoechoic, or echogenic mass lesion, extension into the IVC/periaortic adenopathy in suggestive of the diagnosis. Accurate staging is important for surgical planning.
- *Renal lymphoma:* The most common appearance is a focal renal mass, renal invasion from retroperitoneal mass, and/or infiltrative type. Renal involvement is secondary from either hematogenous or direct extension.
- *Leiomyosarcoma of the IVC with extension to the kidney:* Is an uncommon tumor with poor outcome. Appears as a filling defect in the IVC, with possible extension into the renal vein. The kidney could appear enlarged secondary to limited flow in the renal vein.

Essential facts

- Represent 3% of all adult malignancies and 86% of renal malignancies.
- Associated with von Hippel-Lindau (24 to 45% of patients will develop RCC).
- Appears as solid, hypoechoic, isoechoic, or hyperechoic mass.
- Increase flow on Doppler usually present, lack of flow doesn't exclude malignancy.
- Unilocular cystic RCC will show debris and irregular thick wall.
- Multilocular RCC will show cystic mass with septations. Flow within the septations could be seen on Doppler.

✓ Pearls & × Pitfalls

✓ Doppler and gray scale evaluation of the renal vein and IVC should be performed in the presence of renal mass lesion to exclude extension.

× Unilocular cystic RCC could be misinterpreted as hemorrhagic cyst. The presence of irregular, thick wall is suggestive of malignancy.

Case 4

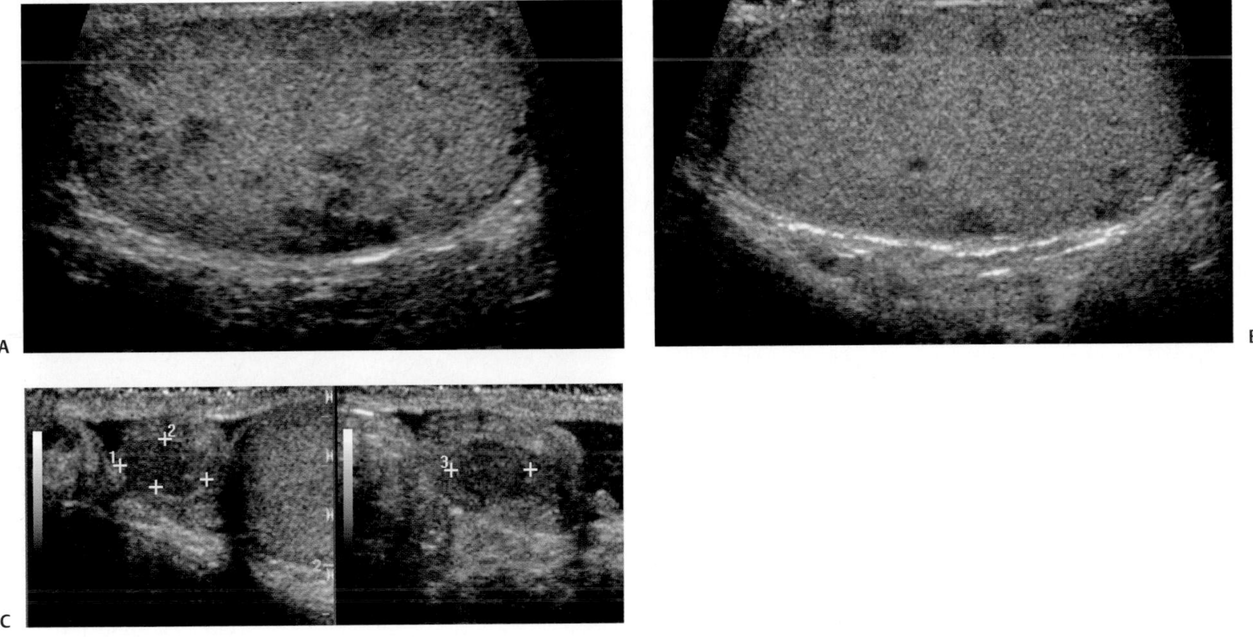

A B C

Clinical Presentation

A 38-year-old black man with nontender scrotal enlargement.

Further Work-up

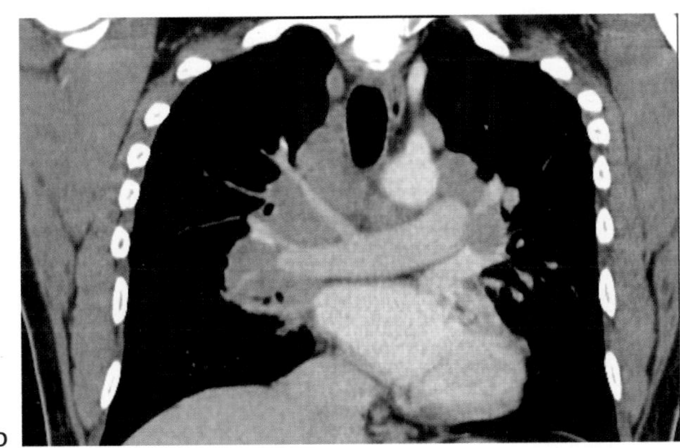

D

Imaging Findings

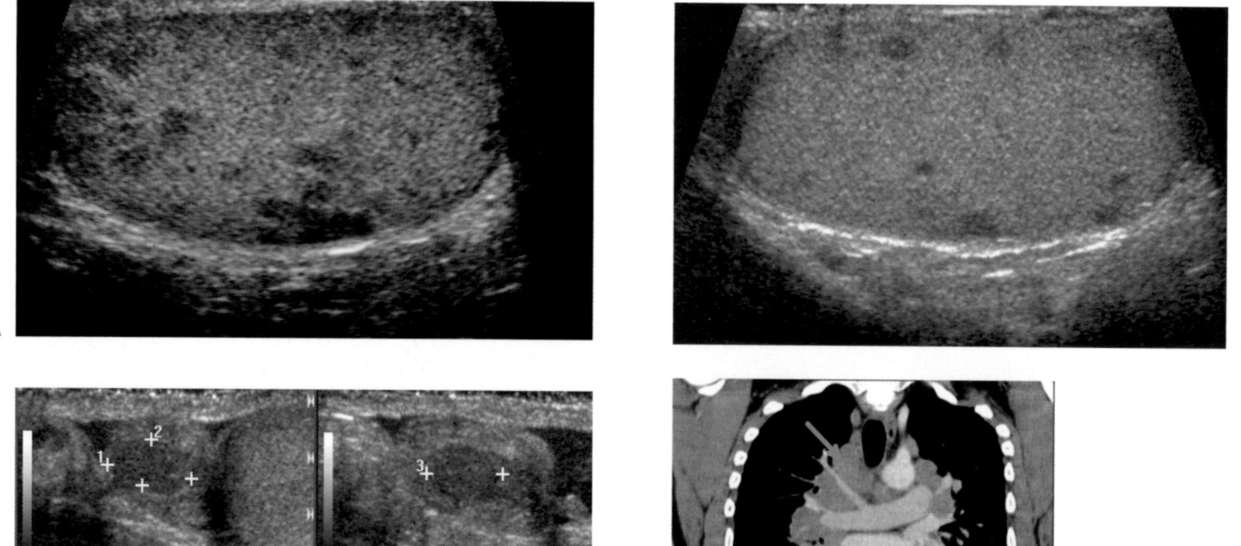

(A, B) Longitudinal gray scale images of each testicle demonstrates innumerable small hypoechoic lesions bilaterally. Similar lesions are present in the epididymis. **(C)** A right epididymal lesion is measured in image. **(D)** Coronal reformatted computed tomography (CT) image of the chest demonstrates bulky hilar and right paratracheal lymphadenopathy. *Arrow* denotes right paratracheal lymphadenopathy.

Differential Diagnosis

- ***Genitourinary sarcoidosis:*** Tuberculosis, fungal infections, syphilis, LGV, Wegeners granulomatous and sarcoidosis can all present with findings in the testicles. The epididymis is the most common site for involvement in genitourinary (GU) sarcoidosis. The bulky mediastinal and particularly right paratracheal lymphadenopathy seen on the subsequent CT of the chest are classic for sarcoidosis.
- *Lymphoma or leukemia:* Statistically, leukemia or lymphoma would be the most common cause for bilateral testicular masses. The testicles contain a barrier to chemotherapeutic agents that allows them to harbor leukemic or lymphomatous cells. Ultrasound findings in the setting of leukemic or lymphomatous infiltration of testicles would be similar to the images above. It usually occurs in older patients with a history of leukemia or lymphoma.
- *Metastatic disease to the testicles:* Usually occurs in the setting of widespread metastatic disease. Metastases to the testicles occur with numerous cancers but lung and prostate are the most frequent. Most testicular metastases are clinically silent and discovered at autopsy.

Essential Facts

- Sarcoidosis is a chronic disease of unknown etiology resulting in noncaseating granulomas involving multiple organ systems.
- Incidence of sarcoidosis in the United States is 1 in 10,000. African Americans have a 3 to 20 times higher incidence; women have a 10 times greater frequency than men.
- Involvement of the GU tract is rare, occurring in $< 1\%$ of patients with sarcoidosis. Sarcoidosis can affect any organ of the GU tract. The most common site of involvement is the epididymis, followed by the testes. It is associated with infertility.
- Sarcoidosis can mimic many conditions that require aggressive or invasive treatments. Biopsy may be required to exclude malignancy.
- Sarcoidosis is generally a self-limited condition and is most commonly treated conservatively with anti-inflammatory medications, including steroids.
- Sarcoidosis is usually diagnosed with bilateral hilar lymphadenopathy on chest radiograph. Patients with sarcoidosis usually present with dyspnea, cough, chest pain, or weight loss.

✓ Pearls & × Pitfalls

✓ In the setting of bilateral testicular masses, involvement of the epididymis will invariably be present with sarcoidosis.

✓ GU involvement of sarcoidosis occurs in the setting of other organ involvement, most typically the lungs with lymphadenopathy, as in this case.

× Testicular sarcoid typically occurs in black men ages 20 to 40, the same age group as testicular cancer.

Case 5

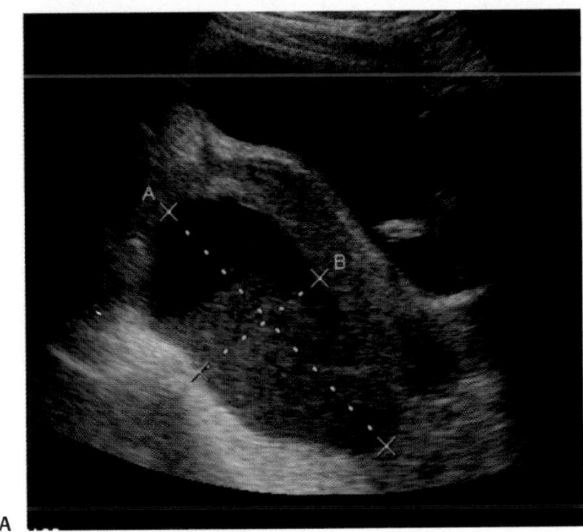

A

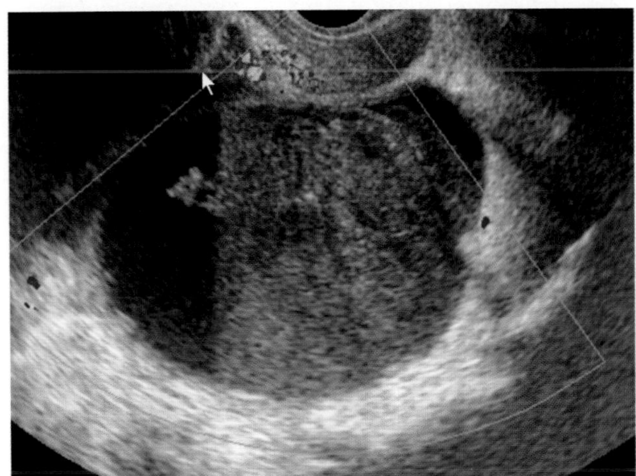

B

Clinical Presentation

A 35-year-old woman presents with pelvic pain and fever.

Further Work-up

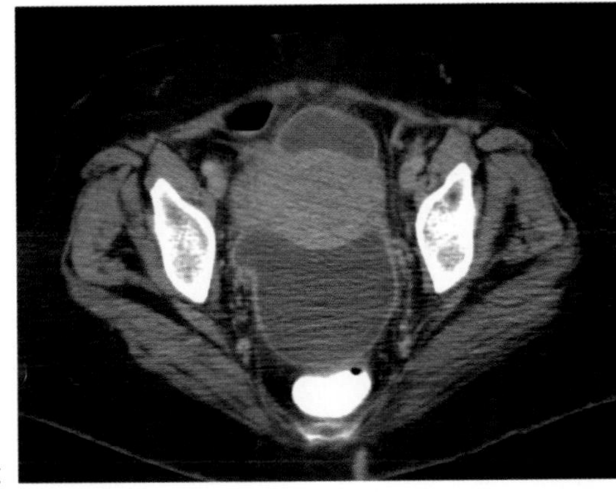

C

Imaging Findings

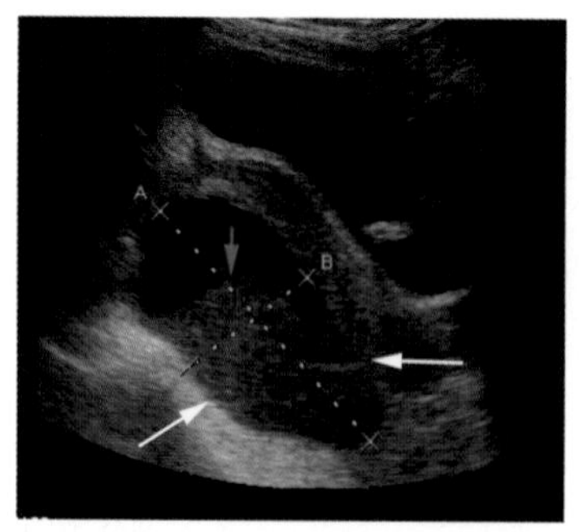
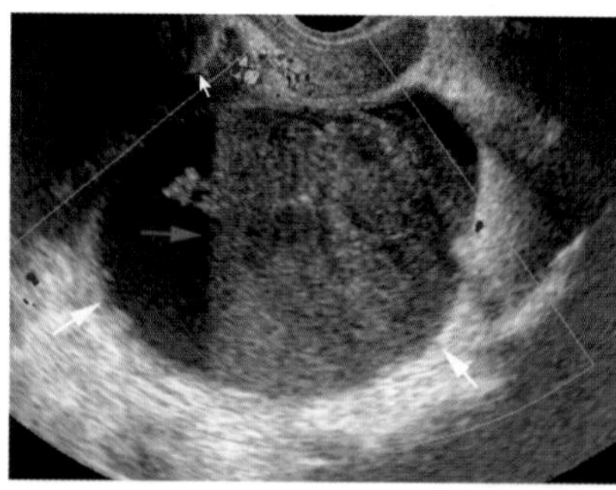
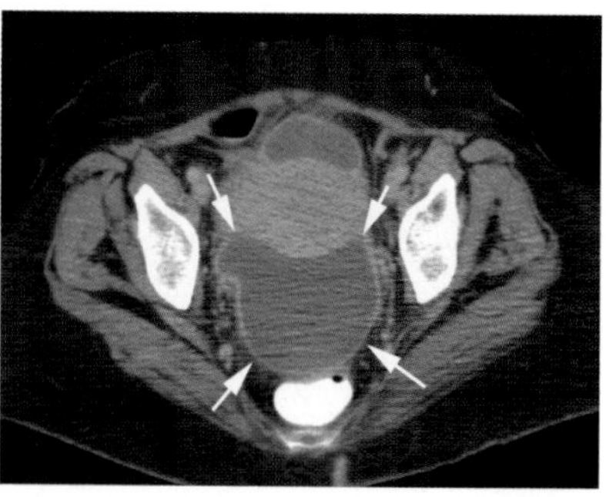

(A, B) Ultrasound images of the pelvis using transabdominal and transvaginal ultrasound show large, complex cystic lesion in the cul-de-sac (*white arrows*) with layering of low-level echoes and fluid-fluid level (*red arrow*). No gross evidence of air is noted on the current study. **(C)** Follow-up computed tomography of the pelvis demonstrates the same lesion with rim enhancement (*white arrows*). No evidence of intraluminal air is noted on the current study.

Differential Diagnosis

- ***Pelvic abscess:*** Appears as complex fluid collection with low-level echoes; no internal flow is seen on color images; peripheral flow occasionally can be seen.
- *Endometrioma:* Diffuse low-level echo with fluid-fluid levels is the typical sonographic appearance. The presence of wall echogenic reflectors/calcifications and multiloculation is suggestive of the diagnosis.
- *Cystic neoplasm:* Appears as complex collection with multiple irregular septations. The presence of arterial flow within the septations and nodularity is suggestive of the diagnosis.

Essential Facts

- The sources of pelvic abscesses include postoperative abscess, perforating appendicitis, diverticulitis, tubo-ovarian inflammation, Crohn disease, and internal bowel fistula due to irradiation.
- Patients present with fever and elevated white blood cells.
- It appears as complex fluid collection with occasional peripheral flow.
- Local tenderness during pelvic ultrasound is suggestive of the diagnosis.
- Imaging-guided drainage and antibiotics provide safe and effective treatment approach.

✓ Pearls & × Pitfalls

✓ Lack of internal arterial flow within a pelvic mass does not exclude cystic neoplasm.

× A necrotic pelvic mass could be misinterpreted as pelvic abscess or endometrioma.

Case 6

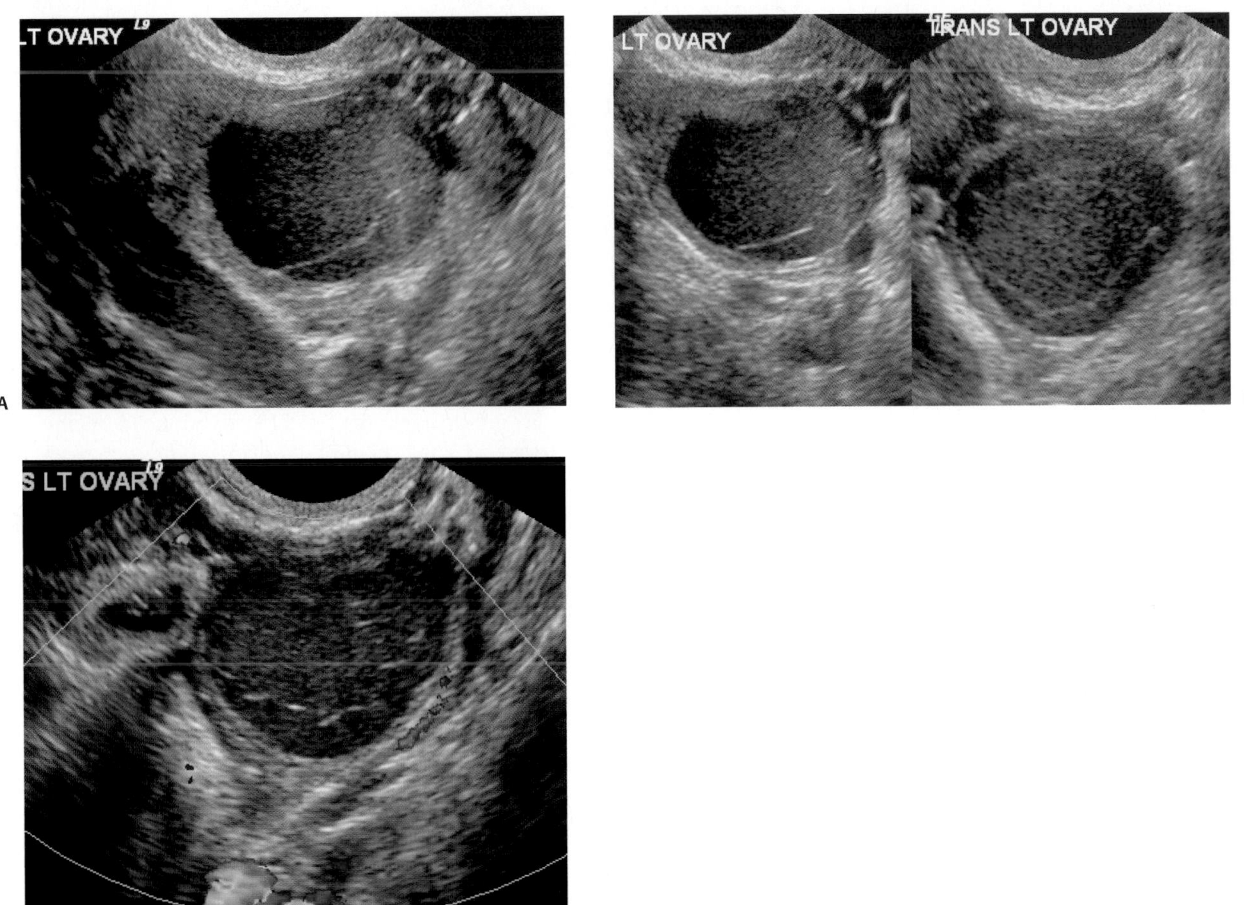

Clinical Presentation

A 32-year-old woman with sudden-onset left lower quadrant pain. Last menstrual period was 3 weeks ago.

Imaging Findings

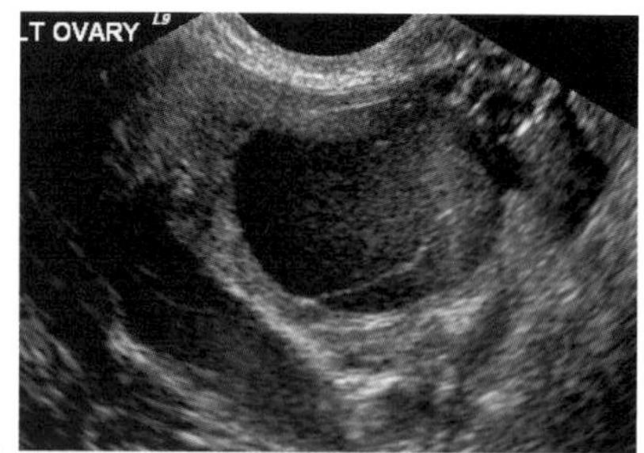

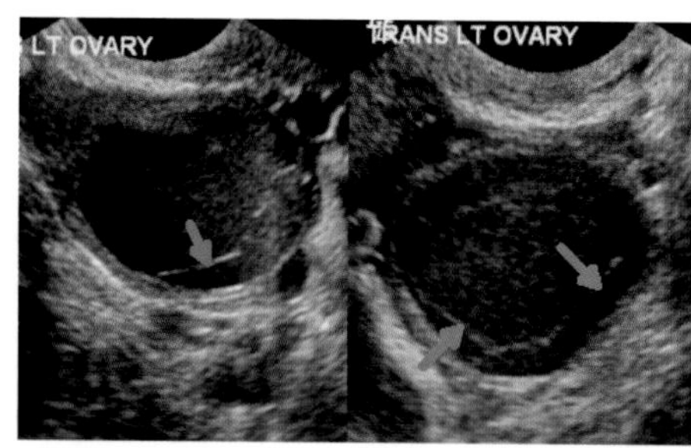

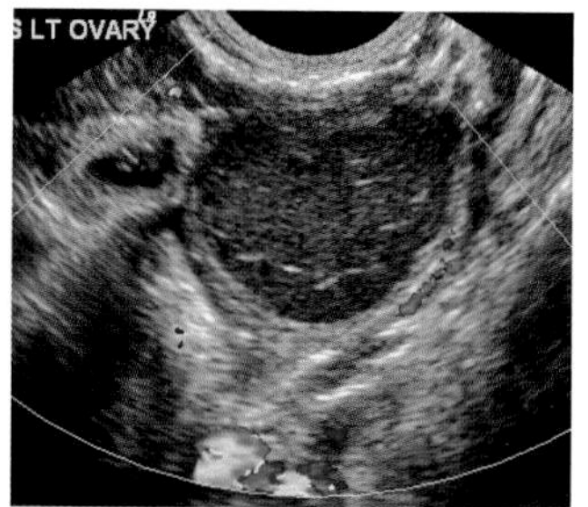

(A–C) The left ovary is enlarged due to a complex cystic lesion. The lesion contains layering debris in the sagittal (or longitudinal) view and fine interdigitating lines seen in both views (*arrows*). With color Doppler imaging, there is no internal vascularity. The lesion resolved on a follow-up study.

Differential Diagnosis

- ***Hemorrhagic cyst:*** Hemorrhagic cysts often have internal echoes with a pattern of fine interdigitating lines as seen in the above lesion. The debris is hemorrhage within the cyst. Because the lesion resolved on a follow-up study, it is consistent with a hemorrhagic cyst.
- *Endometrioma:* Low-level echoes typical of an endometrioma are present in the dependent portion of the lesion. Fine interdigitating lines are not typical of an endometrioma. An endometrioma would persist on a follow-up study.
- *Dermoid or teratoma:* Dermoids can contain a fluid layer. These layers are more distinct than the dependent debris in the above lesion. The more echogenic layering fat would be in the nondependent position in a dermoid.

Essential Facts

- Hemorrhagic cysts are the most common etiology for a complex cystic ovarian lesion. They are usually a result of hemorrhage into a corpus luteum or a ruptured follicle and can cause acute pain.
- The appearance of acute hemorrhage within a cyst is varied. The fine interdigitating lines are typical of hemorrhage. A retracting clot is also classic for hemorrhage.
- No flow is present within a hemorrhagic cyst with color or spectral Doppler imaging.
- Classic hemorrhagic cysts < 5 cm do not need to be followed up. They should be considered physiologic in a premenopausal woman.
- Hemorrhagic cysts typically resolve within 6 to 8 weeks. Therefore, if a complex cystic lesion is > 5 cm, a follow-up ultrasound in 6 to 12 weeks should be performed.
- Hemoperitoneum can result with rupture and hemorrhage of a cyst. Rarely, this requires surgical intervention.

Other Imaging Findings

- Computed tomography (CT) is not as sensitive as ultrasound in detection of a hemorrhagic cyst. The reticular pattern is not seen on CT. A hemorrhagic cyst can be isodense with the ovary and therefore not visible on CT.

✓ Pearls & × Pitfalls

✓ If a lesion is not classic for hemorrhage, recommend follow-up. A hemorrhagic cyst will resolve (or decrease considerably in size).

× The thin fibrin strands seen with hemorrhage can be confused with septations seen in other lesions including malignancy. Septations are usually thicker and may demonstrate flow with color.

Case 7

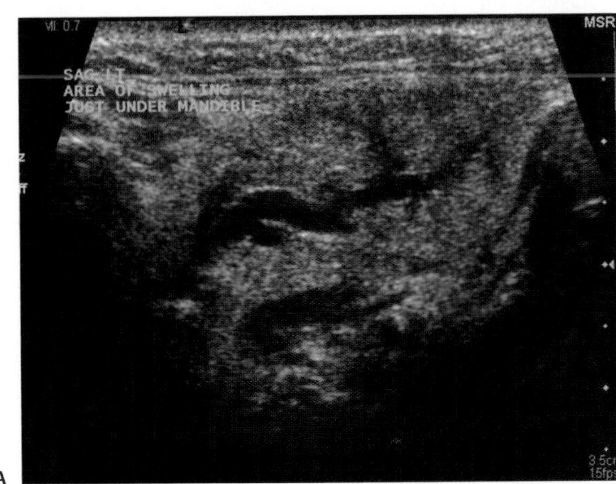

A

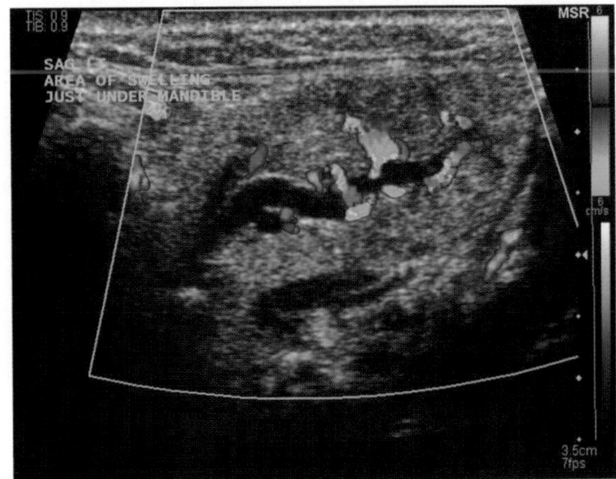

B

■ Clinical Presentation

A 45-year-old woman presents with left mandibular swelling.

■ Further Work-up

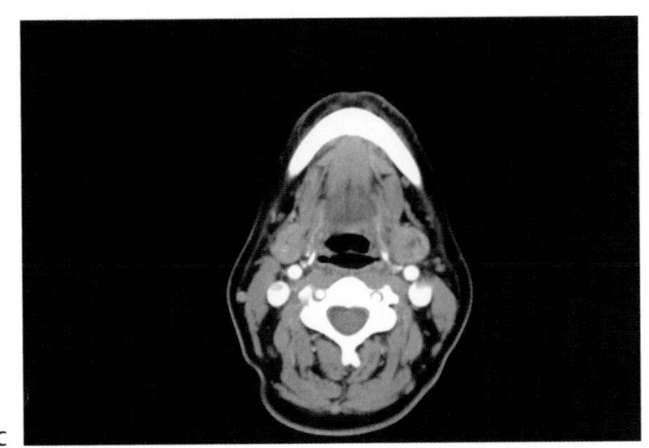
C

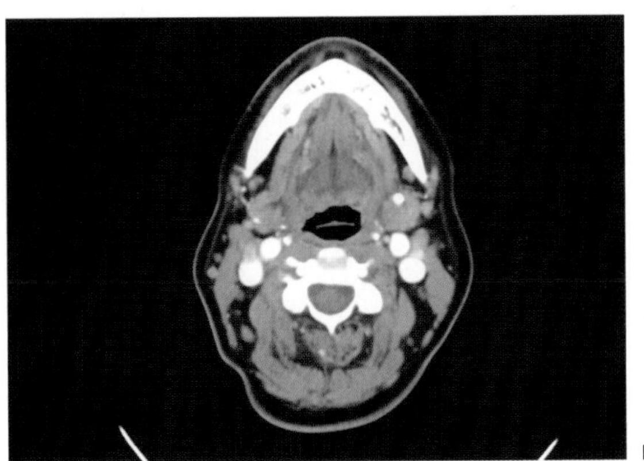
D

Imaging Findings

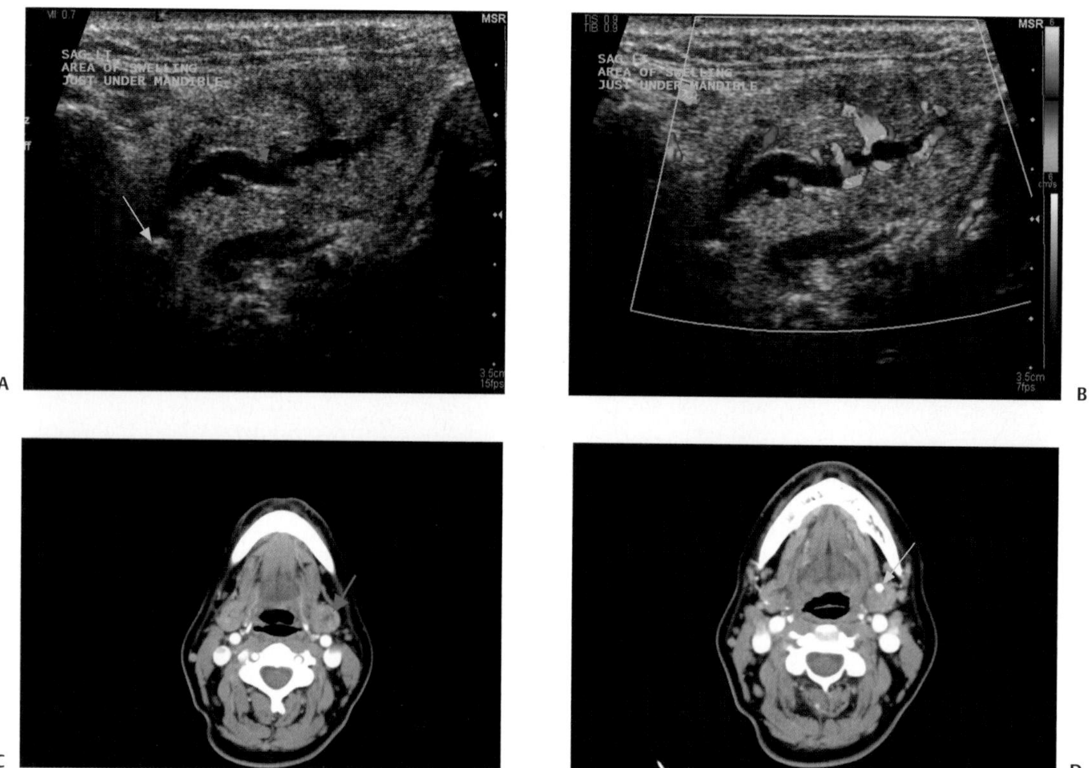

(A, B) Ultrasound image near the left angle of the mandible demonstrates a prominent and serpiginous anechoic structure (*red arrow*) within the submandibular gland with small echogenic focus (*yellow arrow*) that presents posterior shadowing. Color Doppler assessment reveals flow surrounding this tortuous structure. Findings are consistent with a dilated submandibular gland duct (Wharton duct) with central obstructing sialolith. **(C, D)** Follow-up contrast-enhanced computed tomography imaging of the neck demonstrates again a dilated left submandibular gland duct (*red arrow*) and a 5 mm sialolith (*yellow arrow*).

Differential Diagnosis

- ***Sialolithiasis:*** Commonly seen in the submandibular gland. A bright echogenic focus with distal shadowing is noted in 94% of cases with associated ductal dilatation.
- *Submandibular acute inflammation:* The etiology can be viral or bacterial. Ultrasound shows diffuse enlargement of the gland with a decrease in echogenicity. Associated lymph node enlargement can be seen sonographically.
- *Chronic inflammation:* The patients present with intermittent, painless swelling of the gland.

Essential Facts

- Seventy to 95% of salivary gland stones occur in the submandibular gland.
- Both the main duct and intraglandular ductules can be affected
- Common symptoms include mandibular swelling triggered by eating.
- Echogenic rim with posterior acoustic shadow is the main sonographic feature of a calculus.
- The stone is identified in 60 to 80% on plain films and in almost 100% of CTs.
- Chronic obstruction might cause cystic degeneration in the gland.
- In the case of chronic painful swelling, Sjogren's syndrome should be considered.

✓ Pearls & × Pitfalls

✓ The swollen gland can become heterogeneously hypoechoic due to edema.

× A stone impacted at the ductal ostium may not be well depicted on sonography, but many cases have associated main duct dilation.

Case 8

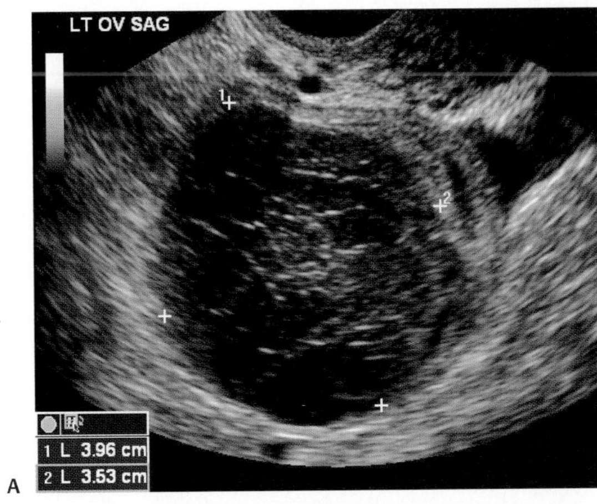

A

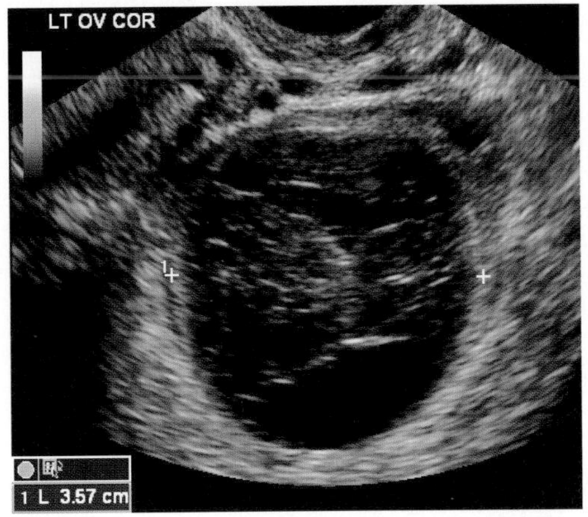

B

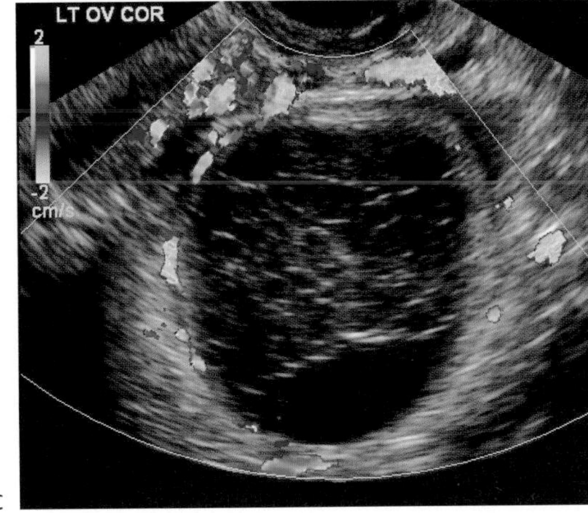

C

Clinical Presentation

A 31-year-old woman with left lower quadrant pain. Last menstrual period was 3 weeks ago.

Imaging Findings

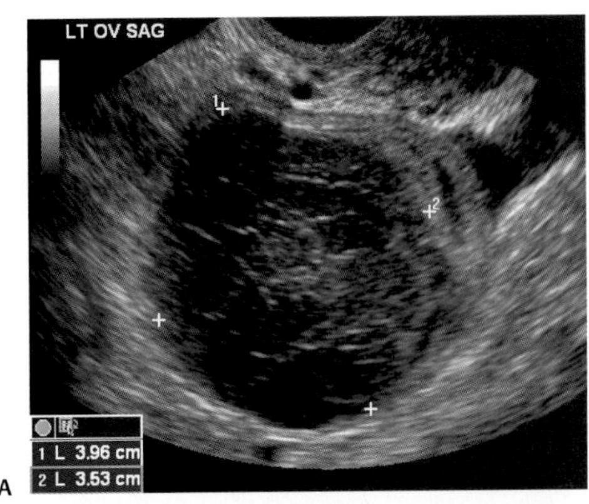

A

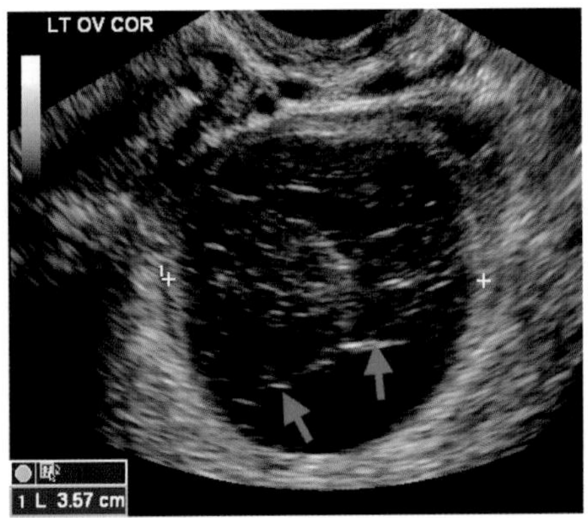

B

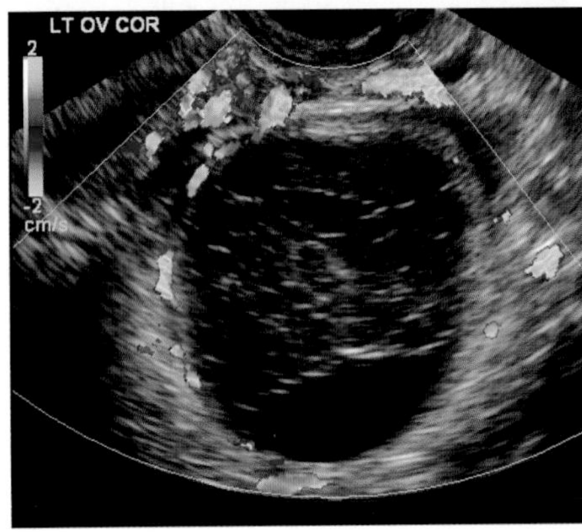

C

(A, B) Longitudinal and transverse gray scale images of the left ovary demonstrate a complex cystic lesion measuring 4 × 3.5 × 3.6 cm. The lesion contains a central region of fine lacelike septations with concave borders (*arrows*). **(C)** With color Doppler imaging there is intense peripheral vascularity surrounding the lesion.

Differential Diagnosis

- ***Hemorrhagic corpus luteum:*** The lacelike appearance of this lesion centrally is typical for hemorrhage. The intense peripheral vascularity surrounding the lesion is classic for a corpus luteum ("luteal flow").
- *Endometrioma:* The peripheral vascularity demonstrated in the lesion above would not be seen in the setting of an endometrioma. Endometriomas are usually homogenous with low-level echoes that result from cyclical bleeding.
- *Cystic ovarian malignancy:* Septations in a malignancy would be thicker and more irregular and may demonstrate color Doppler signal indicating flow with the septations.

Essential Facts

- Hemorrhagic cysts are the most common etiology for a complex cystic ovarian lesion. They are usually a result of hemorrhage into a corpus luteum.
- The term *hemorrhagic corpus luteum cyst* is reserved for lesions > 5 cm.
- A hemorrhagic corpus luteum is often symptomatic, causing pain. They should be mentioned in the setting of ipsilateral pain.
- A corpus luteum is seen during the luteal phase of the menstrual cycle (the second half of the menstrual cycle).
- If a classic hemorrhagic corpus luteum is < 5 cm in size (as in our patient above), no follow-up is needed.
- Lesions > 5 cm should undergo follow-up ultrasound in 6 to 12 weeks.
- A corpus luteum develops within a dominant follicle after rupture (ovulation). A corpus luteum should not be seen in postmenopausal patients.

Other Imaging Findings

- A corpus luteum is a common incidental finding on computed tomography (CT). The intense peripheral vascularity of a corpus luteum is confirmed with a dense peripheral rind on a post contrast CT of the pelvis.
- Positron emission tomography (PET): A corpus luteum is positive on PET. Due to its increased metabolic activity it will demonstrate uptake of FDG.

✓ Pearls & × Pitfalls

× A corpus luteum is PET positive and therefore will mimic a pelvic mass or lymphadenopathy.

× A corpus luteum should not be present in a postmenopausal patient. However in the early postmenopausal period, the ovaries may produce a corpus luteum. Regardless of its size, a presumed corpus luteum in a postmenopausal or perimenopausal patient warrants follow-up.

✓ The intense peripheral vascular rind seen with color Doppler imaging is classic for a corpus luteum.

Case 9

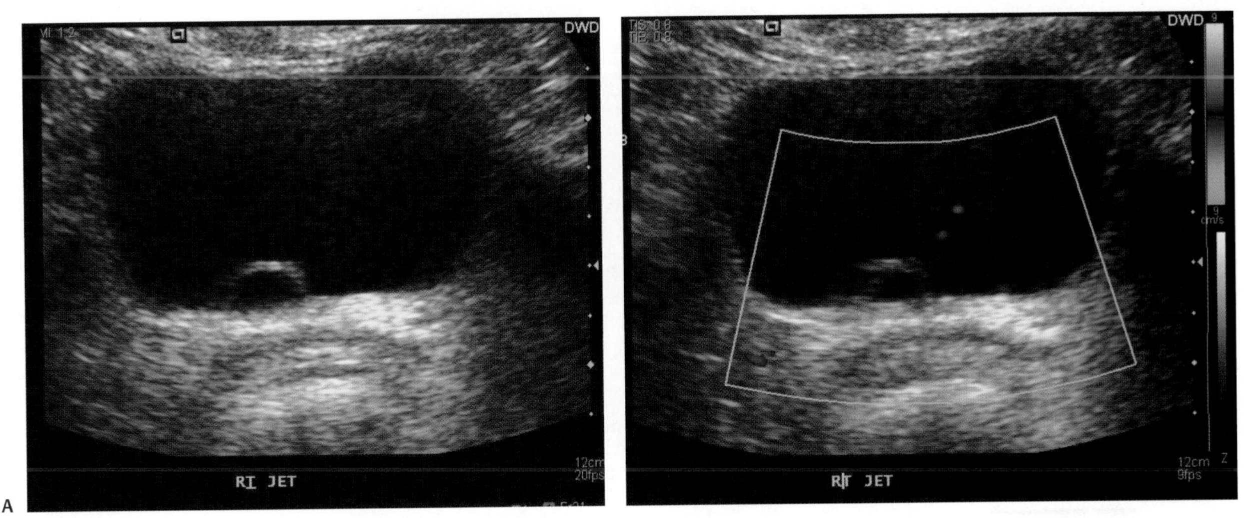

A B

Clinical Presentation

A 34-year-old woman presents with history of recurrent urinary tract infection.

Further Work-up

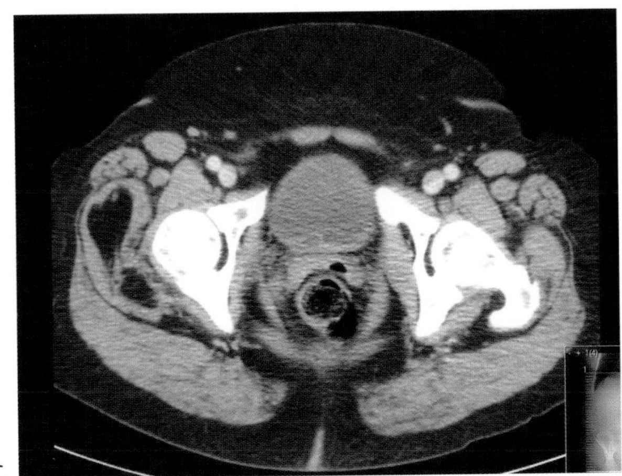

C

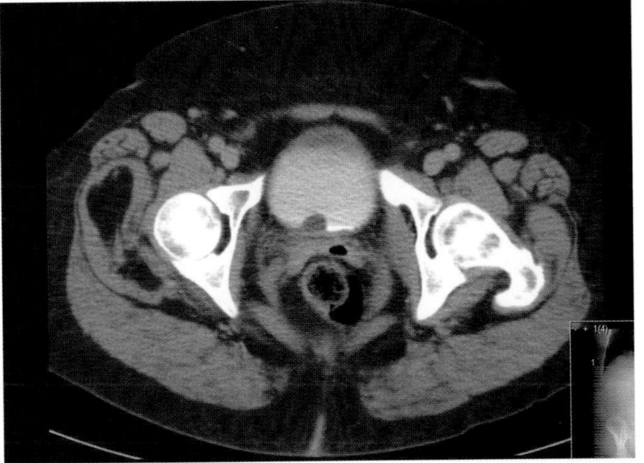

D

Imaging Findings

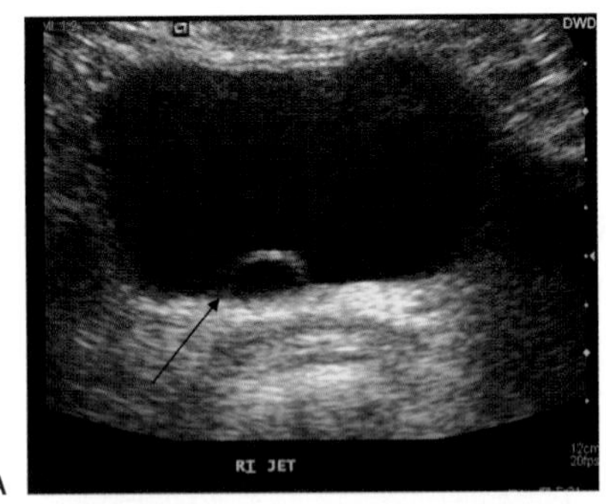

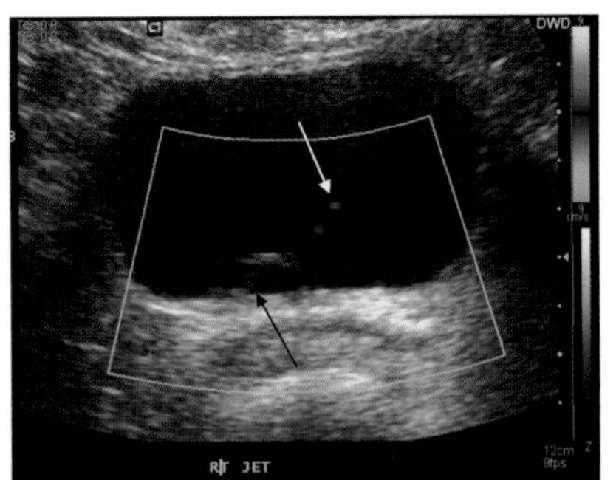

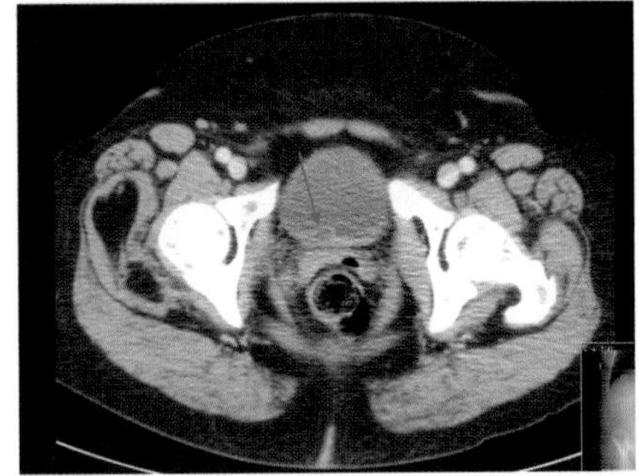

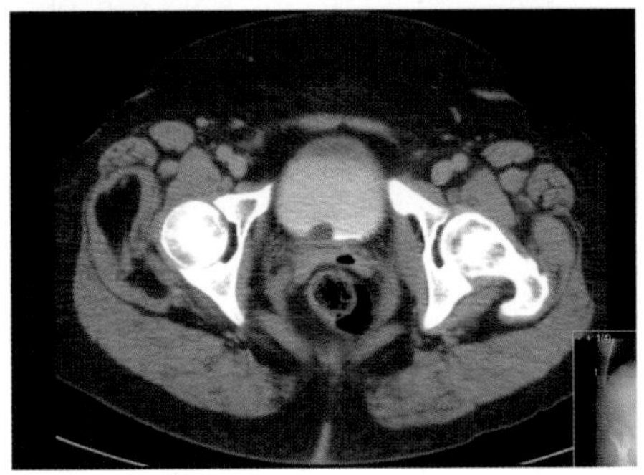

(A, B) Ultrasound images show a well-circumscribed cystic-like structure (*black arrow*) near the expected location of the right ureterovesical junction demonstrating thin uniform wall. Mild to moderate hydronephrosis was evident on evaluation of the kidneys (*not shown*). Color Doppler assessment reveals an attenuated right ureteral jet (*white arrow*). **(C, D)** Follow-up nephrographic phase computed tomography imaging shows a small wall-enhancing cystic structure (*red arrow*) at the right ureterovesical junction. Excretory phase imaging demonstrates no significant enhancement of this cystic lesion.

Differential Diagnosis

- ***Orthotopic ureterocele:*** Appears as an anechoic cystic lesion at the level of the normal ureterovesical junction.
- *Pseudoureterocele*: Cystic dilation of the intravesical portion of the ureter due to obstruction of the ureteral orifice by different etiologies such as invasion of the floor of the bladder by transitional cell carcinoma and cervical cancer, radiation cystitis, or calculus within the intravesical portion of the ureter. Could have similar appearance, usually larger. More common in young women with oral contraceptives usage (> 2 years).

Essential Facts

- Cystic dilation of submucosal segment of the intravesical ureter with prolapse into bladder lumen.
- Orthotopic ureterocele demonstrates normal insertion at the trigone.
- Ectopic ureterocele inserts below trigone and is associated with duplicated systems in 80%.
- Most commonly in females and asymptomatic.
- May evert during voiding and present as a vaginal or, less likely, urethral mass: prolapsing ureterocele.

✓ Pearls & × Pitfalls

✓ Thin-walled, cystic intravesical structure near ipsilateral ureter.
✓ Evaluate the ipsilateral kidney to assess for hydronephrosis.
× Check for mucosal irregularity to rule out tumor.

Case 10

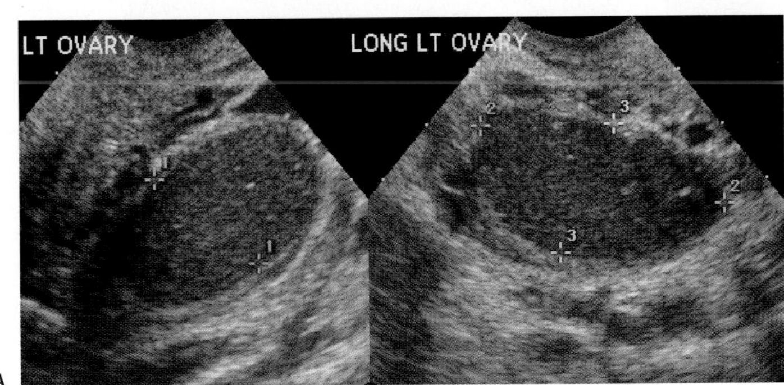

A

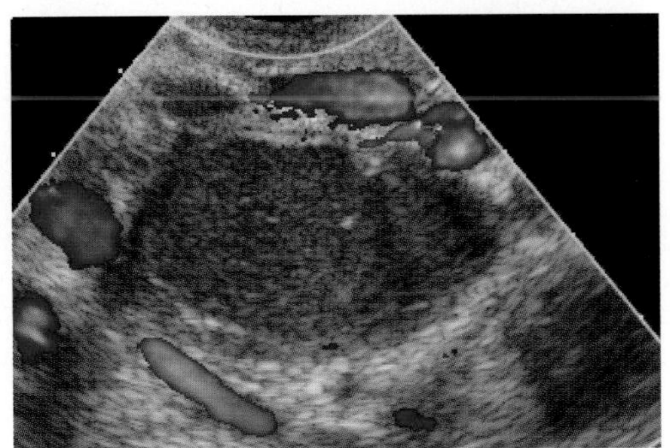

B

Clinical Presentation

A 36-year-old woman being worked up for infertility.

Imaging Findings

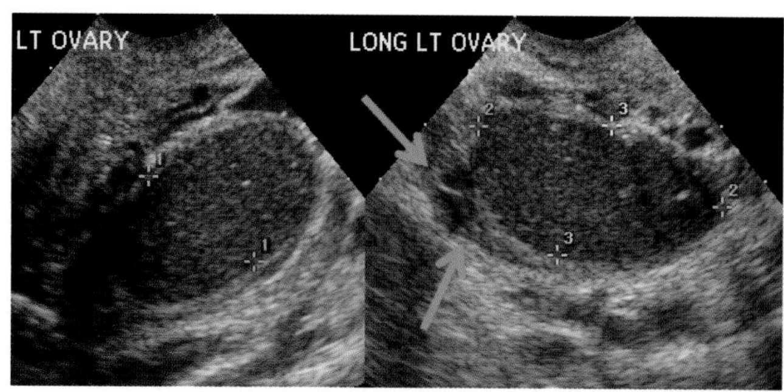

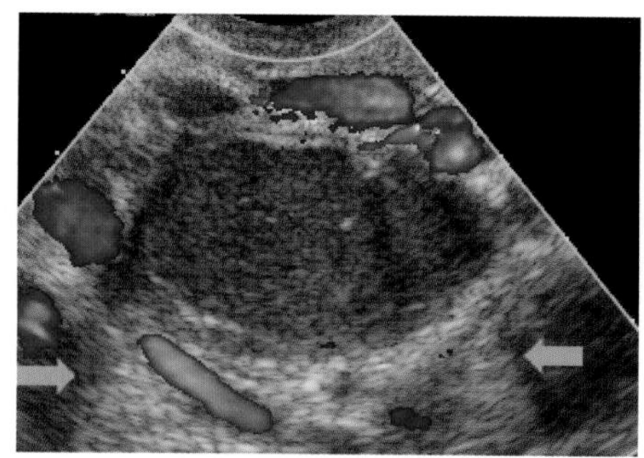

(A, B) The left ovary is almost completely replaced by a homogeneous lesion that contains low-level echoes and no internal vascularity and demonstrates acoustic enhancement (*arrows*). The lesion contains tiny echogenic foci that are predominantly peripheral. A thin rind of ovarian tissue and follicles (*arrows*) surrounds the lesion.

Differential Diagnosis

- ***Endometrioma:*** The tiny echogenic foci within a lesion that is otherwise homogeneous with low-level echoes and no internal vascularity is classic for an endometrioma.
- *Hemorrhagic cyst:* Although a hemorrhagic cyst will occasionally contain low-level echoes, the punctate echogenic foci are not seen with acute hemorrhage.
- *Dermoid or teratoma:* Although a dermoid can contain echogenic lines and dots (hair on face and on end), the above lesion contains only punctate foci.

Essential Facts

- Endometriomas, also known as *chocolate cysts* because of their appearance at surgery, result from ectopic endometrial implants in the ovaries.
- The homogeneous low-level echoes within the lesion result from cyclical bleeding.
- Endometriosis occurs in 5 to 10% of menstruating women. Thirty to 50% of patients with endometriosis have infertility. Only 20% of infertile women have endometriosis.
- Endometriomas are often incidental, as they can be asymptomatic as in this patient.
- Symptomatic endometriosis is usually the result of endometrial implants of the peritoneum that are not usually visible with ultrasound. These implants can be seen with magnetic resonance imaging (MRI).
- A classic endometrioma such as this is often treated conservatively without surgery.
- If endometriomas are not treated surgically, annual follow-up is recommended.
- One percent of endometriomas are believed to undergo malignant transformation. Most malignancies occur in large lesions (> 9 cm) and in older women (> 45 years old).

Other Imaging Findings

- On computed tomography, endometriomas will appear similar to simple cysts or may be of greater density due to the blood products.
- MRI: Endometriomas are high signal on T1-weighted images and may demonstrate T2 shading. They do not enhance.

✓ Pearls & × Pitfalls

✓ Endometriomas should never demonstrate internal vascularity.

× Endometriomas can contain features similar to malignancy. MRI is helpful to distinguish atypical endometriomas from neoplastic lesions.

Case 11

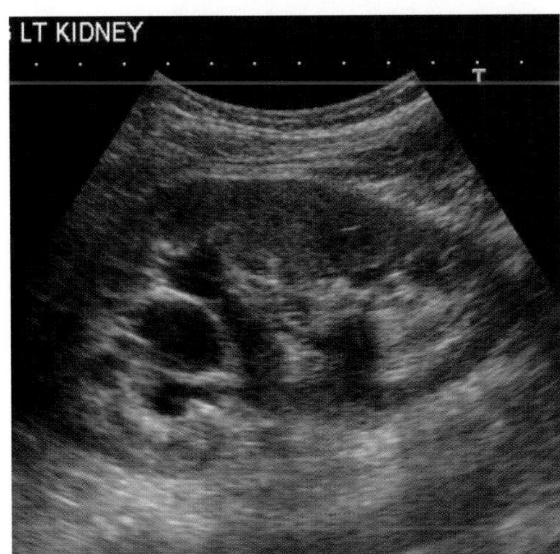

A

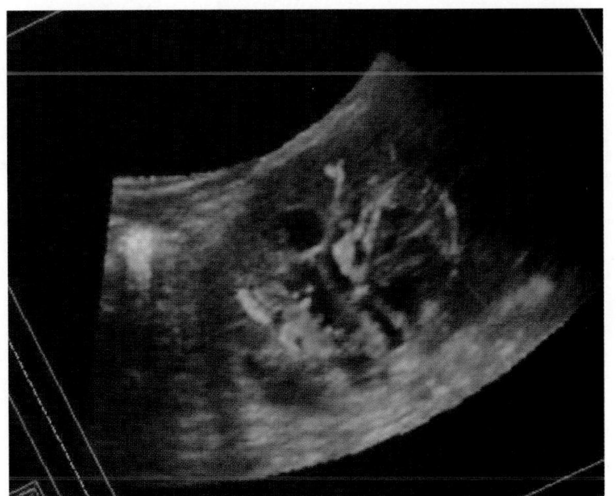

B

Clinical Presentation

A 35-year-old woman with hypertension presents for assessment.

Further Work-up

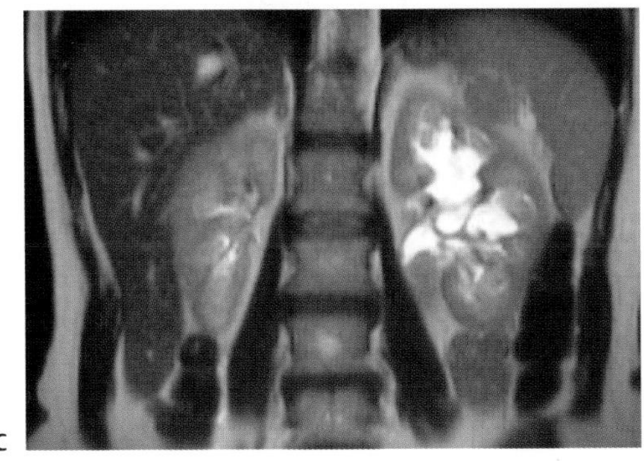

C

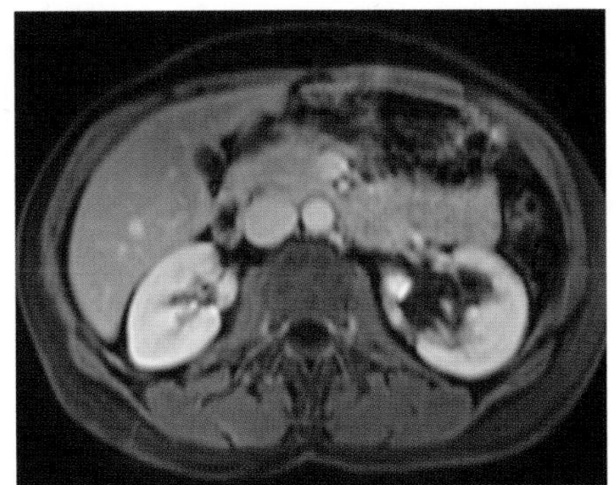

D

Imaging Findings

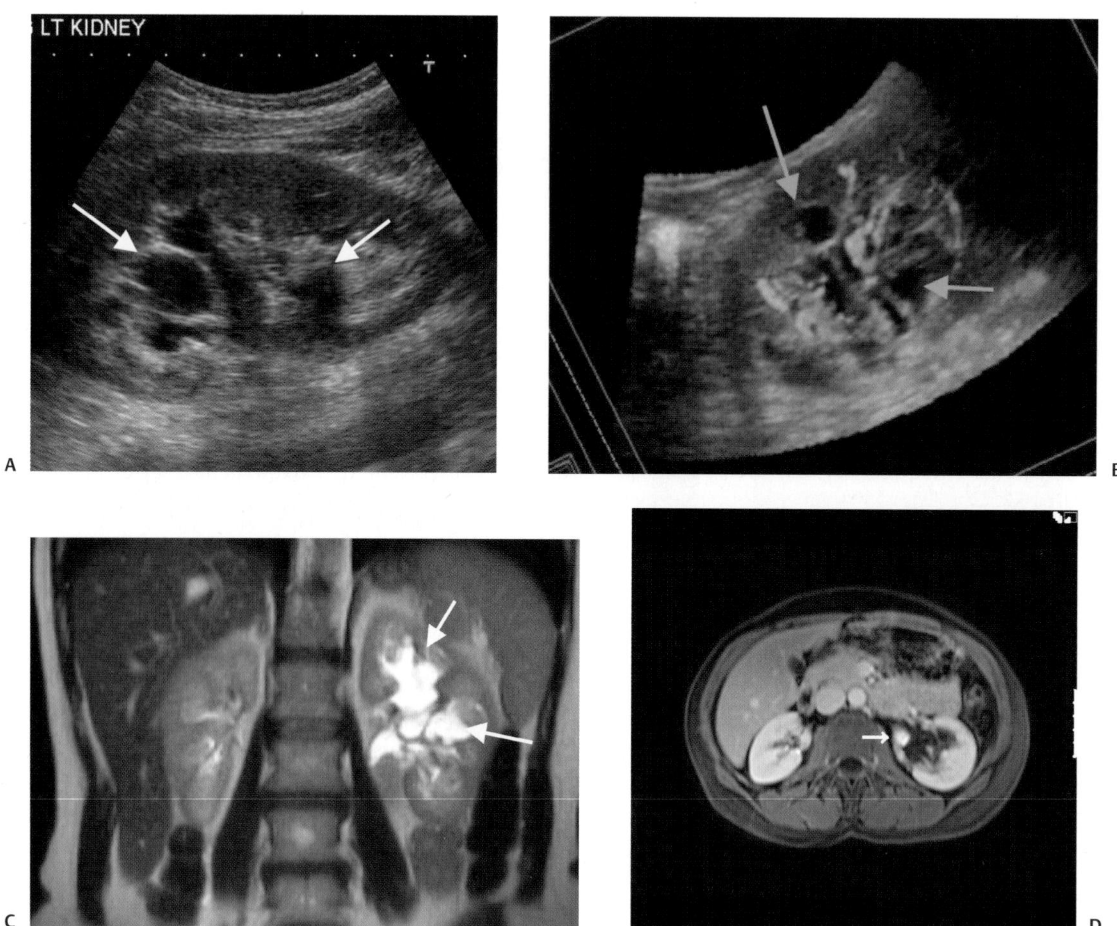

(A) Ultrasound images show cystic lesions in the left renal pelvis, the relation to the renal pelvis is indeterminate (*white arrows*). **(B)** Volume image with color Doppler raise the question of separation of the cystic lesions from the renal pelvis (*orange arrows*). Coronal T2 and axial post contrast MRI images **(C, D)** show multiple cystic lesions in the renal pelvis (*white arrows*), separate from the renal collecting system (*white arrow*).

Differential Diagnosis

- ***Parapelvic Cysts:*** ultrasound shows a cluster of cystic lesions in the renal pelvis with no evidence of communication with renal pelvis. The patient usually is asymptomatic and the finding is incidental.
- *Hydronephrosis:* The presence of documented communication of a cluster of cystic lesions in the renal pelvis suggests hydronephrosis; the presence of hydroureter favors this diagnosis.
- *Cystic Neoplasm:* Is uncommon presentation in the renal pelvis, a thick irregular septation is noted on ultrasound, clear differentiation could be made using computed tomography or MRI.

Essential Facts

- Found in ~ 1.25 to 1.50%.
- Thought to be lymphatic in origin and may be congenital.
- Most are asymptomatic, though they may cause hematuria, hypertension, and hydronephrosis.
- Dilated renal pelvis may present as a cauliflower appearance, whereas a parapelvic cyst is more spherical.
- 3-D ultrasound is a valuable method to document communication/separation of cystic lesions in the renal pelvis.

✓ Pearls & × Pitfalls

✓ Three-dimensional ultrasound is a valuable method to document communication/separation of cystic lesions in the renal pelvis.

× A cluster of parapelvic cysts could cause mass effect on adjacent cysts mimicking the appearance of hydronephrosis.

Case 12

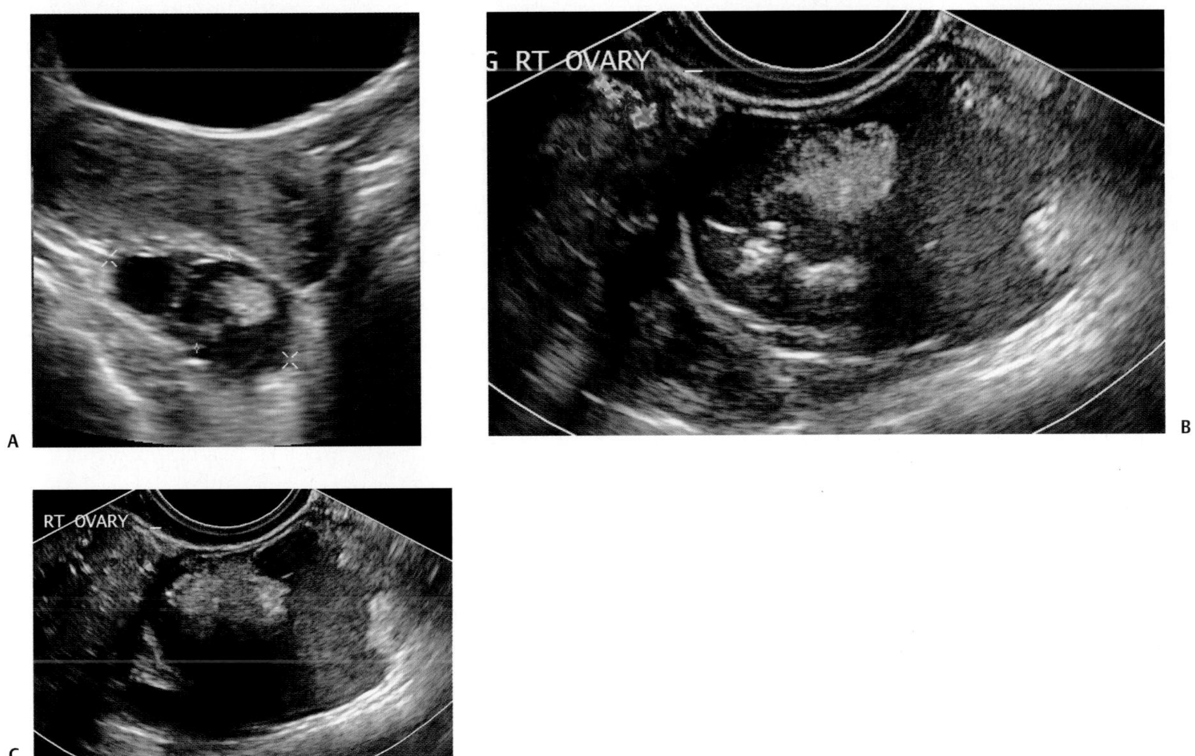

Clinical Presentation

A 32-year-old woman with chronic right lower quadrant pain, normal menses.

Imaging Findings

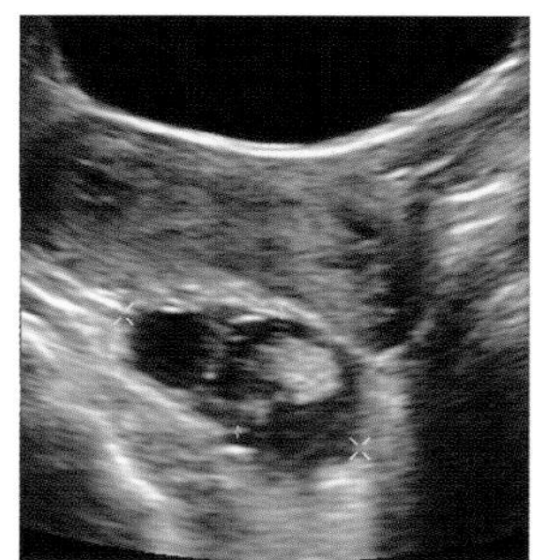
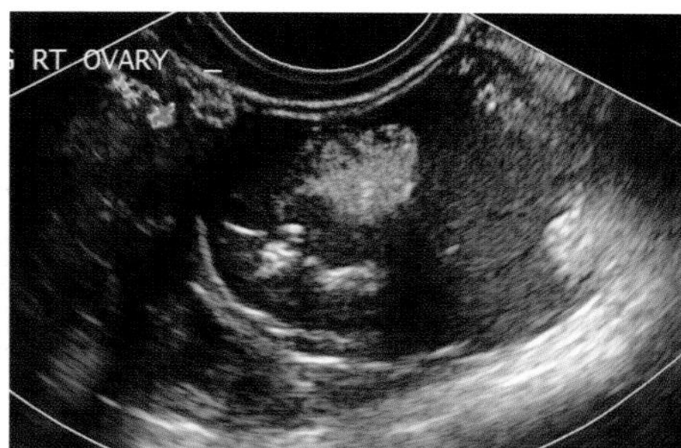

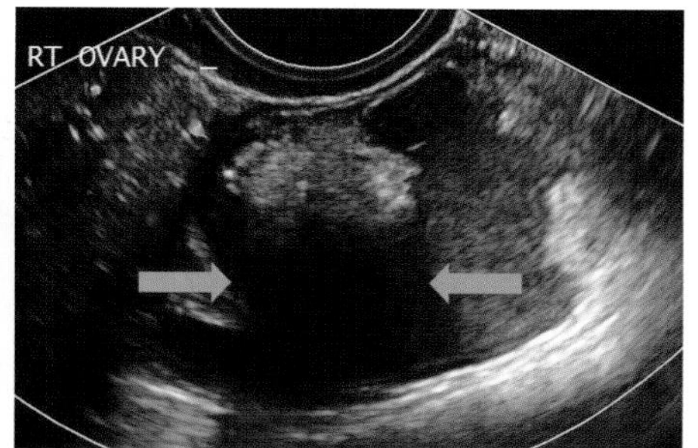

(A–C) The right ovary is enlarged and completely replaced by a complex lesion. The lesion contains multiple echogenic nodules. The largest nodule causes dirty shadowing (*arrows*). There is no internal vascularity with color Doppler imaging.

Differential Diagnosis

- ***Dermoid:*** Multiple echogenic nodules are classic for a dermoid. The nodules are fat globules and therefore nonvascular and cause dirty shadowing.
- *Endometriomas:* The homogenous low-level echoes seen in this lesion are suggestive of an endometrioma. Additionally, endometriomas can contain echogenic nodules. But the nodules seen in endometriomas are due to fibrin or clot and would not cause dirty shadowing like fat does.
- *Complex cystic neoplasm:* Cystic neoplasms can contain solid components that may be echogenic. Solid components of a neoplasm are often vascular and will demonstrate flow with color. Solid components of a neoplasm would not cause shadowing.

Essential Facts

- Mature cystic teratomas, often referred to as dermoids, are the most common ovarian neoplasm. They are bilateral in 12 to 20% of cases.
- Most dermoids are benign. They are usually removed, as they can rupture or cause torsion. Dermoids can grow slowly and destroy the ovary.
- Dermoids can usually be accurately characterized by ultrasound (US). Classic US features of a dermoid include:
  - Focal or diffuse hyperechoic component (fat or oil)
  - Hyperechoic line and dots (hair on face or on end)
  - Calcifications with dense shadowing
  - No internal flow
- Rare but pathognomic feature:
  1. Floating echogenic spherules in a cystic mass
  2. Fluid-filled layer
- Malignant transformation in up to 2% occurs in older women (> 50 years of age) and in large dermoids (> 10 cm).

Other Imaging Findings

- US is usually sufficient to make the diagnosis. The diagnosis of a dermoid on computed tomography or magnetic resonance imaging is usually obvious due to a region of fat.

✓ Pearls & × Pitfalls

- ✓ A geographic area of increased echogenicity that causes dirty shadowing is pathognomonic of a dermoid.
- ✓ Dermoids do not have internal vascularity. If you demonstrate internal vascularity in solid components, it is not a benign dermoid.
- ✓ *Tip of the iceberg* is a term used to described dermoids. Dermoids can contain large fatty components that distort the sound beam. Only the anterior margin of a lesion is imaged. The posterior margin is obscured. Hence, large lesions are often undermeasured.
- ✓ If free fluid is present in a patient with a dermoid and acute pain, consider rupture.
- × Mural nodules seen in malignancy can mimic a fat nodule of a dermoid.

Case 13

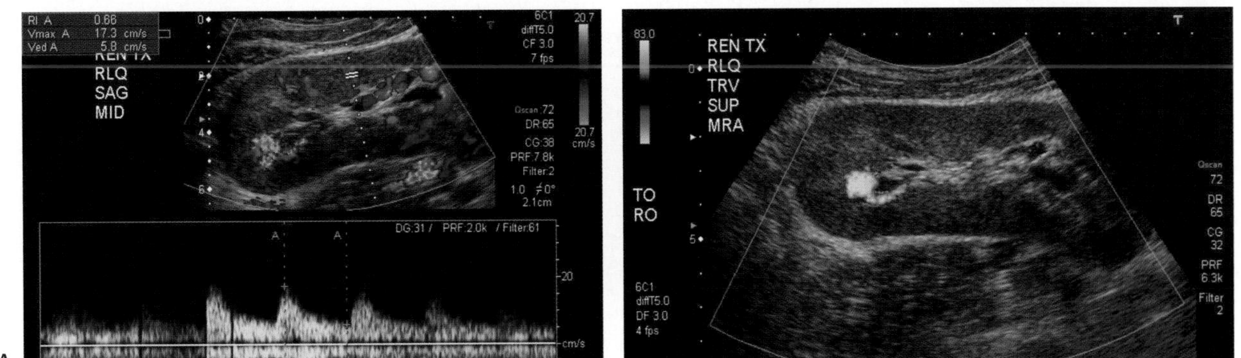

A B

Clinical Presentation

A 45-year-old woman with a history of renal transplant presents with worsening renal function after ultrasound-guided renal biopsy.

Further Work-up

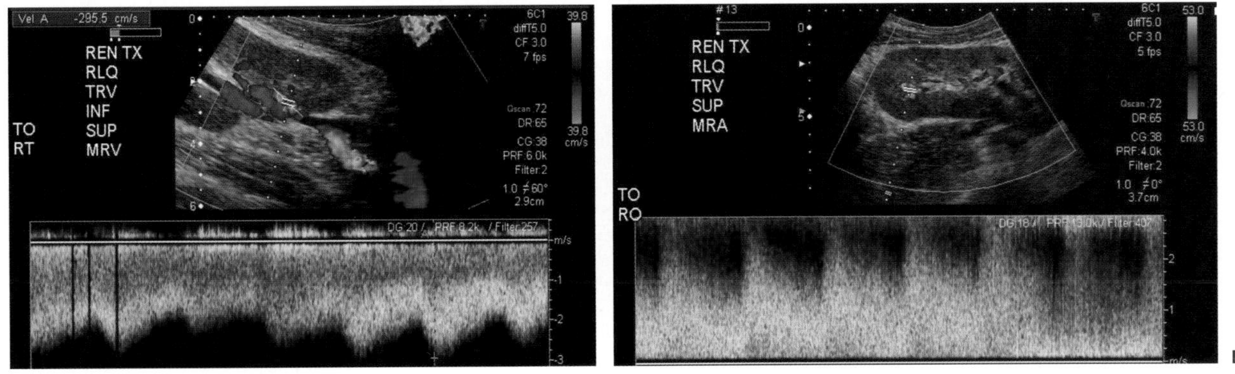

C D

Imaging Findings

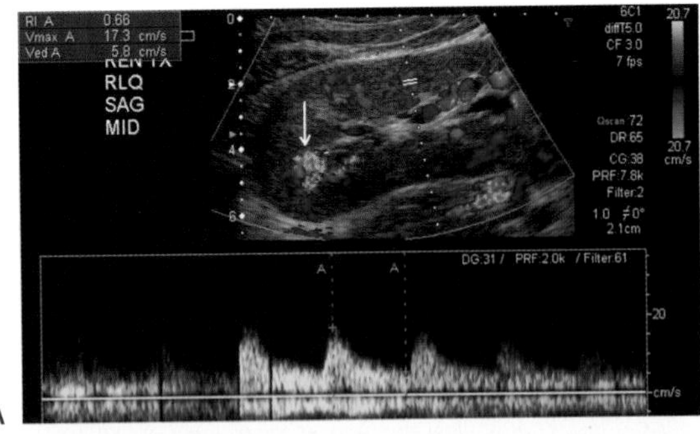

A

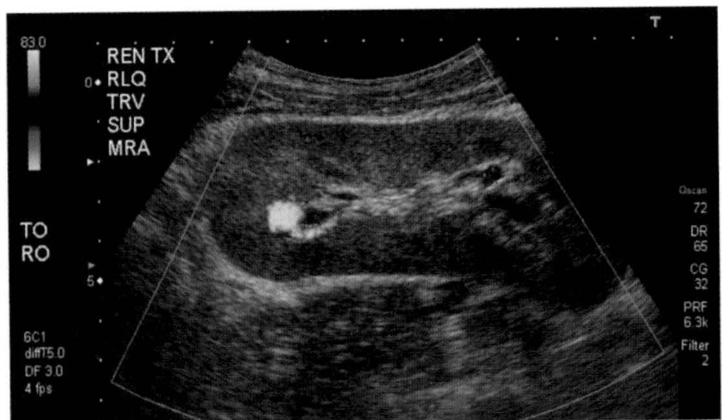

B

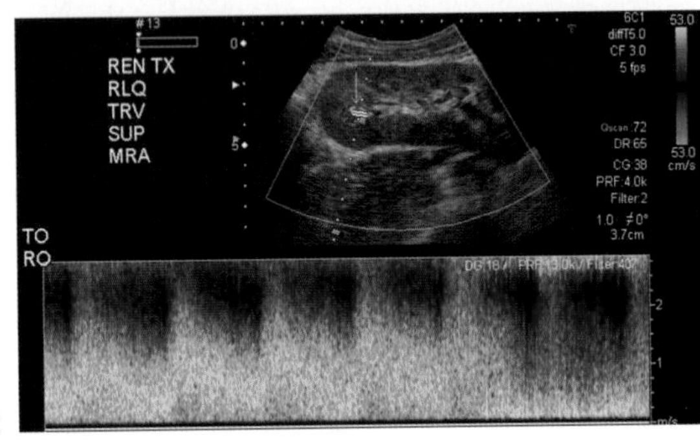

C

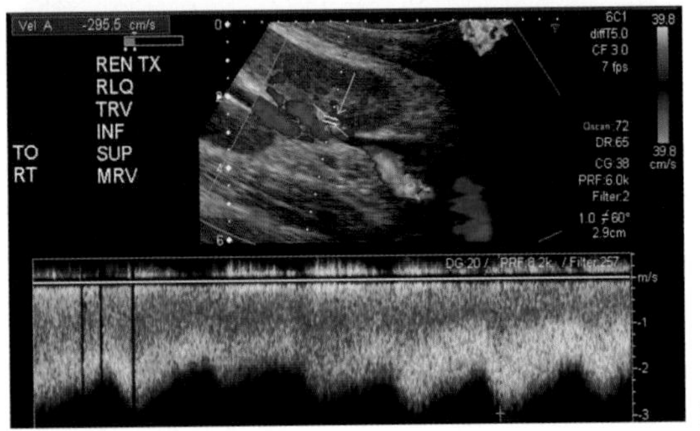

D

(A, B) Doppler ultrasound shows area of markedly increased velocity in the upper pole of the transplanted kidney on image A (*arrow*). Doppler tracing using high Doppler scale setting of that area confirms increased velocity at the questionable area **(B)**. **(C)** Doppler tracing shows low resistance, high velocity flow at that location. **(D)** Doppler tracing of the renal vein shows increased velocity with arterialization of the venous waveform suggestive of arteriovenous communication.

Differential Diagnosis

- ***Arteriovenous fistula:*** Common complication after renal transplant biopsy. Present with focal increased velocity, low RI in the feeding artery, and arterialization of the vein. Spontaneous closure is common, however embolization may be required.
- *Intrarenal pseudoaneurysm:* Usually traumatic (biopsy) or could be infectious. To-and-fro spectral Doppler is present; usually closes spontaneously.
- *Arteriovenous malformation:* Rare congenital condition, usually seen in cadaver kidneys. Present with abnormal communications between arteries and veins; the involved vessels are usually serpiginous and tortuous.

Essential Facts

- Reported in 18% of renal transplant biopsy.
- Waveform with high-velocity, low-resistance flow, and arterialized venous waveform is specific for the diagnosis of an arteriovenous fistula.
- Arteriovenous fistula drives the blood away from the transplant kidney, causing renal impairment. Blood in the collecting system can cause hydronephrosis.
- Spontaneous closure is common in the first 30 minutes after biopsy.
- The treatment of choice is embolization in persistent, symptomatic cases.

✓ Pearls & × Pitfalls

✓ Arteriovenous fistula should be excluded in cases of deterioration of renal function tests after a renal biopsy.

× During closure of arteriovenous fistula, a transient increase in velocity is present; however, there will be less arterialization of the vein.

Case 14

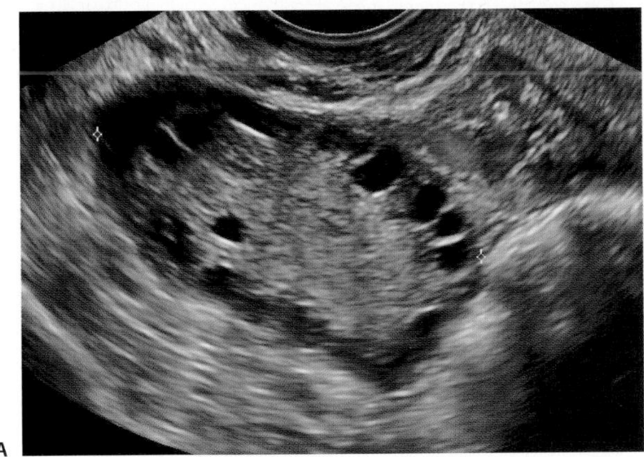
A

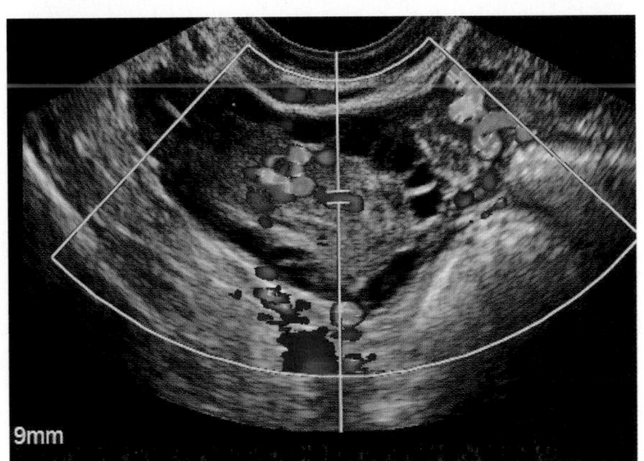

B

Clinical Presentation

A 32-year-old obese woman with irregular menses.

Imaging Findings

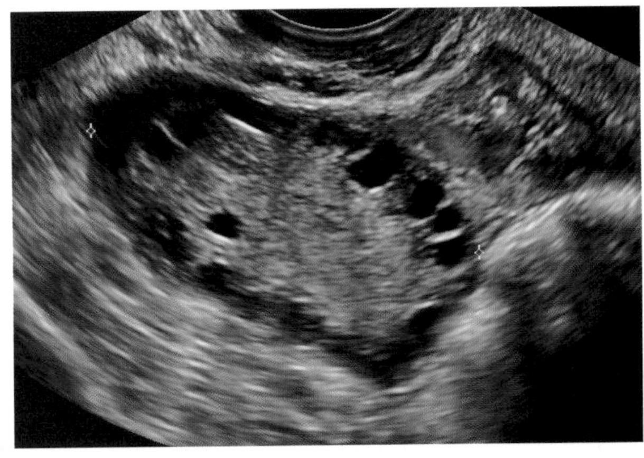

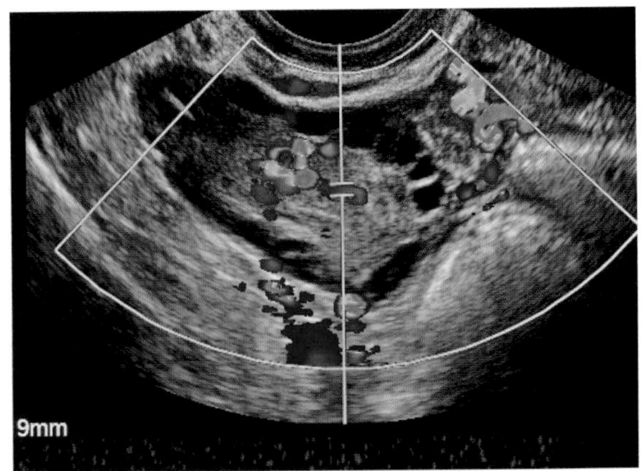

(A, B) The right ovary contains numerous small peripheral follicles. The left ovary is not shown; its appearance was similar to the right. Both color and spectral Doppler waveforms demonstrate flow within the ovary.

Differential Diagnosis

- ***Polycystic ovarian syndrome (PCOS):*** In PCOS, an ovary will contain > 12 follicles per image (Rotterdam criteria). The follicles range in size between 2 and 9 mm. A dominant follicle is not usually present. The central stroma may be echogenic.
- *Oral contraceptive use:* Women taking birth control pills will have numerous arrested follicles within the ovaries. These are usually larger and distributed throughout the entire ovary.
- *Ovarian torsion:* In the setting of torsion, the ovary is edematous and enlarged (due to edema) with peripheral follicles. Color and spectral tracings are not usually identifiable in the setting of torsion. Patients with torsion are acutely symptomatic with pain.

Essential Facts

- PCOS is the most frequent endocrine problem in women of reproductive age. It was originally referred to as *Stein-Leventhal syndrome.*
- It occurs in 5 to 10% of women of reproductive age and is one of the leading causes of subfertility. There is a wide spectrum of involvement.
- The etiology is not known but it is believed to be partially genetic. The diagnosis of PCOS is a consensus of:
  - Clinical: Amenorrhea or oligomenorrhea, hirsutism, acne, obesity
  - Biochemical: Elevated androgens and other endocrine imbalances
  - Ultrasound (US) findings: Often enlarged ovaries with small peripheral follicles (> 12) and echogenic central stroma
- Patients with PCOS are often obese and have insulin resistance, type 2 diabetes, and high cholesterol levels.

✓ Pearls & × Pitfalls

✓ The peripheral follicles have been described as "string of pearls."

✓ US criteria for PCOS is 12 or more follicles per ovary on one image. Often, the intervening ovarian stroma is echogenic.

× The tiny peripheral follicles seen in polycystic ovaries may be too small to decipher from one another. The tiny peripheral cysts can appear as a hypoechoic peripheral region.

× PCOS-appearing ovaries can be seen in normal patients without clinical or biochemical evidence of the disease.

× PCOS ovaries may be normal in size. It is the abnormal appearance of the ovary that is seen with PCOS.

× There is a tremendous spectrum of involvement of the disease.

× PCOS can be unilateral.

Case 15

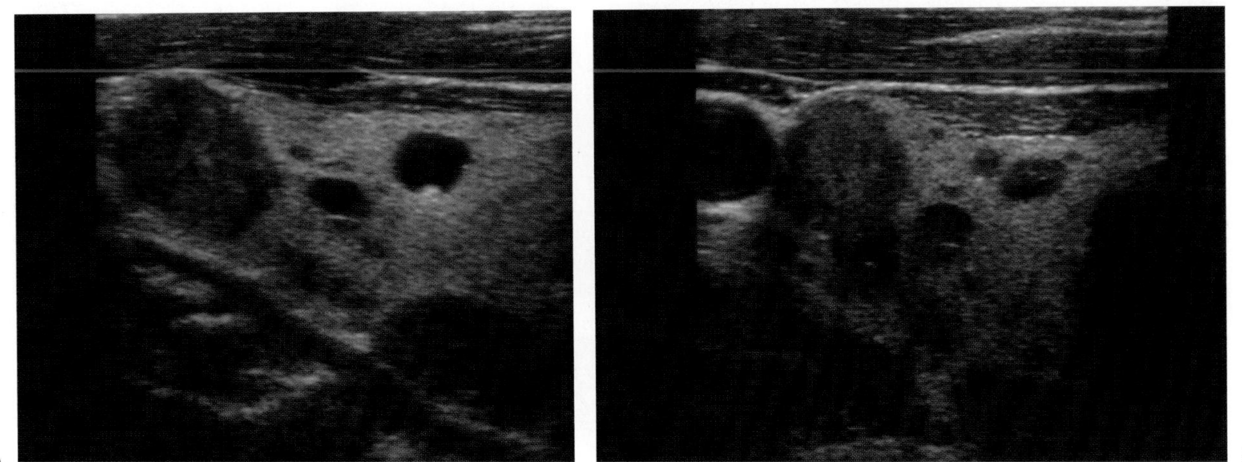

A B

Clinical Presentation

A 45-year-old male with a thyroid nodule seen on computed tomography (CT) of the chest.

Further Work-up

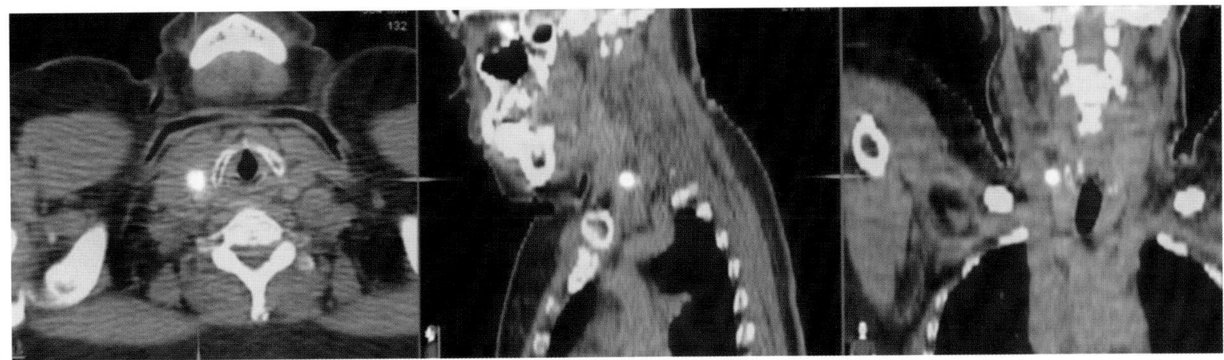

C

Imaging Findings

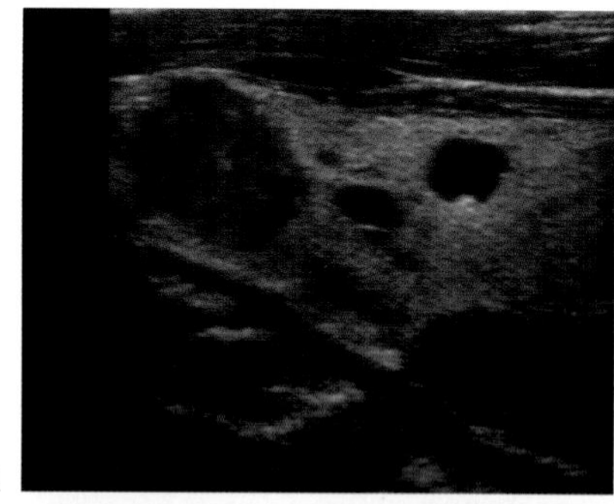

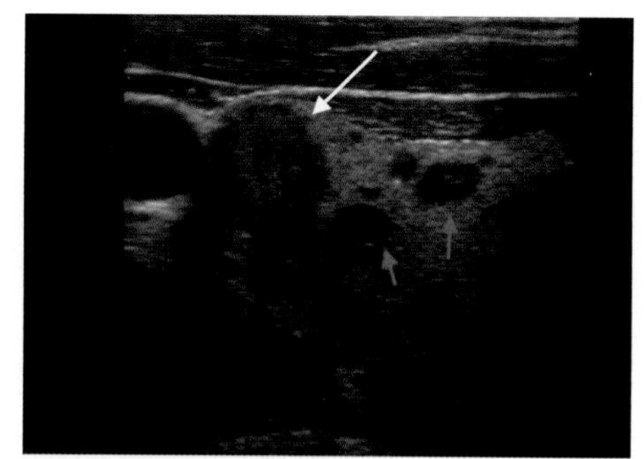

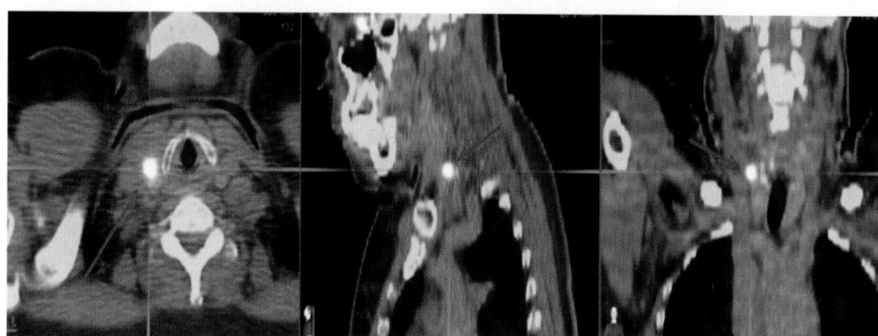

(A, B) Ultrasound evaluation of the thyroid right lobe shows hypoechoic, solid nodule that corresponds to prior imaging findings (*white arrow*); small cysts and small hypoechoic nodules in the right lobe are also seen (*red arrows*). **(C)** Positron emission tomography (PET) scan demonstrates intense uptake of fluorodeoxyglucose (FDG) within the lesion seen on CT and ultrasound (*red arrow*).

Differential Diagnosis

- ***Thyroid malignancy:*** Sonographically appears hypoechoic in 90% of cases. Microcalcifications and hypervascularity are common findings on ultrasound. Increased uptake on PET scan is suggestive of malignancy.
- *Hyperplastic adenomatous (colloid nodule):* On ultrasound it appears as an isoechoic, hyperechoic, and/or hypoechoic nodule; a honeycomb pattern could also be seen. The nodule may undergo cystic degeneration.
- *Lymphoma:* Non-Hodgkin lymphoma represents 4% of all thyroid malignancies. Appears as hypoechoic lobulated mass. Increased uptake on PET is common.

Essential Facts

- Has two peaks, the third and seventh decades.
- Seventy to 90% have mixed papillary and follicular.
- Lymphatic spread
- Distant metastases are rare (3%), mainly in the mediastinum.
- Appears hypoechoic on ultrasound. Microcalcifications and hypervascularity with cervical lymph enlargement is suggestive of malignancy.
- Focal PET uptake is suggestive of primary or secondary malignancies. Diffuse uptake could be seen with thyroiditis.

✓ Pearls & × Pitfalls

✓ The presence of focal uptake on PET in the thyroid gland requires fine-needle aspiration to exclude malignancy.

× Fine-needle aspiration and cytology are not reliable for differentiating follicular adenoma from carcinoma; the lesions should be surgically removed.

Case 16

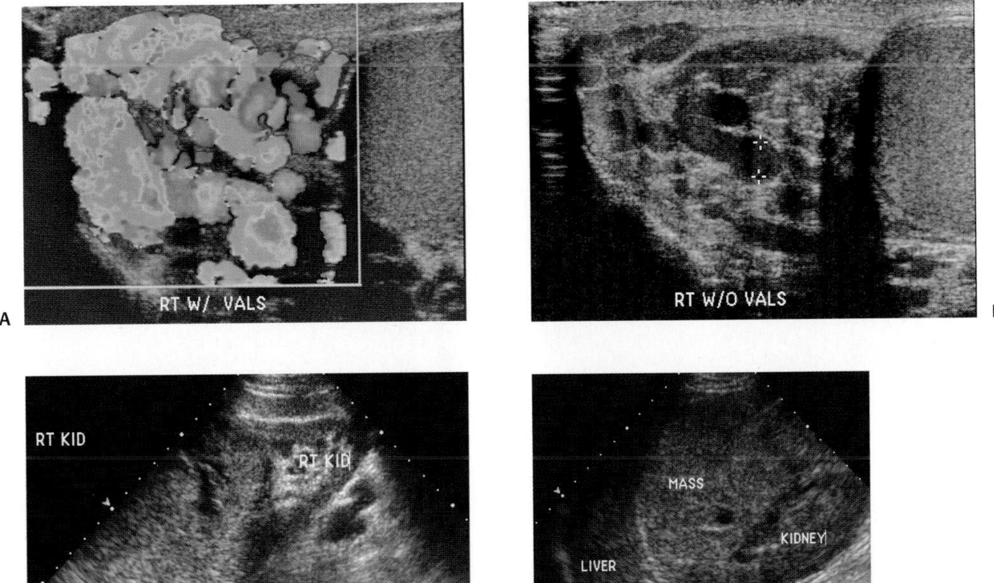

A B C D

Clinical Presentation

A 26-year-old man with right scrotal discomfort.

Further Work-up

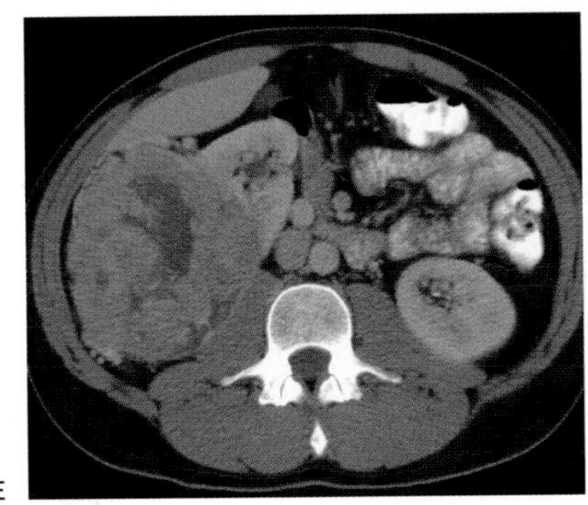

E

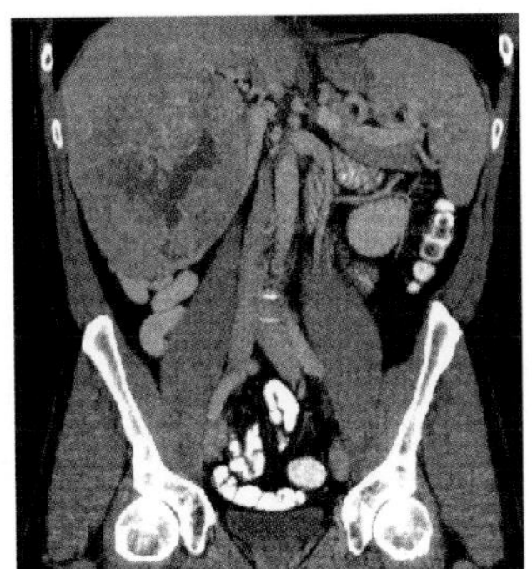

F

Imaging Findings

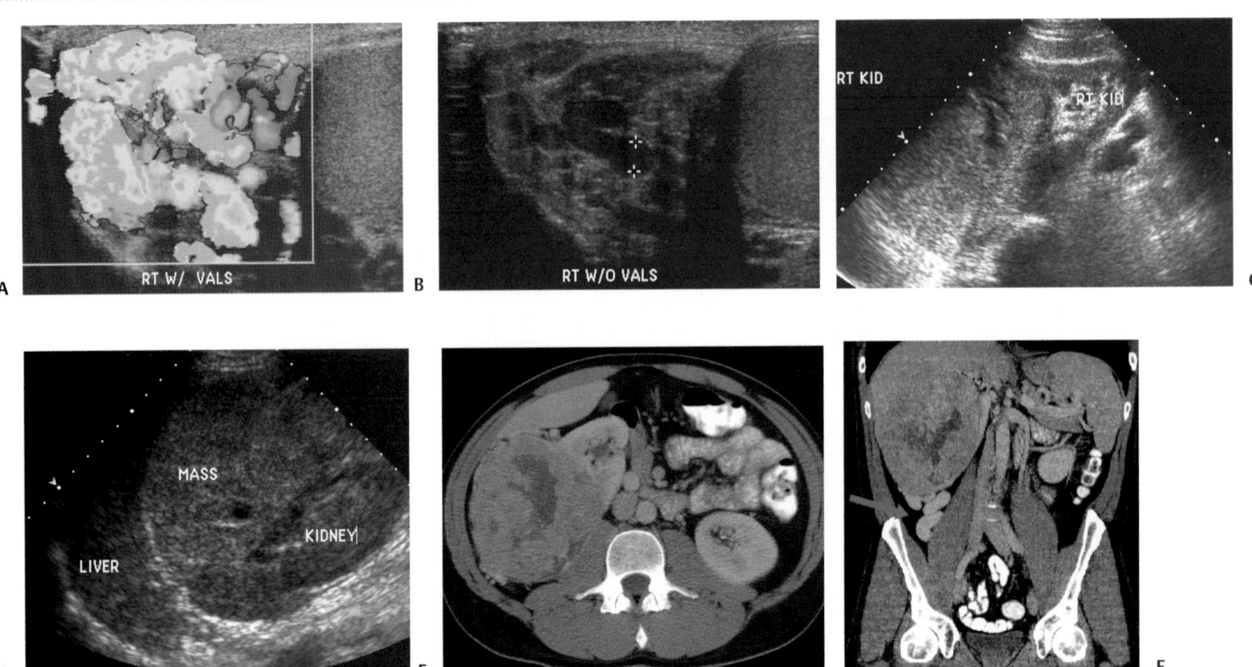

(A-F) On scrotal ultrasound, the testicles are normal in size and homogenous in echotexture without focal lesions. The epididymis is normal bilaterally. Hypoechoic, serpiginous tubular, extratesticular structures are seen in the right hemiscrotum. These demonstrate flow with color Doppler imaging and increase in size with valsalva maneuvering. A large, solid mass occupies the right upper quadrant. Its organ of origin is difficult to delineate given its size. CT reveals a large mass displacing the right kidney. Note the enlarged gonadal vein on image **F** (*arrow*).

Differential Diagnosis

- ***Unilateral right varicocele:*** The presence of color Doppler confirms vascular structures. The veins increase in size with Valsalva maneuver.
- *Ectasia of the rete tubules:* Would not demonstrate flow with color Doppler imaging. Ectatic rete tubules often extend into the testicular mediastinum.
- *Epididymitis:* Usually more echogenic and not tubular, though it also demonstrates increased vascularity.

Essential Facts

- Varicoceles occur from increased venous pressure or venous reflux and are isolated abnormalities occurring in 10 to 15% of men in the United States. Varicoceles are most commonly left sided (80%), bilateral 15% of the time, and only occur on the right in 5% of patients.
- Unilateral left varicocele is due to the discrepant venous drainage between the right and left sides. The left gonadal vein forms a 90-degree angle as it drains into the left renal vein and the right drains into the IVC.
- Unilateral right varicocele can result from intra-abdominal pathology, most commonly a renal mass, affecting drainage of the gonadal vein. As in this case, a large mass is seen in the right upper quadrant.
- Criteria for diagnosis: veins measure > 2 to 3 mm and increase in size with Valsalva maneuver. Dilated veins are seen posterolateral and superior to the testicle.

✓ Pearls & × Pitfalls

✓ Varicoceles are usually bilateral or more prominent on the left.

✓ Unilateral right varicocele can be the result of a retroperitoneal or abdominal mass.

✓ Varicoceles are the most frequent cause of male infertility.

✓ Right-sided varicoceles are uncommon and should raise suspicion of a right abdominal mass.

Case 17

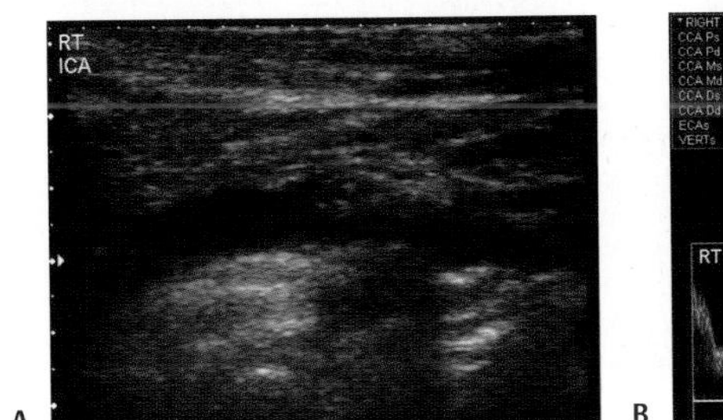

A

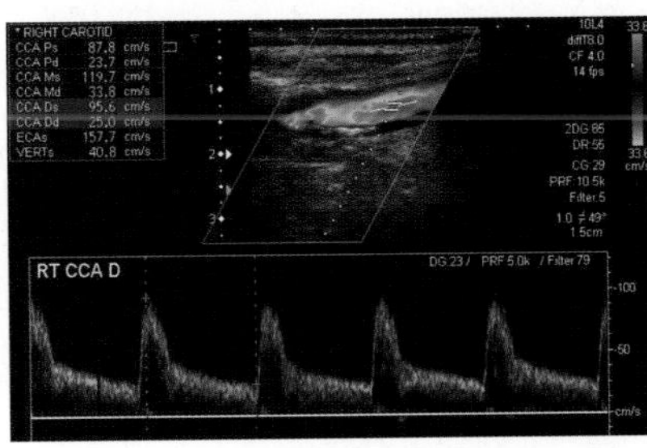

B

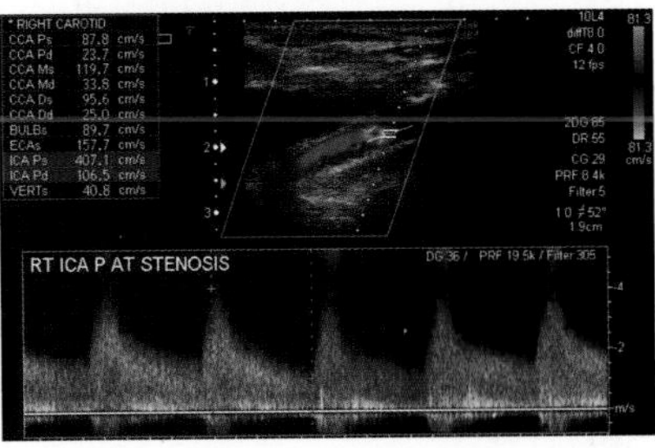

C

Clinical Presentation

A 79-year-old man presents with a history of transient ischemic attack.

Further Work-up

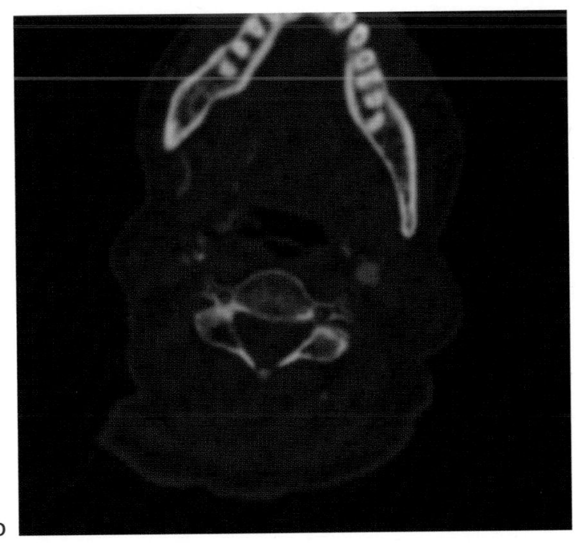
D

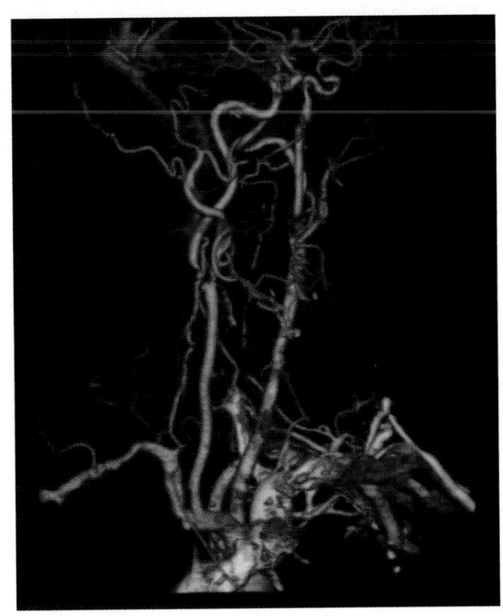
E

Imaging Findings

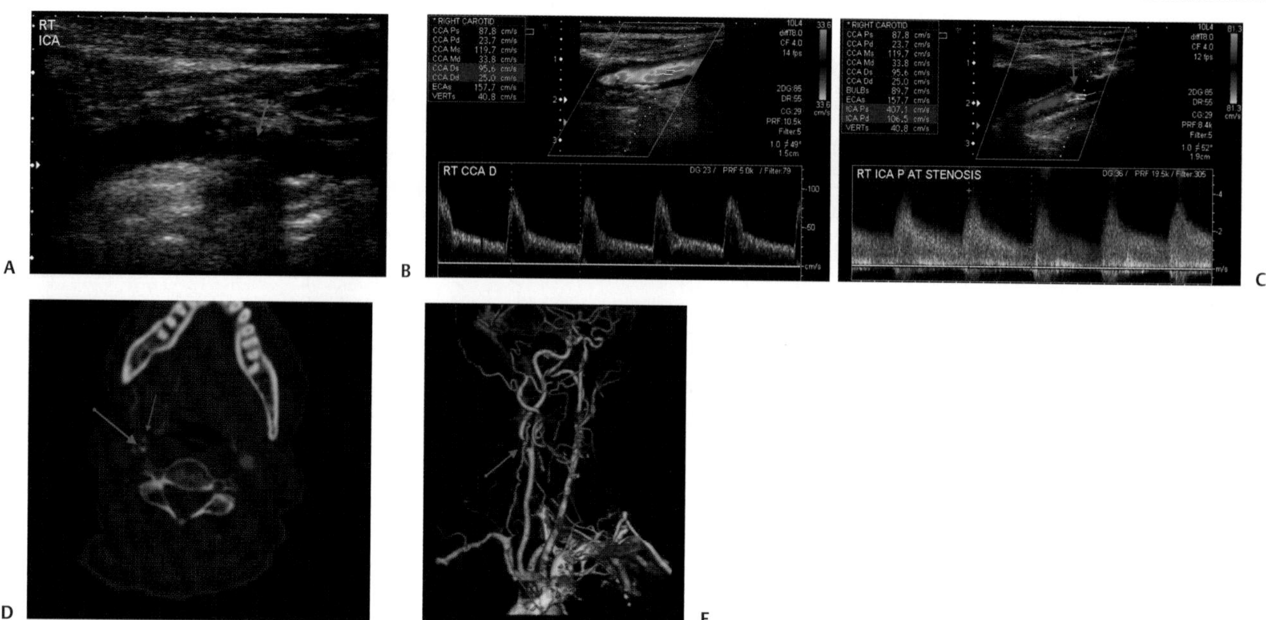

(A–C) Gray scale ultrasound images of the right carotid artery at its origin demonstrate > 50% luminal narrowing with plaque (*green arrow*). Doppler evaluation of the common carotid artery demonstrates normal flow without evidence of turbulence and/or increased velocity. Further evaluation with Doppler tracing at the origin of the right internal carotid artery demonstrates marked increased velocity with turbulence of waveform. The internal carotid artery/common carotid artery (ICA/CCA) ratio is more than 4. **(D, E)** Further evaluation with contrast-enhanced computed tomography (CT) angiography demonstrates large calcified plaque at the origin of the right internal carotid artery (*green arrow*). The external carotid artery appears grossly unremarkable (*red arrow*). Three-dimensional volume rendering confirmed the finding of narrowing at the origin of the right internal carotid artery.

Differential Diagnosis

- ***More than 70% stenosis at the origin of the right internal carotid artery:*** The systolic velocity is markedly elevated exceeding 230 cm/sec. Gray scale images demonstrate > 50% narrowing in the lumen. The ICA/CCA ratio is markedly elevated, exceeding 4. Surgical treatment might be indicated.
- *Atherosclerotic plaque at the origin of the internal carotid artery without significant stenosis:* Defined as a stenosis < 50% in diameter, considered not clinically significant. The peak systolic velocity within the internal carotid artery is < 125 cm/sec. The ICA/CCA ratio is less than 2.
- *Fifty to 69% stenosis at the origin of the right internal carotid artery:* Sonographically defined as > 50% narrowing of the diameter. The peak systolic velocity is elevated at 125 to 230 cm/sec. The ICA/CCA ratio is estimated elevated at 2 to 4. Turbulence of flow at and post stenosis could also be seen.

Essential Facts

- Strokes are more common in blacks and Hispanics
- Increased incidence in diabetes, smoking, and hypertension.
- Patients with carotid artery disease are classified into symptomatic and asymptomatic groups.
- The asymptomatic groups include patients with stroke, transient ischemic attack, or amaurosis fugax.
- Doppler is inaccurate for grading stenosis < 50%; these patients should be included under a single category.
- Seventy percent stenosis is believed to be the threshold used for surgical intervention.
- The internal carotid artery is considered normal when the velocity is < 125 cm/sec.
- Fifty to 69% ICA stenosis is diagnosed when the systolic velocity is 125 to 230 cm/sec, with plaque visible causing ~ 50% stenosis. The ICA/CCA ratio is 2 to 4.
- More than 70% stenosis is diagnosed when the velocities exceed 230 cm/sec with plaque causing significant narrowing on gray scale imaging. The ICA/CCA ratio is more than 4.
- Near occlusion is diagnosed when the lumen is markedly narrowed on color or power ultrasound.
- Total occlusion is diagnosed when there is no flow in the internal carotid artery.

✓ Pearls & × Pitfalls

✓ A combination of gray scale finding, color Doppler, and tracing should be used to categorize the degree of internal carotid artery stenosis.

× In case of near occlusion, the velocity parameters should not be used since the velocity could be high and/or low. The diagnosis should be made by demonstrating markedly narrowed lumen.

Case 18

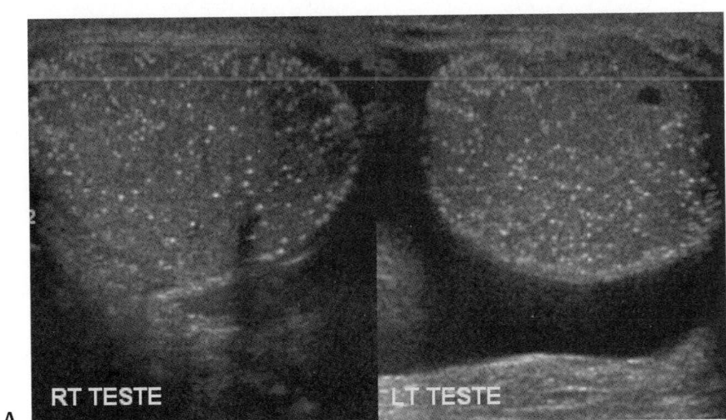

A

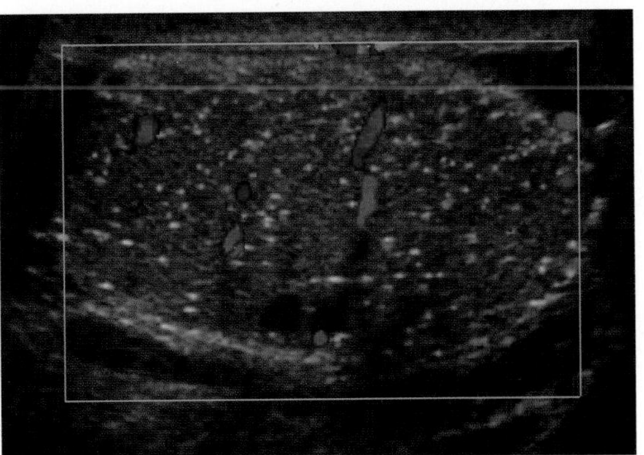

B

Clinical Presentation

A 25-year-old man with vague scrotal pain, but no swelling.

Imaging Findings

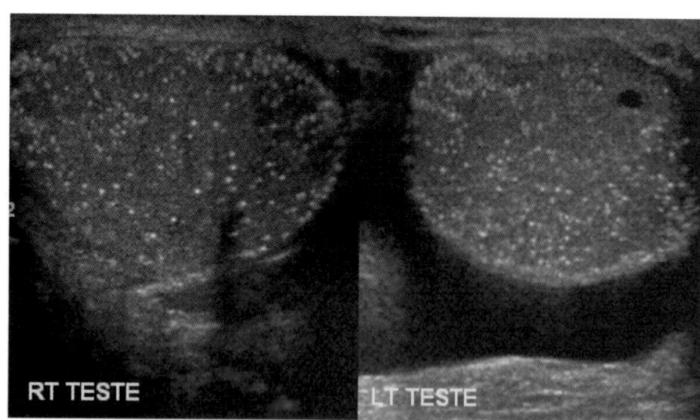

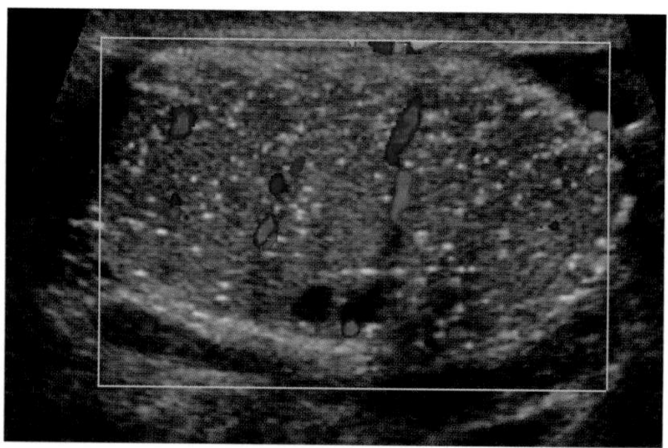

(A, B) Scrotal ultrasound demonstrates punctate echogenic foci in the testicles bilaterally.

Differential Diagnosis

- ***Testicular microlithiasis:*** Multiple punctate nonshadowing echogenic foci, often more numerous in the periphery of the testicles. Calcifications measure 2 to 3 mm. These tiny calcifications do not shadow with gray scale imaging or cause twinkle artifact with color Doppler imaging.
- *Dystrophic calcifications from prior infection or injury:* These calcifications are larger, causing shadowing, and are less numerous.
- *Testicular cancers:* Can contain calcifications but would be associated with a mass.

Essential Facts

- Diagnosis requires five or more echogenic foci per image in one or both testicles. Usually bilateral (80%).
- Occurs in 1.5 to 5% of normal males and may be found in up to 20% of patients with subfertility.
- Usually asymptomatic and nonprogressive
- Association with malignancy is controversial.

✓ Pearls & × Pitfalls

✓ Microlithiasis can be subtle or marked.
✓ The degree of microlithiasis is not relevant.
✓ With improved imaging and higher frequency transducers, microliths are more commonly noted.

Case 19

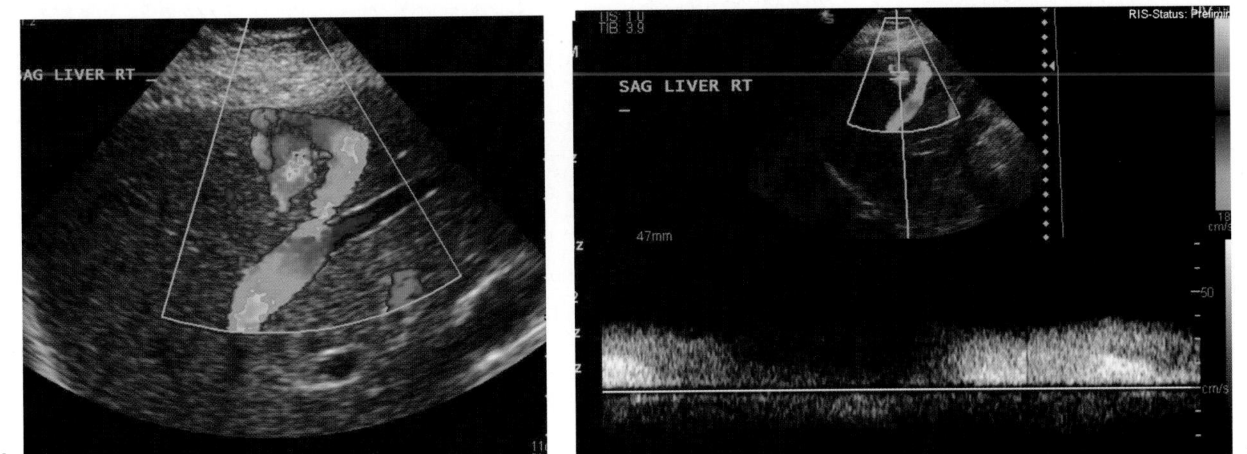

■ Clinical Presentation

A 45-year-old man with history of prior liver surgeries presents with right upper quadrant discomfort.

■ Further Work-up

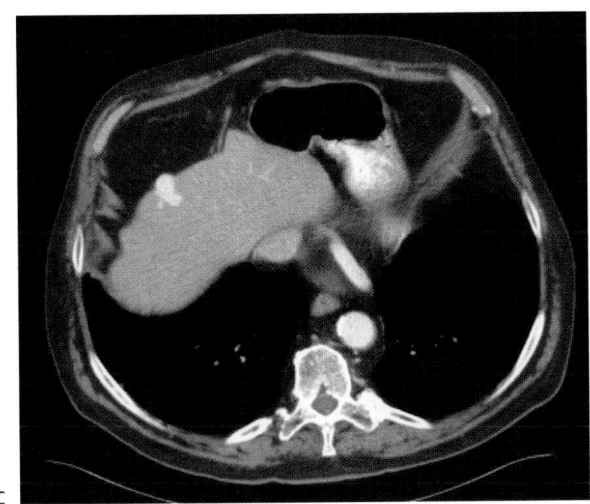

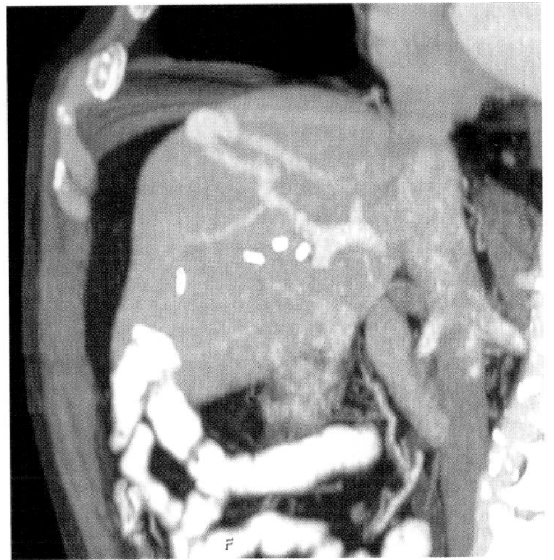

Imaging Findings

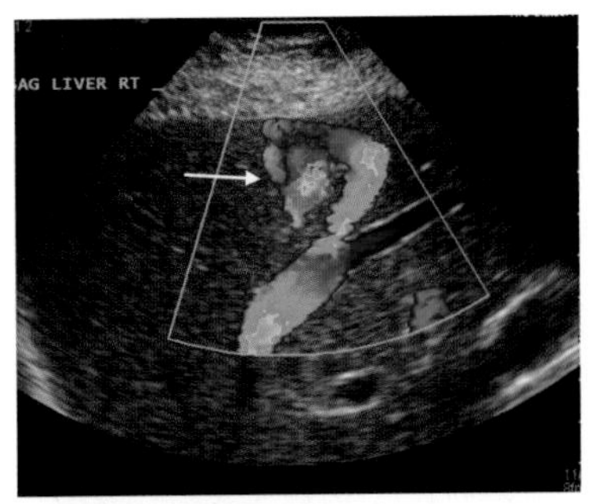

A

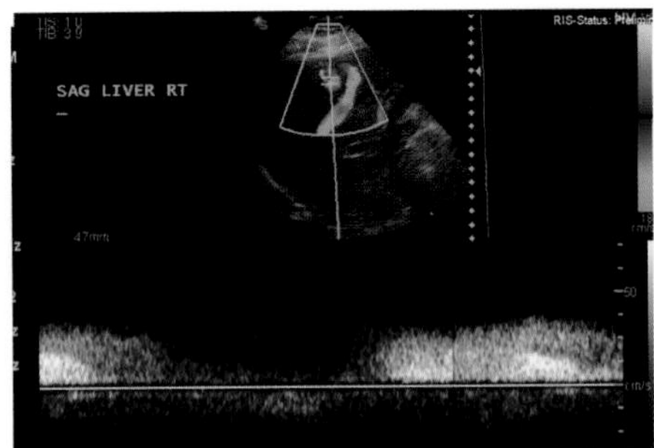

B

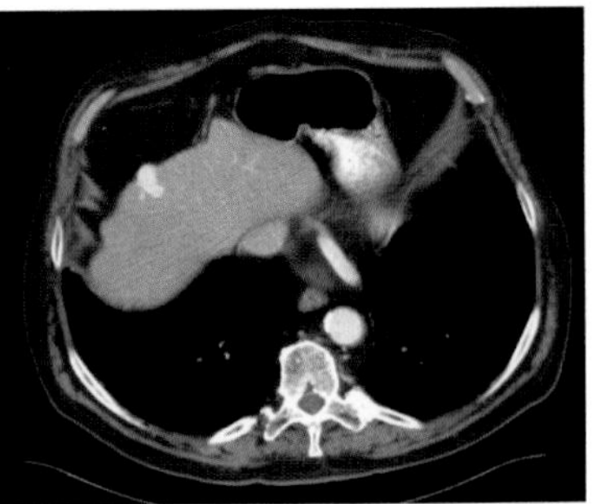

C

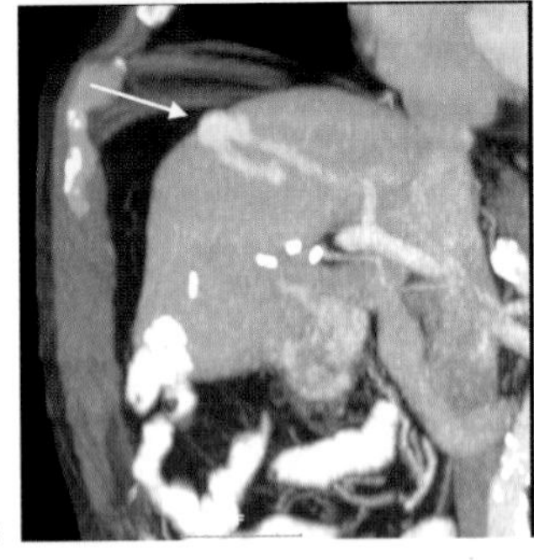

D

(A, B) Ultrasound images of the liver with Doppler demonstrate abnormal communication between the anterior branch, right portal vein, and the middle hepatic vein (*white arrow*); the waveform is predominantly monophasic with respiratory variation. **(C, D)** Computed tomography (CT) of the liver after intravenous contrast with coronal reconstruction confirms the presence of abnormal communication between the right portal and middle hepatic vein (*white arrow*).

Differential Diagnosis

- ***Portovenous malformation:*** A developmental diversion of portal venous blood into a systemic vein without passage of blood through the liver. Usually is detected as incidental finding on Doppler ultrasound and/or cross-sectional angiography (in asymptomatic patients).
- *Arterio-portal fistula:* Abnormal communication between the hepatic artery and portal vein. Could be related to trauma/intervention, hepatitis, liver cirrhosis, neoplasm, and infections. On ultrasound, arterialization of the portal system is noted with potential signs of portal hypertension.
- *Hypervascular mass lesion:* Primary liver lesions (benign and/or malignant) or hypervascular metastatic lesion could present with similar appearance on dynamic CT angiography or magnetic resonance angiography.

Essential Facts

- Can be either extrahepatic or intrahepatic.
- Occasionally associated with congenital cardiac defects, lobulation of the liver, hepatoblastoma, extrahepatic biliary atresia, and hyperammonemia.
- On imaging, could be seen as single tubular, peripheral shunt; aneurysmal communication; or multiple communications.
- Doppler is capable of ascertaining the presence of shunt, quantifying shunt flow, and determining shunt topography and morphology.
- The presence of monophasic flow is suggestive of the diagnosis.
- Hepatic encephalopathy is the most common complication in large communications. There is increased incidence of septic emboli.

✓ Pearls & × Pitfalls

✓ In case of abnormal intrahepatic vascularity, the presence of arterialization of the portal vein is suggestive of arterio-portal fistula. A monophasic flow is suggestive of portovenous malformation.

× The presence of shunt on cross-sectional imaging could be misinterpreted as an enhancing mass lesion.

Case 20

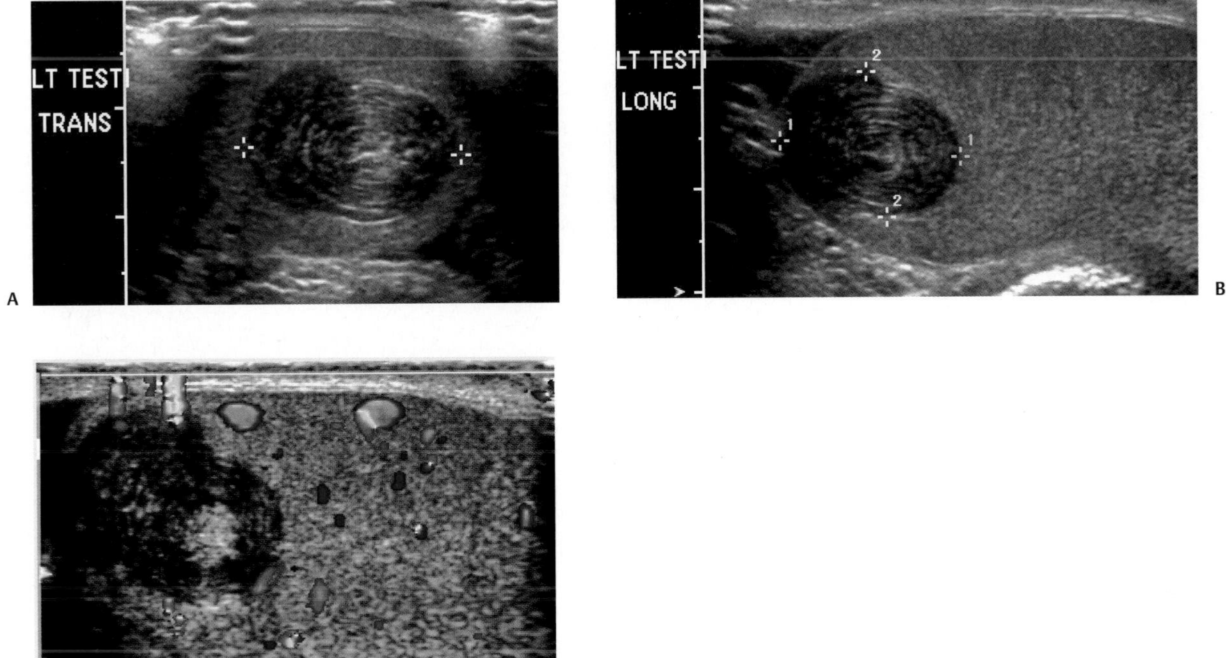

Clinical Presentation

A 40-year-old man presents with a palpable abnormality of the left testicle noted on physical exam performed 2 days ago. No scrotal pain or swelling.

Imaging Findings

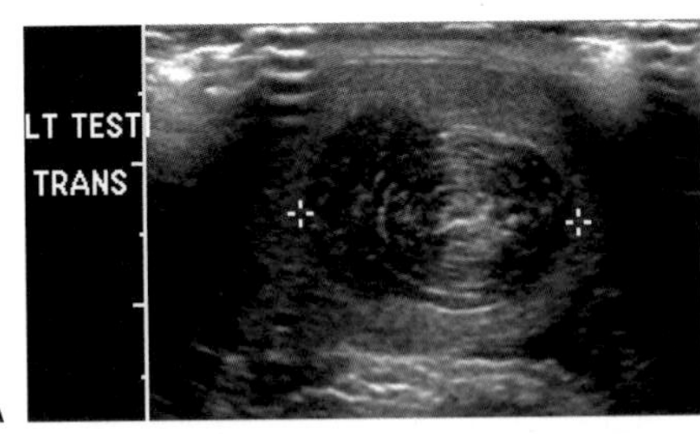

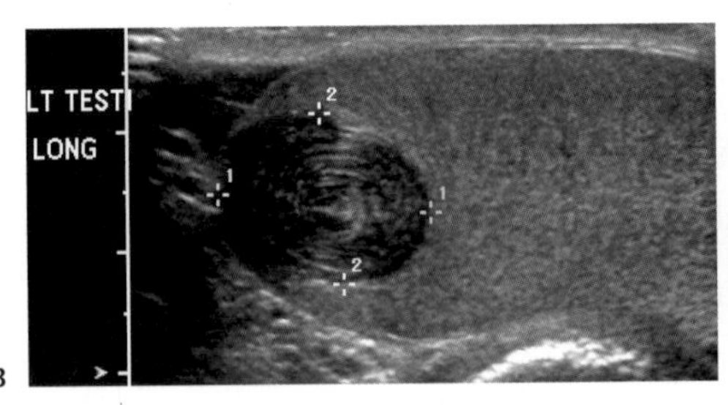

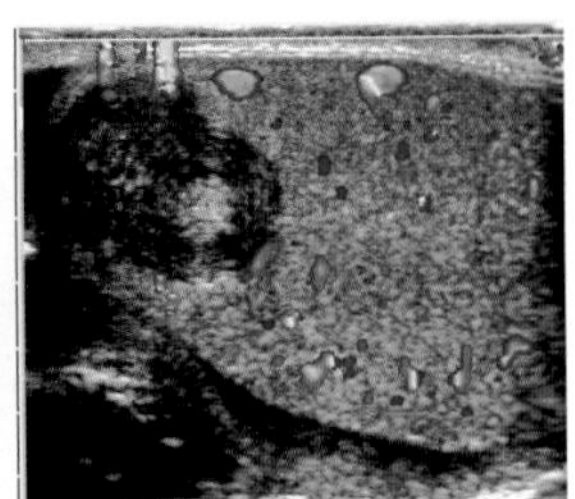

(A–C) Transverse and longitudinal gray scale images of the testicles demonstrate a 1.8 × 1.4 × 2 cm lesion located superiorly within the testicle. The lesion is well circumscribed and hypoechoic with a hyperechoic center surrounded by whirling lines. Color Doppler imaging indicates that there is no internal vascularity.

Differential Diagnosis

- ***Epidermoid:*** The alternating rings of hyperechogenicity and hypoechogenicity ("onion skin" appearance) and the lack of internal vascularity are classic of an epidermoid.
- *Testicular tumors:* Testicular tumors are vascular and therefore demonstrate color tagging with color Doppler imaging. Testicular tumors are usually solid and therefore more echogenic than an epidermoid. Testicular neoplasms are not usually as well circumscribed or smoothly marginated as an epidermoid.
- *Testicular cysts:* Testicular cysts are simple. They are anechoic and cause acoustical enhancement unlike an epidermoid. Testicular cysts are much less common than frequently encountered epididymal cysts.

Essential Facts

- Epidermoids can demonstrate a pathognomonic appearance of "onion skinning."
- Rare, constitute < 1% of tumors
- Benign, often removed via local resection or enucleation
- Can calcify
- At pathology, they are encapsulated and contain alternating rings of white-yellow paste-like material that corresponds to the layers of keratinizing squamous epithelium. The keratin debris seen at both gross and histologic examination corresponded to the echogenic center seen at ultrasound.
- Can occur at any age but most common in second to fourth decade.

✓ Pearls & × Pitfalls

× Epidermoids occasionally densely calcify and can be difficult to differentiate from a teratoma.

✓ The whorled appearance or onion skinning of the lesion is pathognomonic.

Case 21

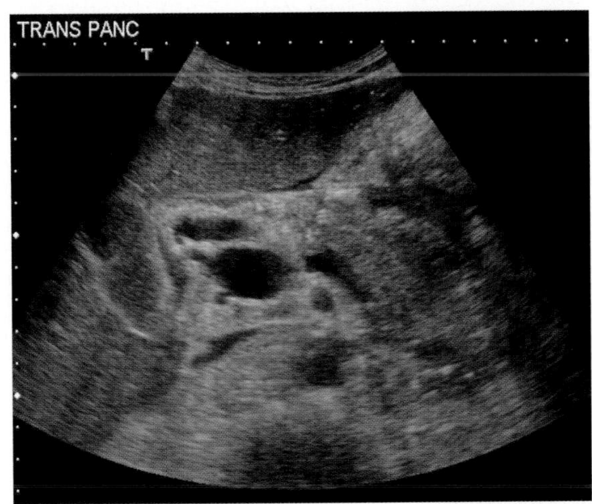

A

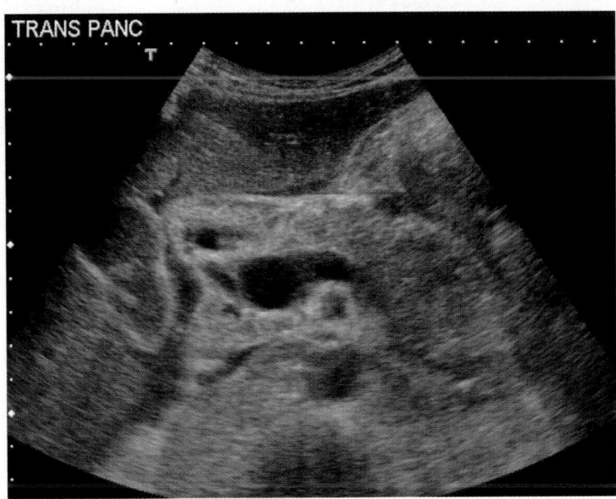

B

Clinical Presentation

A 65-year-old woman with multiple underlying medical problems complains of epigastric pain and weight loss.

Further Work-up

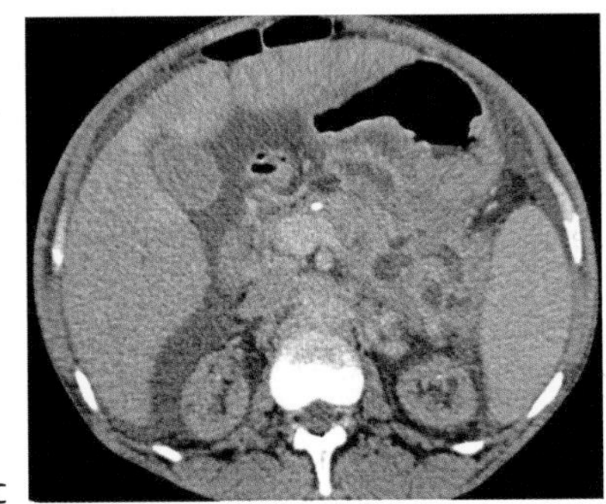

C

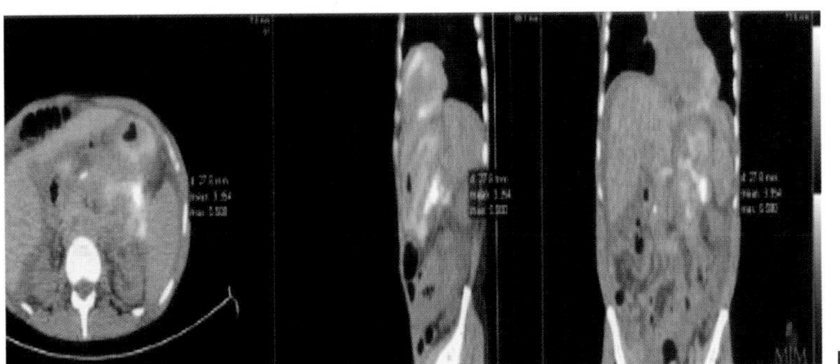

D

Imaging Findings

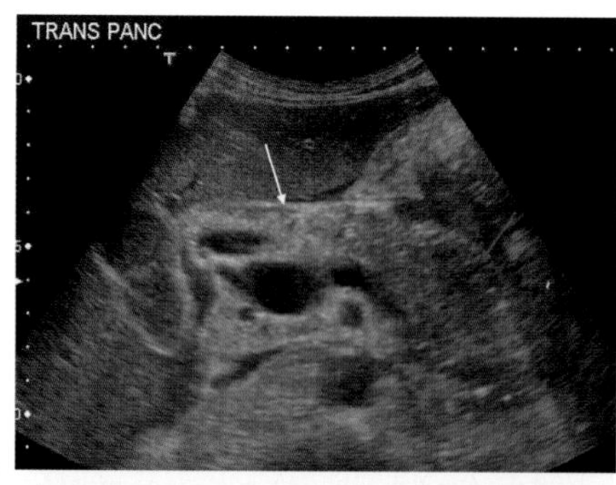

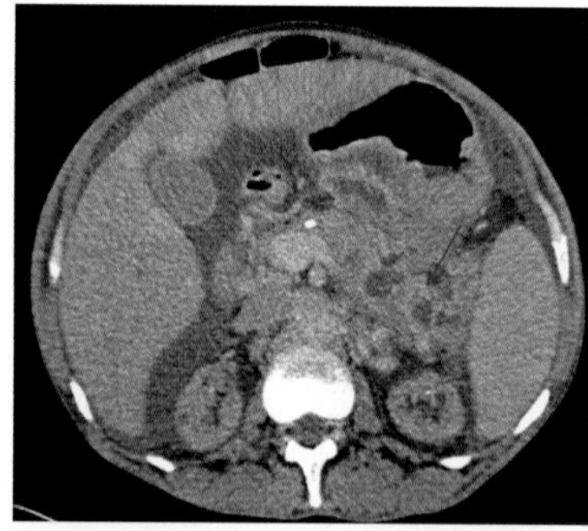

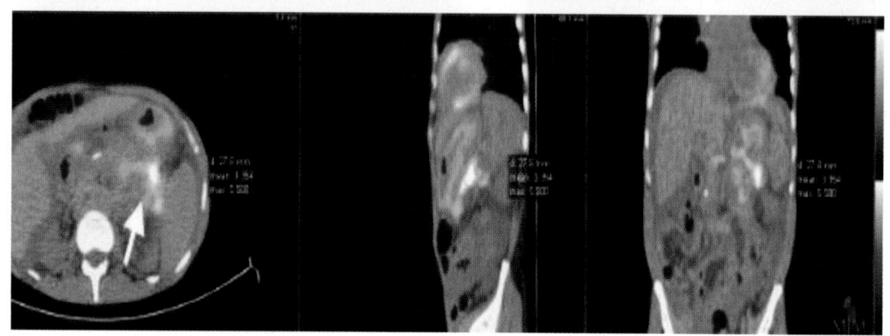

(A) Ultrasound (US) shows poorly defined hypoechoic area in the tail of the pancreas (*red arrow*). The proximal body and head appear normal (*white arrow*). Trace amount of ascites is noted. **(B)** Follow-up computed tomography (CT) scan shows cystic lesions in the tail of the pancreas (*red arrow*) corresponding to the abnormal finding on US. Ascites in the abdomen is also noted on CT. **(C)** Follow-up positron emission tomography (PET) scan shows intense uptake in this tail of the pancreas (*white arrow*) corresponding to the cystic changes in the tail of the pancreas.

Differential Diagnosis

- ***Cystic neoplasm of the pancreas:*** There are two types, microcystic adenoma and macrocystic neoplasm. Sonographically appears as well-circumscribed, unilocular or multilocular cystic lesions; a solid component might be seen.
- *Intraductal papillary mucinous neoplasms:* Intraductal calcifications can be seen, as well as a grapelike cluster of dilated side branches. An echogenic mucin may make the tumor indistinguishable from the surrounding pancreatic parenchyma on US.
- *Acute pancreatitis with pseudocyst formation:* The pancreas appears hypoechoic in the acute form. A pseudocyst occurs in 10 to 20% of patients with acute pancreatitis. It appears as well-defined cystic lesions/lesions with enhanced transmission. The pseudocyst could be complex with multiloculation and calcifications.

Essential Facts

- There are two types microcystic serous cystadenoma/ macrocystic musinous cystadenoma and cystadenocarcinoma.
- The microcystic type occurs in older patients, could have central calcifications, and is benign. The cyst varies in size from 1 mm to 2 cm.
- In the macrocystic type, the cysts measure > 2 cm and could be unilocular or multilocular; the tumor is malignant or premalignant.
- The appearance of macrocystic lesions could be clear cysts, echogenic cysts, cysts with mural nodule, or a solid cyst.
- The presence of a mural nodule in a cystic lesion is suggestive of the mucinous type.

✓ Pearls & × Pitfalls

✓ The ability to establish communication between cystic lesions and the pancreatic duct helps to differentiate intraductal papillary neoplasms from cystic neoplasm of the pancreas.

× Necrotic adenocarcinoma and cystic islet cell tumors could have imaging appearance overlapping with cystic neoplasm of the pancreas.

Case 22

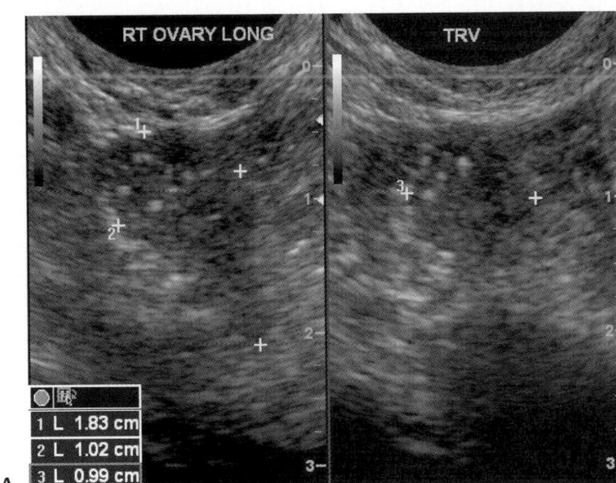

A

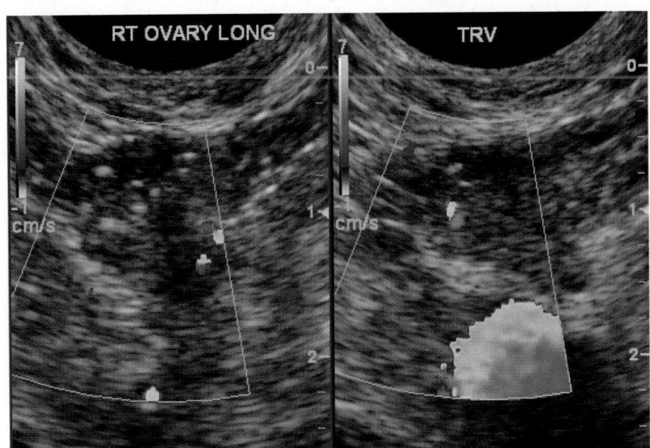

B

■ Clinical Presentation

A 72-year-old woman with pelvic pain, no postmenopausal bleeding.

Imaging Findings

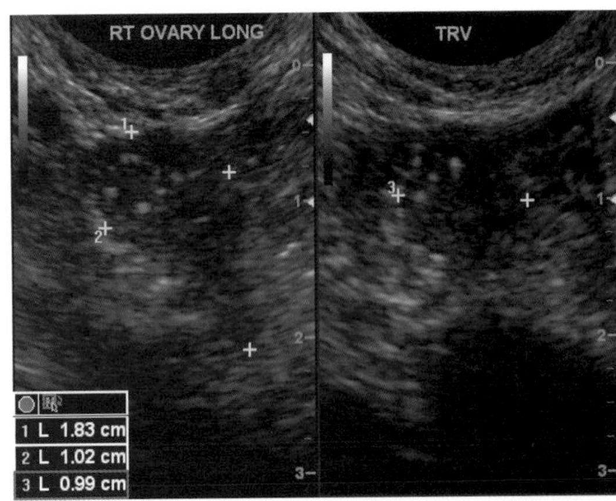

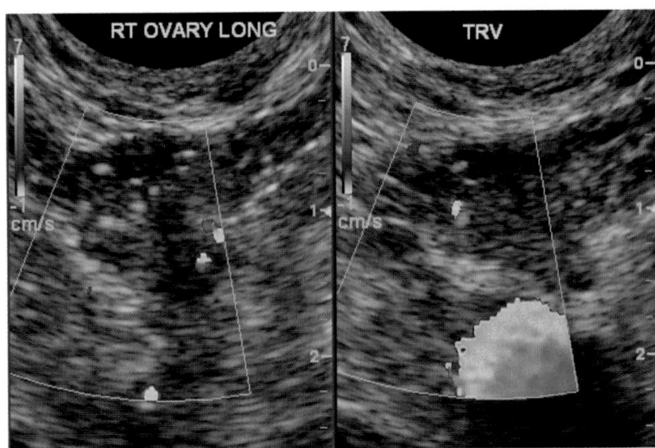

(A, B) Longitudinal and transverse images of the ovaries demonstrate several punctate echogenic foci (this was present bilaterally). With color Doppler there is no twinkle artifact. The ovaries are atrophic as expected in a patient of this age.

Differential Diagnosis

- ***Echogenic ovarian foci (EOF):*** Multiple echogenic foci are not shadowing and do not twinkle with color Doppler ultrasound. They are consistent with EOF and are a frequent incidental finding of no clinical significance. The specular reflection is from the walls of tiny unresolved benign cysts.
- *Dystrophic calcifications:* Dystrophic calcifications in the ovaries are larger and less numerous. They would shadow and cause twinkle artifact.
- *Dermoid:* Calcifications associated with dermoids are larger. They are usually associated with a cystic mass.

Essential Facts

- EOF can occur in both premenopausal and postmenopausal women.
- The specular reflection is caused by the walls of a tiny cyst. These cysts are comparable in size to the ultrasound (US) wavelength (0.50 mm) and therefore too small to decipher with US.
- EOF are more frequently peripheral in location and usually mulitiple. EOF are frequently bilateral.

✓ Pearls & × Pitfalls

- ✓ As gray scale image optimization continues to improve with high-frequency transducers, harmonic imaging, etc., EOF is a more frequently imaged finding.
- ✓ EOF is unrelated to psammomatous calcifications or microlithiasis. These are true calcifications that are associated with malignancy.
- ✓ True calcifications in the ovaries usually exhibit twinkle artifact regardless of size.
- × EOF are often not recognized in premenopausal women whose ovaries contain multiple follicles and a corpus luteum.
- ✓ EOF are more obvious in the postmenopausal ovary, which is usually homogenous and atrophic.

Case 23

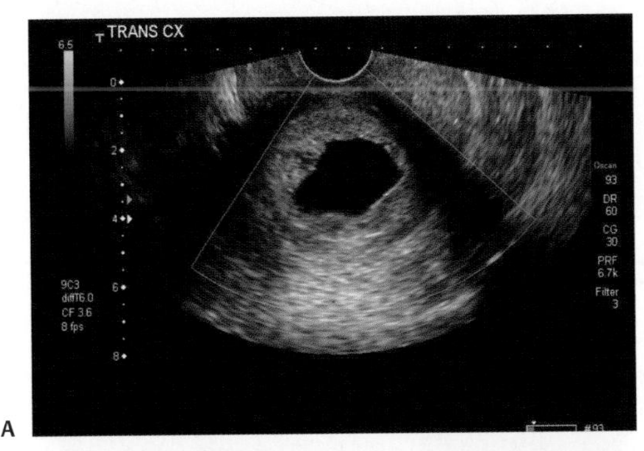

A

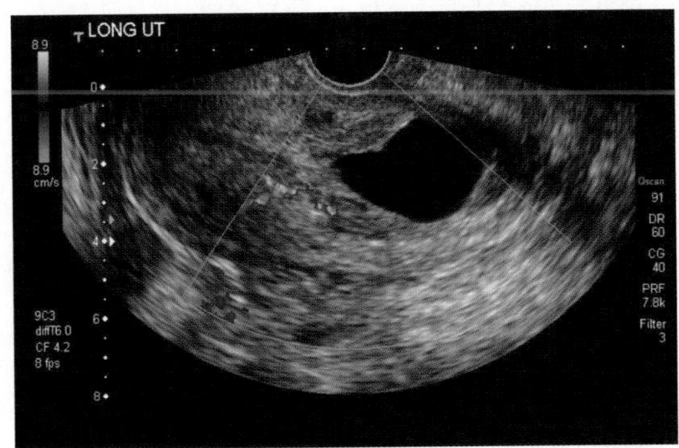

B

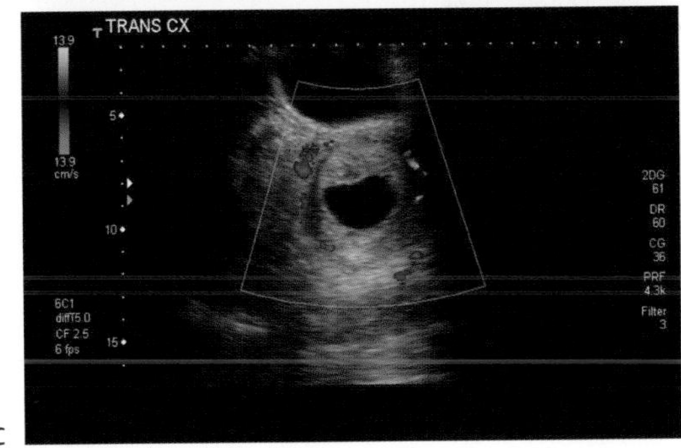

C

Clinical Presentation

A 25-year-old woman with positive pregnancy test presents with vaginal bleeding.

Further Work-up

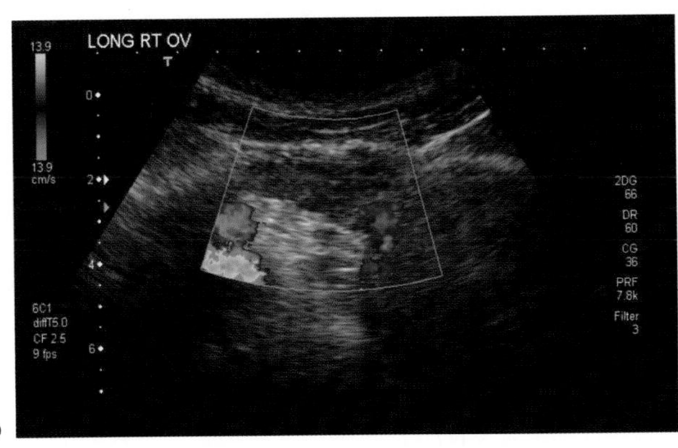

D

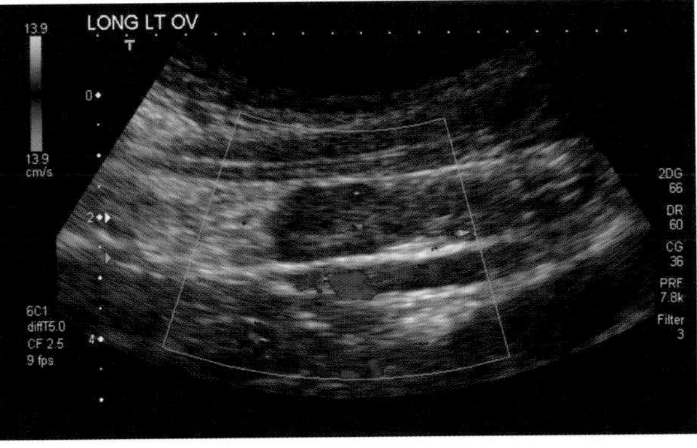

E

Imaging Findings

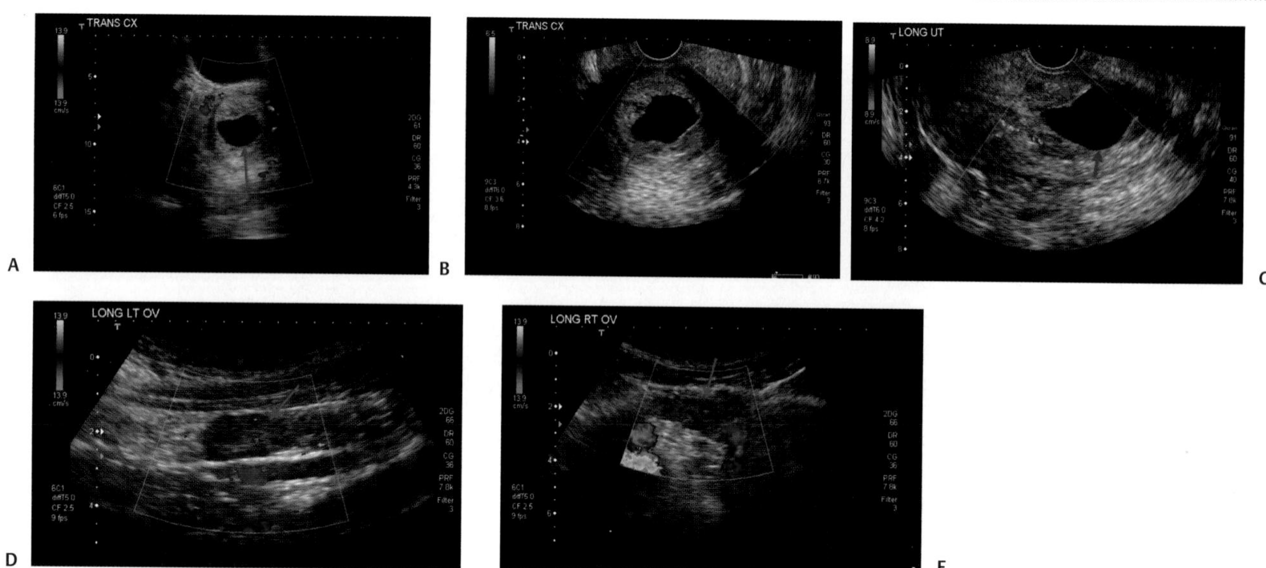

(A–C) Ultrasound (US) of the pelvis using transvaginal and transabdominal approach demonstrates an irregularly shaped cystic lesion within the lower uterine segment/cervical canal (*red arrows*). No significant flow is appreciated within the described cystic structure on color or power Doppler US. No definite evidence of fetal pole and/or yolk sac is visualized within the sac. **(D, E)** Further evaluation of the adnexa demonstrate normal-appearing right and left ovary (*green arrow*). No definite evidence of adnexal masses are seen.

Differential Diagnosis

- ***Miscarriage in progress:*** Miscarriage could be complete and/or missed. Sonographically, an irregularly shaped gestational sac is visualized with absent embryonic pole and/or fetal pole without cardiac activity. Subchorionic hemorrhage and or active bleeding could be visualized on real-time US.
- *Cervical ectopic pregnancy:* Cervical ectopic pregnancy is rare, more frequently associated with assisted reproductive techniques. The patient presents with excessive pelvic pain and vaginal bleeding. The bleeding could be life-threatening. Sonographically, gestational sac in the cervix is noted. Yolk sac and embryo could be visualized. The presence of thick echogenic hypervascular rim around the sac is highly suggestive of cervical ectopic pregnancy. Visualization of embryo with cardiac activity within the cervical sac is diagnostic of cervical ectopic.
- *Pseudosac secondary to ectopic pregnancy:* A pseudosac is sloughing of the decidua producing a fluid collection in the endometrial cavity. Approximately 20% of patients with ectopic pregnancy have a pseudosac seen on transvaginal ultrasound. Sonographically, a pseudosac is centric in location and a true gestation is eccentric. The presence of a double decidual sac sign is diagnostic of true gestational sac.

Essential Facts

- The incidence is difficult to assess accurately but ranges from 5 to 10% of total pregnancies.
- Miscarriage can be related to fetal, maternal, and/or paternal factors.
- The clinical presentation includes vaginal bleeding, cramps, and pelvic pain.
- The sonographic findings include a large, empty gestational sac; irregular sac margins; a sac with a yolk sac only; and smaller than expected gestational sac.
- On follow-up examinations, lack of growth or development is suggestive of the diagnosis.
- Fetal pole is seen without cardiac activity.
- When the gestational sac is smaller than the expected gestational age, the possibility of incorrect date should be considered.
- In complete miscarriage, the conception has completely lost; only endometrial blood is seen.
- In missed miscarriage, the pregnancy has stopped developing; however, the gestational sac remains within the uterus.
- US should be performed in all patient presenting with first-trimester vaginal bleeding.

✓ Pearls & × Pitfalls

✓ A gestational sac of mean diameter > 20 mm with no evidence of a yolk sac or an embryo is suggestive of nonviable pregnancy.

× When the mean gestational sac diameter is < 15 mm or the crown-rump length is < 10 mm, lack of visualization of cardiac motion should not be presumed to be fetal demise. Follow-up examination in 1 week is indicated.

Case 24

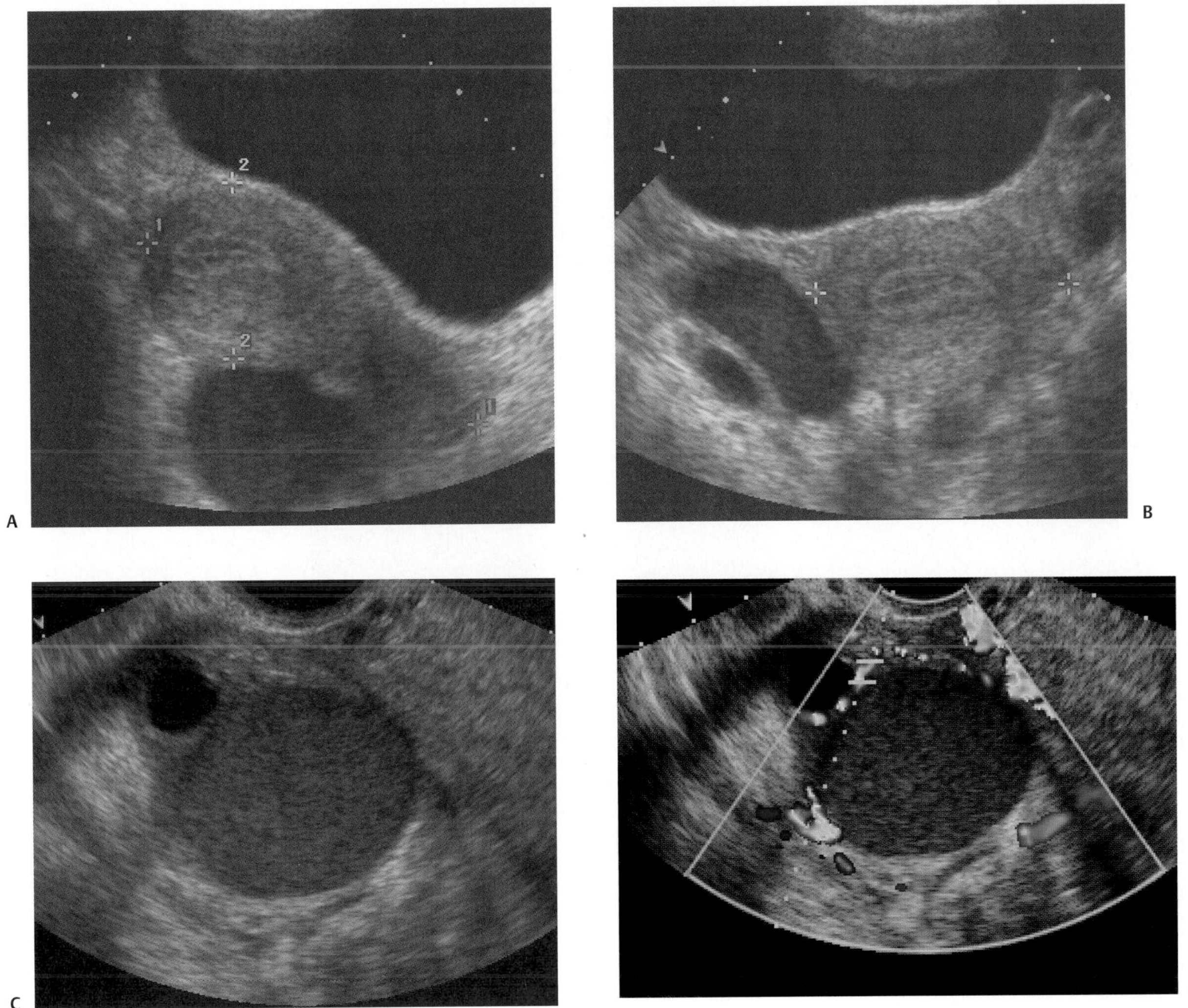

■ Clinical Presentation

A 30-year-old woman with pelvic mass on exam.

Imaging Findings

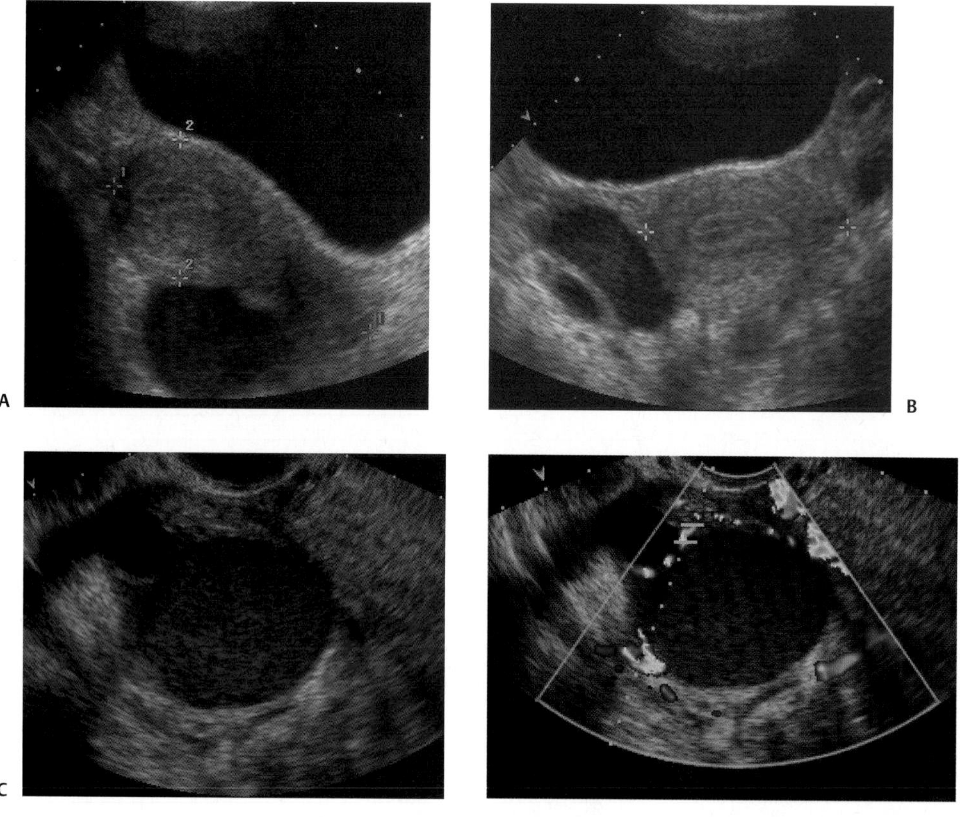

(A–D) The right ovary contains a well-circumscribed homogeneously isoechoic lesion that demonstrates acoustic enhancement. The internal echoes are more obvious on transvaginal scanning. No flow is identified within the lesion with color or spectral Doppler imaging.

Differential Diagnosis

- ***Classic endometrioma:*** A cystic lesion with homogeneous low-level echoes and no internal vascularity is most consistent with an endometrioma.
- *Hemorrhagic cyst:* Hemorrhagic cysts are usually heterogeneous. They often contain lacelike reticulations or retracting clot. Like an endometrioma, they do not demonstrate internal vascularity with color Doppler imaging.
- *Solid ovarian neoplasm:* A solid lesion in the ovary can be homogeneous with low-level echoes similar to an endometrioma. However, solid lesions are usually vascular and would therefore demonstrate flow with color Doppler.

Essential Facts

- Endometriomas, also known as *chocolate cysts* because of their appearance at surgery, result from endometrial implants in the ovaries.
- The homogeneous low-level echoes within the lesion result from cyclical bleeding.
- Endometriomas are often incidental as they can be asymptomatic, as in this patient.
- Symptomatic endometriosis is usually the result of endometrial implants of the peritoneum and are not usually visible with ultrasound. These implants can be seen with magnetic resonance imaging (MRI).
- A classic endometrioma such as this is often treated conservatively without surgery.
- If endometriomas are not treated surgically, annual follow-up is recommended.
- One percent of endometriomas are believed to undergo malignant transformation. Most malignancies occur in large lesions (> 9 cm) and in older women (> 45 years old).

Other Imaging Findings

- On computed tomography, endometriomas appear similar to simple cysts or may be of greater density due to the blood products.
- On MRI, endometriomas are high signal on T1-weighted images and may demonstrate T2 shading. They do not enhance.

✓ Pearls & ✗ Pitfalls

✓ Endometriomas should never demonstrate internal vascularity.

✗ Endometriomas can contain features similar to malignancy. MRI is helpful to distinguish atypical endometriomas from neoplastic lesions.

Case 25

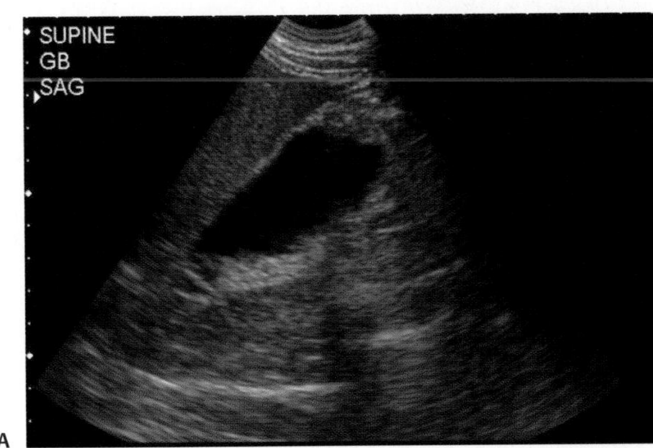

A

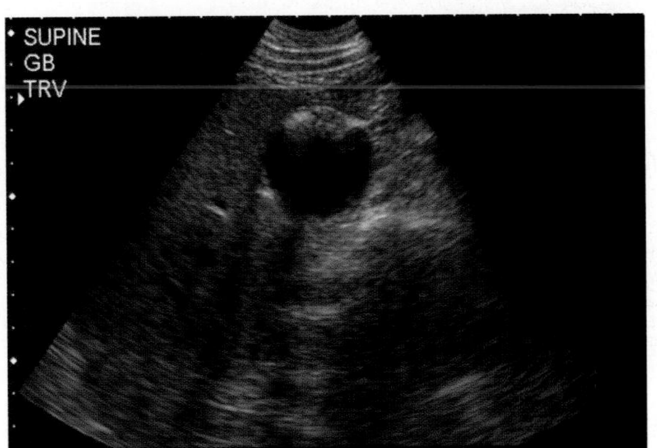

B

Clinical Presentation

A 35-year-old man presents with right upper quadrant pain.

Further Work-up

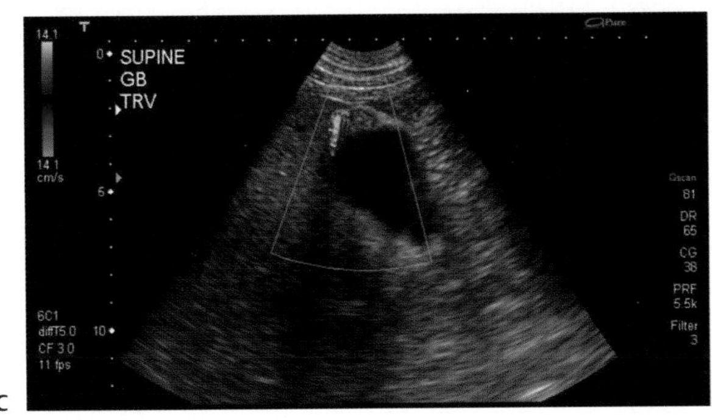

C

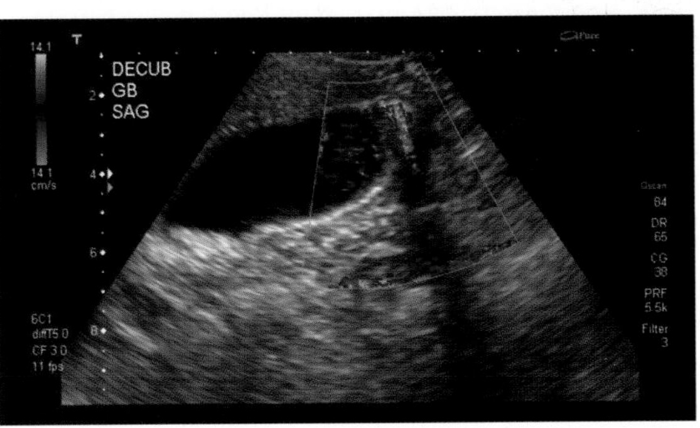

D

Imaging Findings

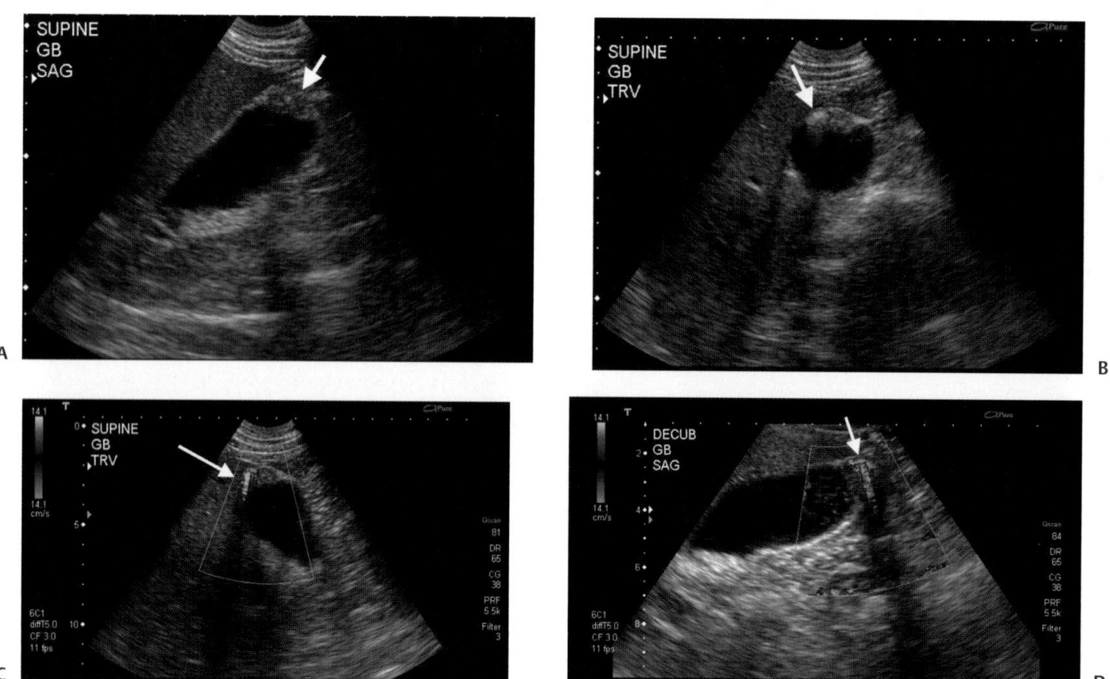

(A, B) Ultrasound (US) images using gray scale show focal thickening of the gallbladder fundus with ring down artifact/v-shape artifact (*white arrow*). **(C, D)** Color Doppler ultrasound images confirm the presence of twinkle artifact in the fundus of the gallbladder (*white arrow*). No gross evidence of arterial or venous flow is noted.

Differential Diagnosis

- ***Focal adenomyomatosis of the gallbladder:*** Hyperplasic process of the gallbladder mucosa. Could be focal or diffuse types. Rokitansky-Aschoff sinuses may contain echogenic foci that cause a reverberation artifact.
- *Gallbladder polyp:* Could be single or multiple. The polyp ranges from 2 to10 mm. Lesions > 10 mm with broad base raise the suspicion for malignancy.
- *Gallbladder cancer:* Usually present as single or multiple intraluminal mass; focal thickening as early presentation is less likely to be diagnosed. The presence of vascular flow and invasion of the liver is suggestive malignancy.

Essential Facts

- Benign epithelial proliferation is seen in 5% of cholecystectomies.
- More common in females.
- It is commonly focal, commonly in the fundus; could be segmental or diffuse.
- Intramural cystic formation, reverberation artifacts, and focal wall thickening of the gallbladder wall are diagnostic of adenomyomatosis on ultrasound.
- The presence of twinkle artifact on color imaging also favors the diagnosis.

✓ Pearls & × Pitfalls

✓ The presence of twinkle artifact with focal thickening favors the diagnosis of adenomyomatosis.

× The presence of focal thickening and twinkle artifact could be misinterpreted as gallbladder mass with vascular flow. The presence of noise on Doppler tracing will help to differentiate this finding from true vascular flow.

Case 26

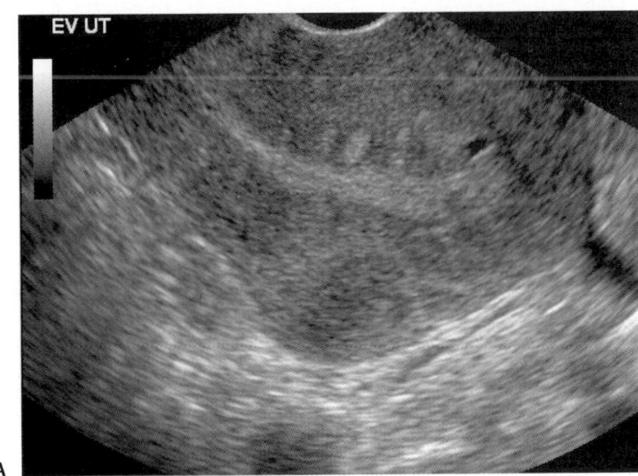

A

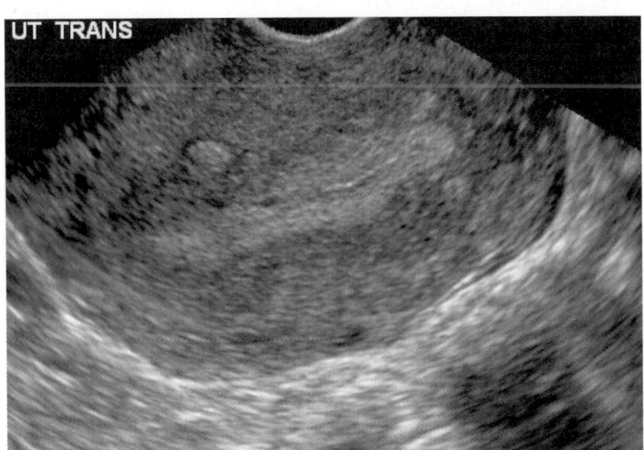

B

Clinical Presentation

A 45-year-old woman with pelvic pain and menorrhagia.

Further Work-up

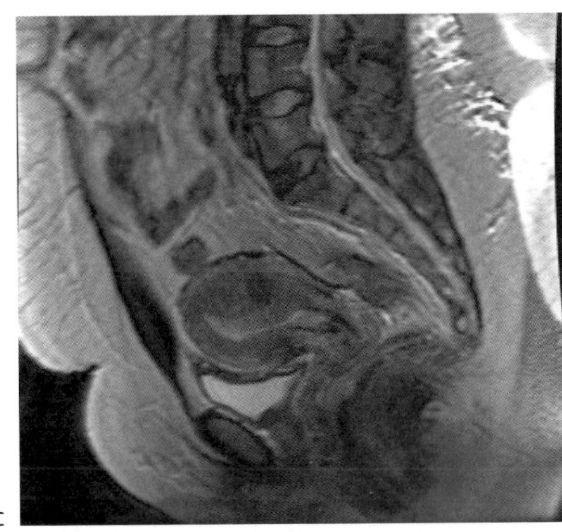
C

Imaging Findings

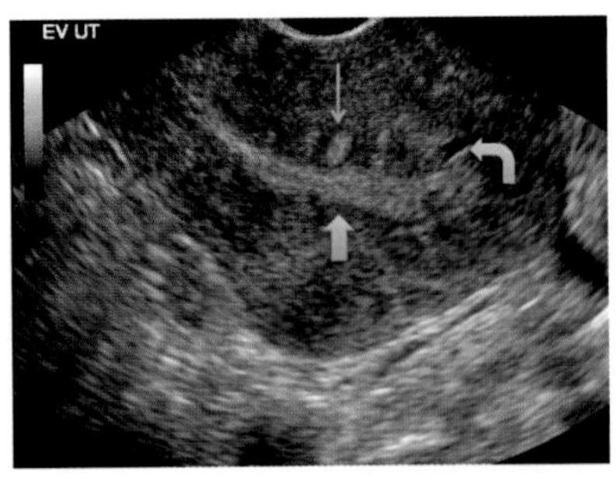

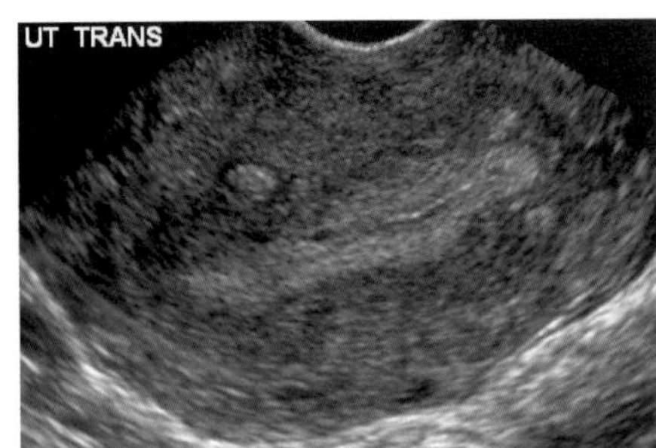

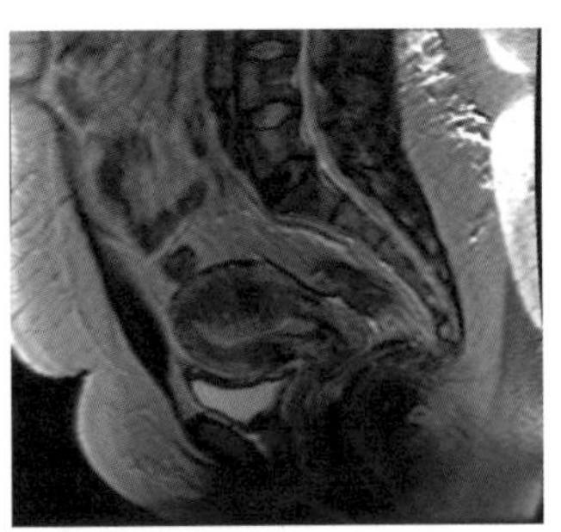

(A, B) Longitudinal and transverse transvaginal images demonstrate a retroflexed uterus. The endometrial myometrial junction along the anterior wall of the uterus (more posterior in the image) is well defined (*thick arrow*). In the posterior uterus, the endometrial myometrial junction is irregular. There are echogenic regions within the inner myometrium (*thin arrow*). A small cyst is seen toward the posterior fundus (*curved arrow*). **(C)** T2 weighted sagittal image demonstrates a thickened junctional zone posteriorly with punctuate foci of increased signal in the posterior myometrium.

Differential Diagnosis

- ***Adenomyosis:*** An ill-defined endometrial myometrial junction with endometrial implants in the myometrium and cystic changes as seen above are classic for adenomyosis.
- *Submucosal myoma:* The endometrial implants in the myometrium may mimic masses such as fibroids. Fibroids are usually hypoechoic and may cause shadowing. The endometrial implants are similar in appearance to the endometrium in adenomyosis.
- *Endometrial carcinoma:* The endometrial myometrial junction in endometrial cancer can be ill defined, indicating invasion. The endometrium would be thicker and heterogenous with endometrial cancer. Cystic changes would be present in the endometrium, not the myometrium as seen with adenomyosis.

Essential Facts

- Adenomyosis is the uterine correlate of endometriosis. It is associated with endometriosis; occurs in 1% of women.
- It presents in the fourth and fifth decade and is more common in multiparous women.
- Ultrasound (US) findings include enlarged uterus, ill-defined endometrium, cystic changes of the myometrium, and heterogeneous myometrium.
- Can be diffuse or focal. If focal, it is more commonly posterior, as in the above case. A focal collection of adenomyosis is referred to as an adenomyoma.
- Clinically, these patients have painful menses with a tender, boggy uterus on exam.
- Historically, treatment was surgical. Uterine artery embolization now plays a role.

Other Imaging Findings

- Magnetic resonance imaging: Thickening of the junctional zone. < 8 mm is normal, 8 to 12 mm is suggestive of adenomyosis, and > 12 mm is diagnostic of adenomyosis. Focal areas if T2 bright signal representing the cystic spaces.

✓ Pearls & × Pitfalls

× Adenomyosis can be difficult to diagnose with US. Classic features not always visible by US.

× Features of adenomyosis are similar to fibroids, particularly diffuse myomatous change.

× MRI is very sensitive for the detection of adenomyosis, US is not.

✓ Both fibroids and adenomyosis cause uterine enlargement. Unlike a myomatous uterus, the uterine contour is smooth in the setting of adenomyosis.

Case 27

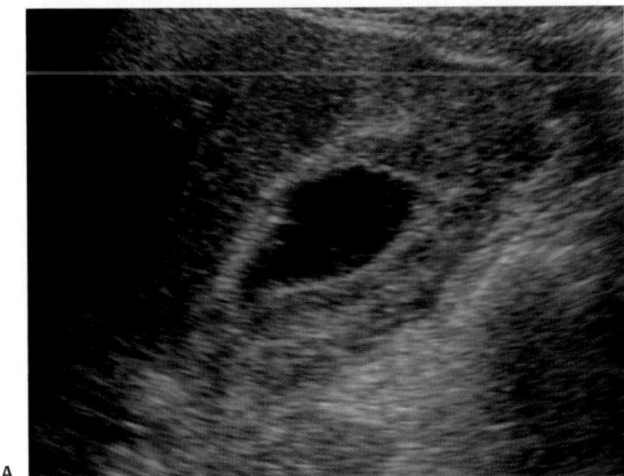
A

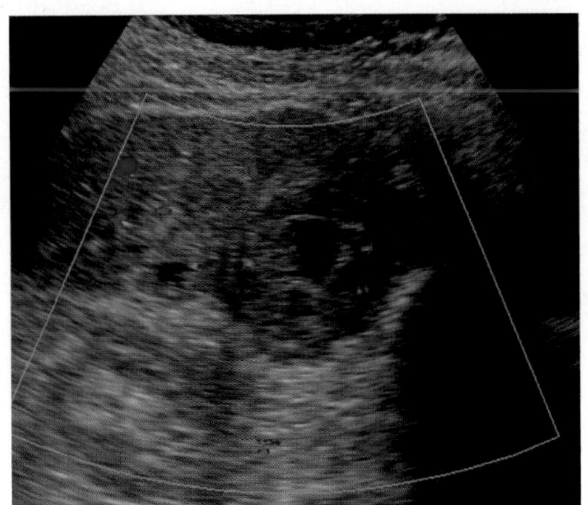
B

Clinical Presentation

A 65-year-old man presents with history of right upper quadrant pain.

Further Work-up

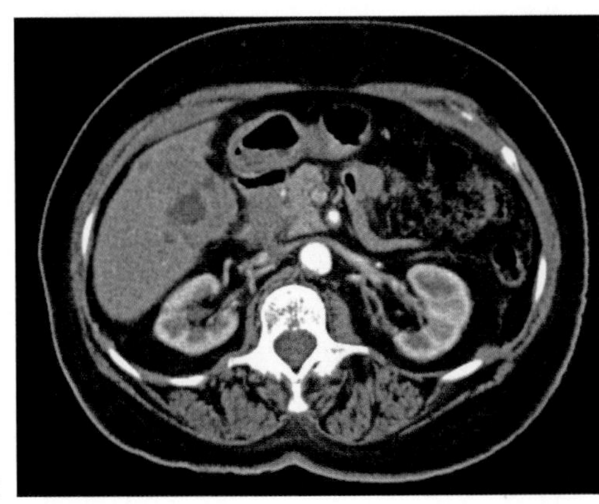
C

Imaging Findings

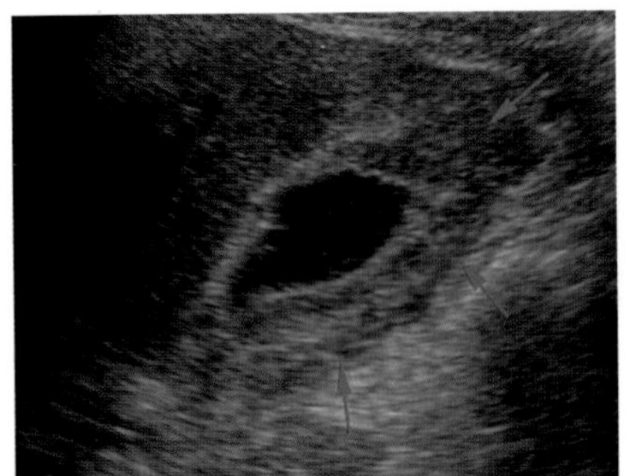

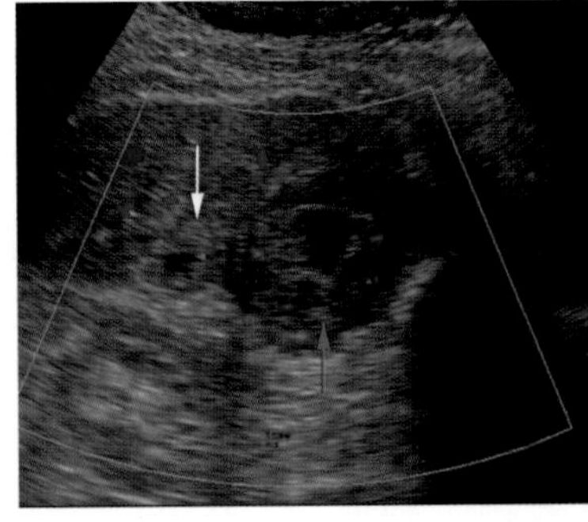

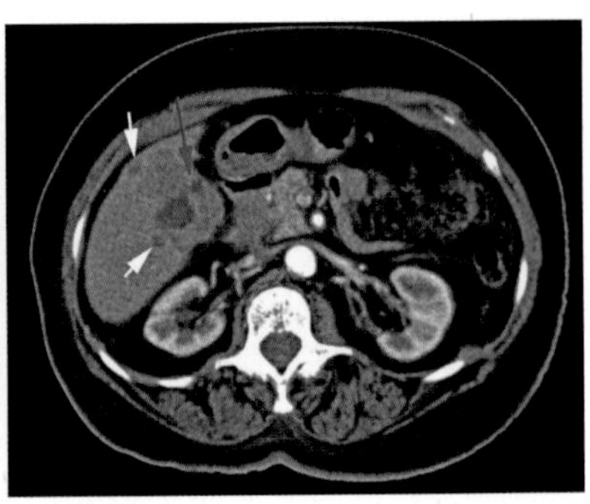

(A, B) Ultrasound (US) images show diffuse, irregular wall thickening of the gallbladder (*red arrows*) with vascular flow. Hypoechoic hepatic lesion abutting the gallbladder is also noted on ultrasound (*white arrow*). **(C)** Computed tomography scan with intravenous contrast confirms the presence of irregular wall thickening of the gallbladder (*red arrow*) with multiple rim-enhancing hepatic lesions (*white arrows*).

Differential Diagnosis

- ***Gallbladder carcinoma:*** Irregular wall thickening with arterial follow, the presence of hepatic invasion favor the diagnosis of malignancy.
- *Metastatic disease to the gallbladder and liver:* Rare manifestation of gallbladder masses seen in 2% of cases. Present on US as multiple hepatic lesions and multiple gallbladder masses, arterial flow usually present especially in hypervascular lesions.
- *Acute cholecystitis with liver abscesses:* Acute cholecystitis could rupture into the liver with subsequent development of a liver abscess. The sonographic appearance could overlap and should be in the differential diagnosis in the proper clinical setting.

Essential Facts

- Gallbladder carcinoma is lethal with local invasion.
- The majorities are adenocarcinoma and rarely squamous cell carcinoma.
- Three times more common in women, epithelial in origin.
- Imaging findings include mass replacing the gallbladder in 40 to 65%, focal or diffuse wall thickening in 20 to 30%, and an intraluminal polypoid mass in 15 to 25%.
- The gallbladder demonstrates irregular margins and heterogeneous echotexture on ultrasonography.
- Gallbladder carcinoma might produce a large amount of mucin with subsequent distention.
- Trapped stone sign represent a nonmobile stone within the tumor. The presence of arterial flow in the mass helps in the diagnosis.

✓ Pearls & × Pitfalls

✓ Inability to visualize the gallbladder without a prior history of cholecystectomy should raise the suspicion of gallbladder mass replacing the normal gallbladder.

× Twinkle artifact secondary to intraluminal stone could be misinterpreted as polypoid intraluminal mass with flow. The presence of noise on Doppler tracing confirms the presence of twinkle artifact.

Case 28

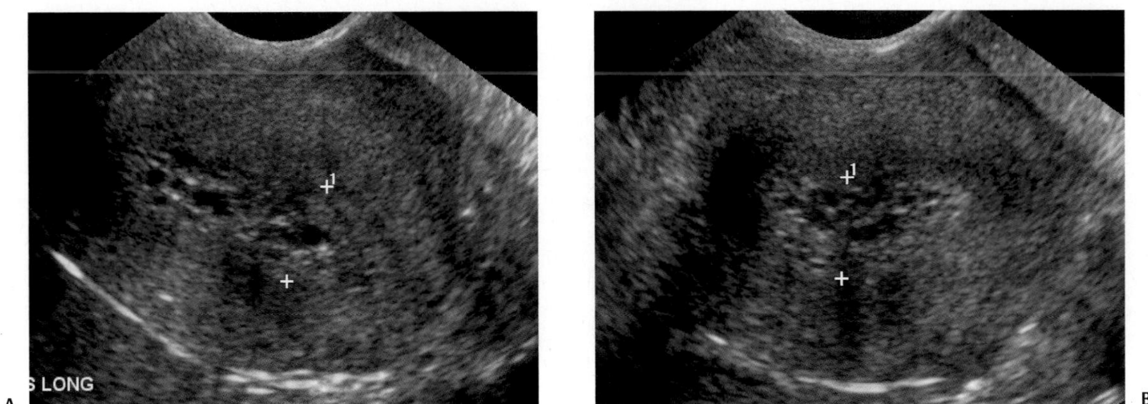

A B

Clinical Presentation

A 55-year-old woman with breast cancer and pelvic pain but no postmenopausal bleeding.

Imaging Findings

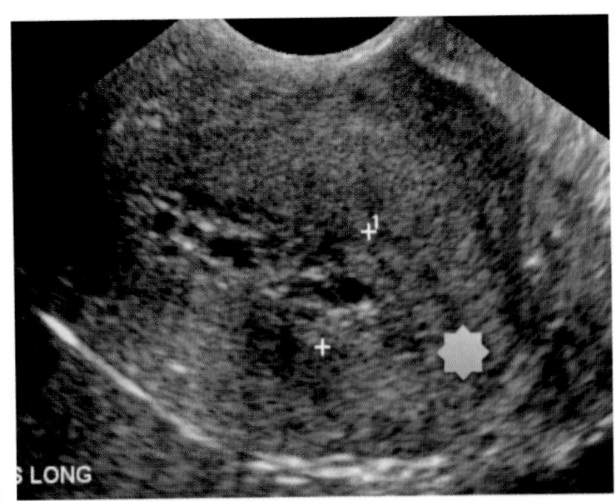

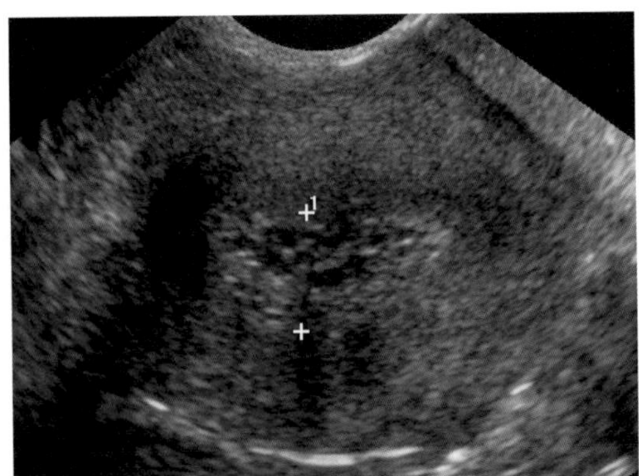

(A, B) Longitudinal and transverse images of the uterus obtained with transvaginal ultrasound (US) demonstrates a retroflexed uterus (*asterisk denotes the fundus*). The endometrium is diffusely thickened (10 mm) with cystic changes. The endometrial myometrial junction is ill defined with subendometrial cysts.

Differential Diagnosis

- ***Tamoxifen-induced cystic changes of the endometrium:*** Tamoxifen therapy results in diffuse thickening of the endometrium with cystic changes.
- *Endometrial polyp:* Endometrial polyps can contain cystic changes but usually contain a solid echogenic component. Polyps usually cause focal, not diffuse, thickening.
- *Endometrial carcinoma:* The endometrium in the setting of endometrial carcinoma is usually thicker and more heterogeneous with solid components. Endometrial fluid is ususally present in the setting of carcinoma. Myometrial invasion can be seen with US.

Essential Facts

- Tamoxifen has an antiestrogen effect in the breast and has been shown to help prevent the original breast cancer from recurring after surgery while also hindering the development of new cancers in the opposite breast.
- Tamoxifen has an estrogenic effect on the endometrium, increasing the risk of endometrial polyps and endometrial cancer. For this reason, tamoxifen is usually only taken for 5 years or less.
- The estrogenic effect of tamoxifen causes cystic changes and thickening of the endometrium. The cystic changes are likely subendometrial.
- Endometrial thickness increases with increasing duration of tamoxifen use. There is no consensus regarding what thickness the endometrium should be to prompt further investigation.
- Following cessation of tamoxifen, the endometrial thickness decreases at a very slow rate. Endometrial thickening can persist for years after discontinuation of tamoxifen.

Other Imaging Findings

- Computed tomography will delineate a thickened endometrium but will not define the cystic changes.
- The cystic changes of the endometrium will demonstrate increased signal with T2-weighted imaging. Magnetic resonance imaging is helpful to detect enhancing solid elements within the endometrium as seen with polyps and endometrial carcinoma.

✓ Pearls & × Pitfalls

× Patients on tamoxifen are at risk for developing endometrial carcinoma, and tamoxifen is known to cause changes in the endometrium that mimic carcinoma.

✓ There is no upper limit of normal measurement of the endometrium in patients on or previously on tamoxifen. By convention, the endometrial measurement is a bilayer measurement including the anterior and posterior layers.

✓ In asymptomatic patients, a thickened cystic endometrium, regardless of diameter, does not warrant intervention.

✓ Patients who develop bleeding while on tamoxifen need tissue sampling.

✓ Endometrial thickening and cystic changes persist long after discontinuation of tamoxifen.

✓ Patients on tamoxifen have an increased incidence of ovarian cysts.

Case 29

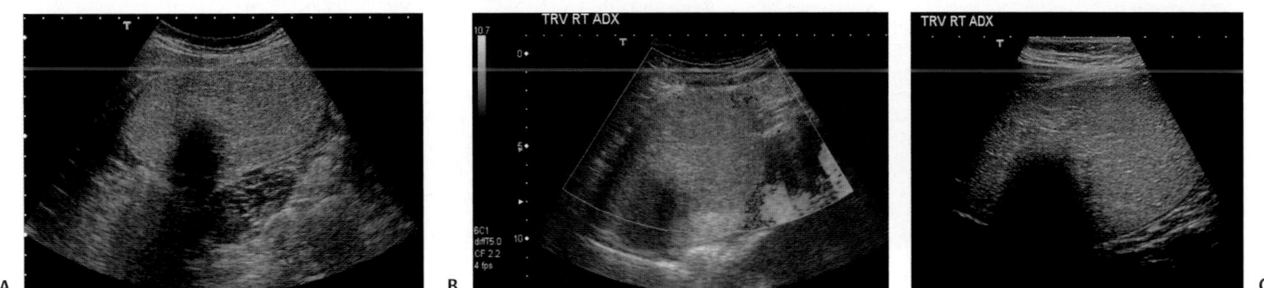

Clinical Presentation

A 25-year-old woman presents with right lower quadrant pain.

Further Work-up

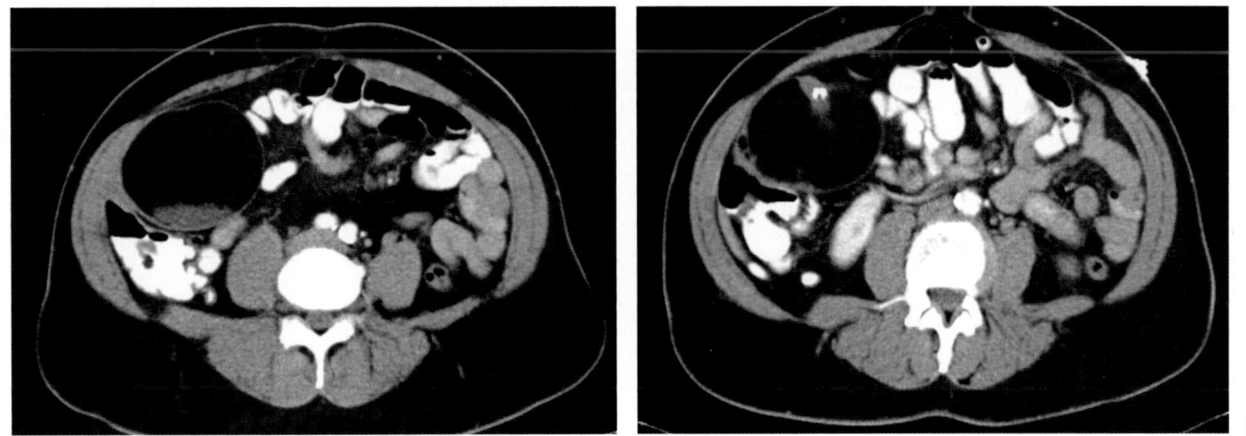

Imaging Finding

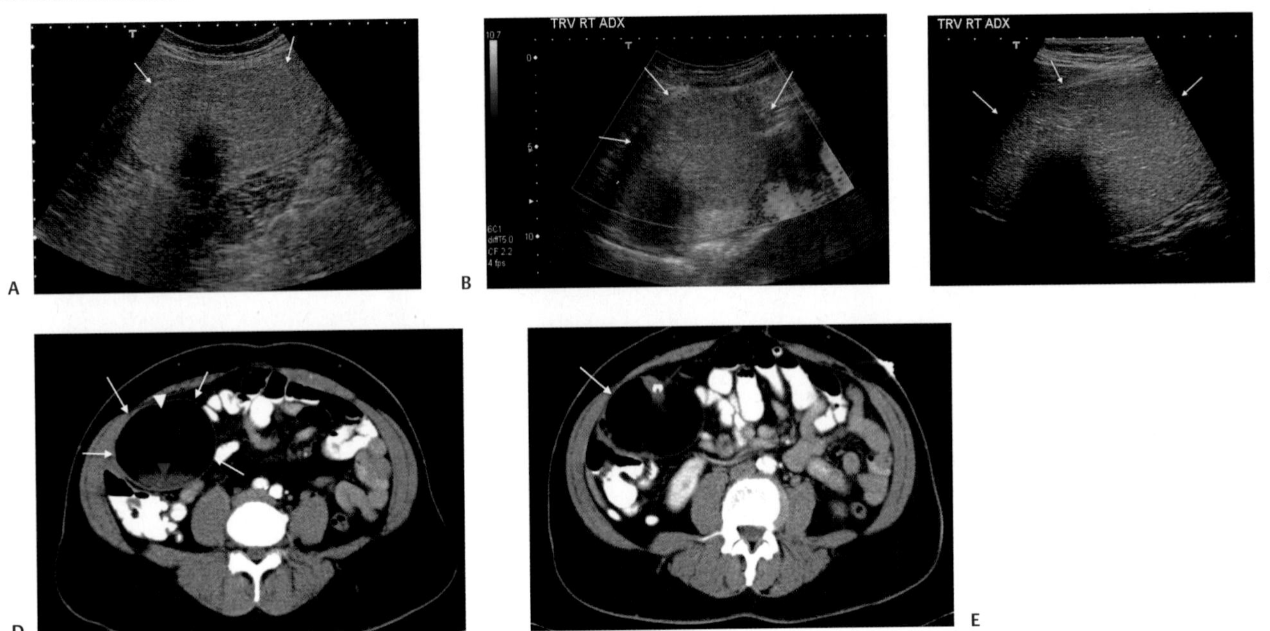

(A–C) Transabdominal ultrasound (US) images of the pelvis demonstrate right-sided echogenic adnexal mass (*white arrows*); no definite evidence of intrinsic flow is seen on Doppler images. An echogenic focus is noted with distal shadowing (*red arrow*), suggesting the presence of calcifications. **(D, E)** Follow-up computed tomography (CT) scan of the pelvis with intravenous contrast shows predominantly fat-containing mass lesion in the expected location of the right adnexa (*white arrows*). It contains fat (*white arrowhead*) and soft tissue (*red arrowhead*). Focal calcification in the mass is also noted (*red arrow*).

Differential Diagnosis

- ***Ovarian mature cystic teratoma:*** Have different sonographic appearance but commonly appears as echogenic mass. No significant intrinsic flow is usually present. Calcifications and soft tissue component might be present, depending on the composition of the tumor.
- *Solid ovarian malignancy:* Granulosa cell tumor, Sertoli-Leydig cell tumors, and fibromas appear as solid adnexal lesions on US. The majority are hypoechoic on US; however, masses with hemorrhage could be echogenic. Vascular flow within the mass and signs of malignancy could be seen.
- *Ovarian torsion:* The patient presents with acute onset of abdominal pain. In missed torsion and/or in case of superimposed hemorrhagic component, the ovaries could appear echogenic without gross evidence of significant internal low. The presence of fat on CT helps to exclude this diagnosis. Additionally, the clinical history is valuable in differentiating dermoid from ovarian torsion.

Essential Fact

- Represents ~ 10 to 20% of ovarian neoplasm.
- Ten to 15% of dermoids are bilateral.
- Usually composed of variable amount of ectoderm, mesoderm, and endoderm.
- More common in the productive years.
- The average diameter growth is 2 mm/year.
- Usually discovered as incidental finding on US or physical examination; majority of patients are asymptomatic.
- Complication includes ovarian torsion, malignant transformation, and rupture with subsequent chemical peritonitis.
- The sonographic appearance ranges from anechoic to echogenic mass lesion in the ovary.
- Fat fluid level, echogenic floating structures, calcifications, and echogenic mural nodules can be seen on ultrasound.

✓ Pearls & × Pitfalls

✓ On US, acute hemorrhage into cyst and/or endometrioma could appear as echogenic mass overlapping with the imaging appearance of mature cystic teratoma. Limited CT scan would be helpful for further differentiation.

× Bowel in the pelvis could have imaging appearance overlapping with mature cystic teratoma; real-time scanning to observe peristalsis will be helpful to differentiate bowel from a real lesion.

Case 30

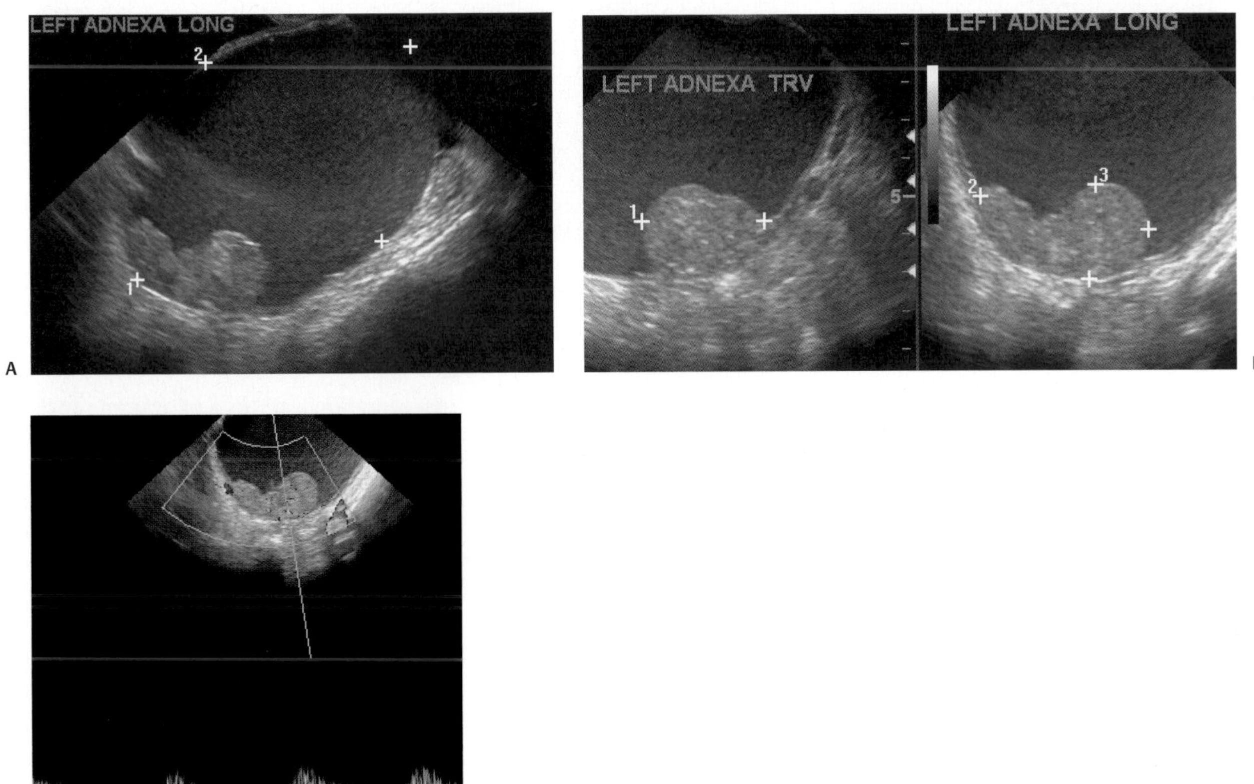

Clinical Presentation

A 35-year-old woman with left lower quadrant pain.

Imaging Findings

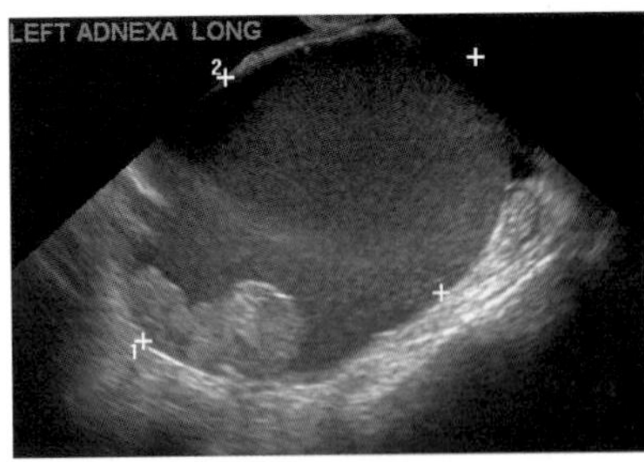

A

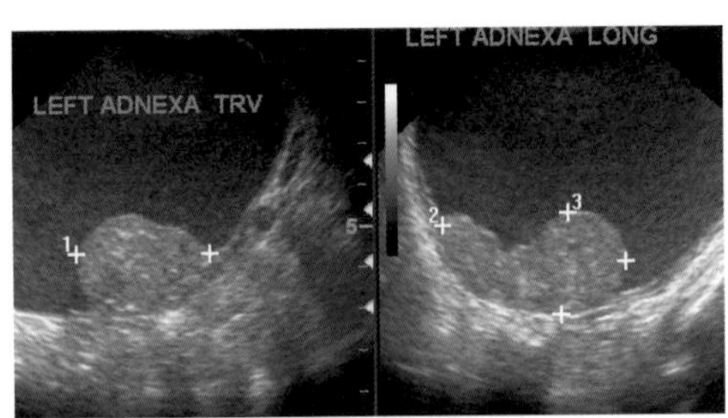

B

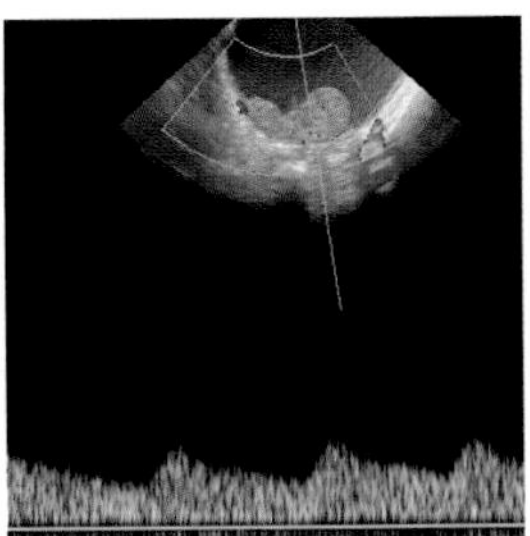
C

(A–C) There is a large complex cystic mass in the left adnexa presumably arising from the left ovary. The lesion contains complex fluid with low-level echoes and an echogenic multilobulated nodule along the posterior wall. Flow is identified within the nodule with color and spectral Doppler imaging.

Differential Diagnosis

- ***Cystic ovarian neoplasms:*** Flow within nodular solid components of a cystic lesion is the most sensitive finding for malignancy.
- *Dermoid:* Echogenic peripheral nodules are seem in dermoids. These nodules do not demonstrate internal vascularity (they are fat).
- *Endometrioma:* Endometriomas contain low-level echoes as seen above and can have echogenic nodules usually in the periphery of a lesion. Flow is not present in these nodules. They represent clot and are avascular.

Essential Facts

- Cystic ovarian lesions containing solid elements that are vascular should be considered malignant until proven otherwise.
- Ovarian cancer is the fifth most common malignancy in women and the leading cause of death from gynecological malignancy.
- Eighty-five percent of ovarian cancers present in stage III or IV. Twenty-five percent ovarian cancer is bilateral.
- Ninety percent of cases are sporadic. Ten percent are associated with hereditary syndromes including BRCA1 and BRCA2 mutation (risk of breast cancer) and Lynch syndrome II (colon cancer). Patients with endometriosis are at increased risk.
- Average age at presentation is 63. Risk of ovarian cancer increases with age and decreases with number of pregnancies. Oral contraceptives have a protective effect.
- Signs and symptoms of ovarian cancer are very vague and include bloating, abdominal or pelvic pain, and pressure.
- Screening for ovarian cancer with pelvic ultrasound is not standard practice. Screening may be indicated in patients with significant family history.
- CA125 is a tumor marker for ovarian cancer. It is nonspecific and can be elevated due to benign entities including fibroids and endometriosis.

✓ Pearls & × Pitfalls

✓ Signs of metastatic disease can be identified with newly diagnosed ovarian cancer. These include ascites and peritoneal implants (most commonly seen in cul-de-sac and paracolic gutters).

✓ Flow within solid components of a cystic ovarian lesion is the most specific sign of malignancy.

× Most ovarian cancer presents with advanced metastatic disease. Screening is not performed in the general population.

✓ Ovarian cancer is felt to arise not in the ovary but from the fimbriated end of the fallopian tube.

✓ The spectrum of appearances of ovarian cancer is very varied from predominantly cystic to completely solid.

Case 31

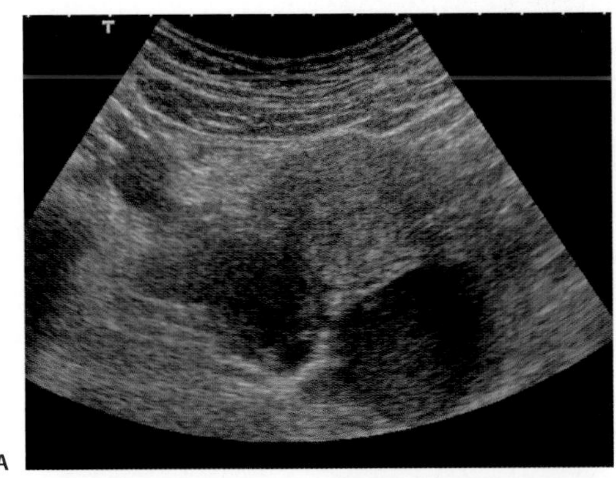

A

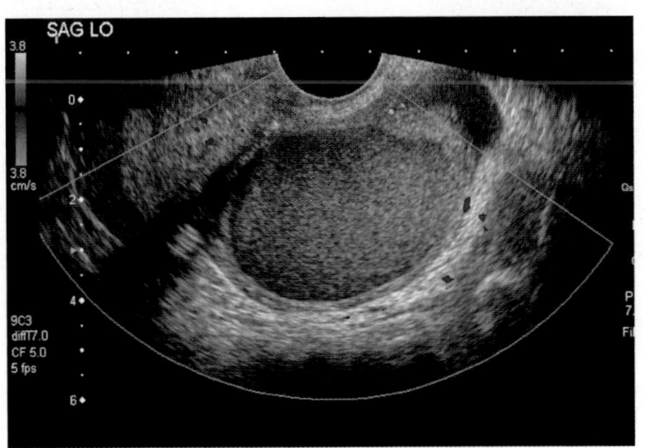

B

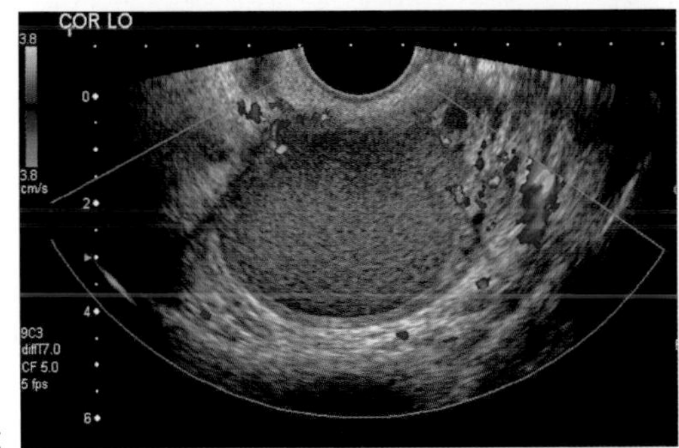

C

Clinical Presentation

A 25-year-old woman presents with pelvic pain.

Further Work-up

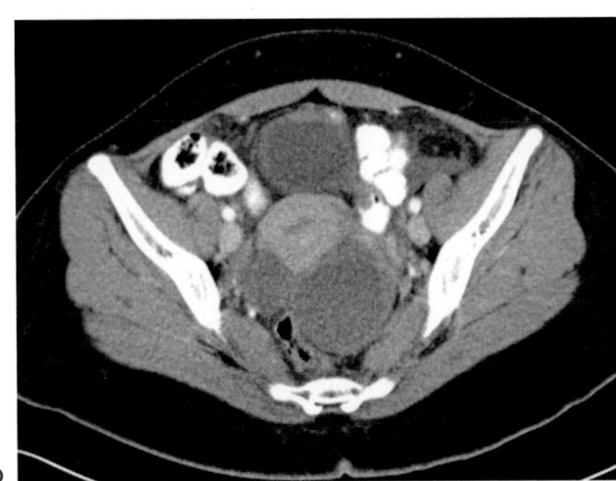

D

Imaging Findings

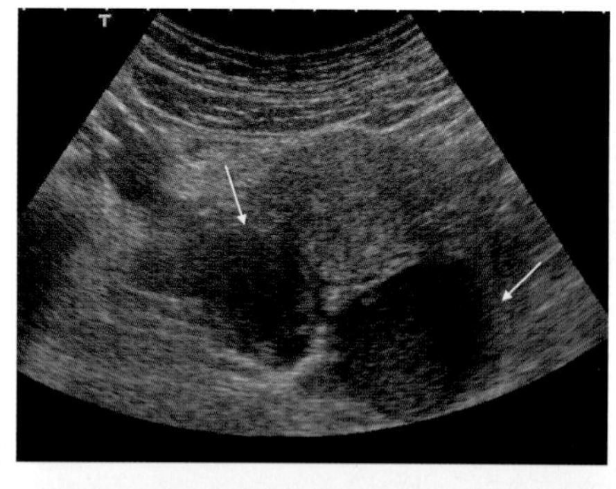

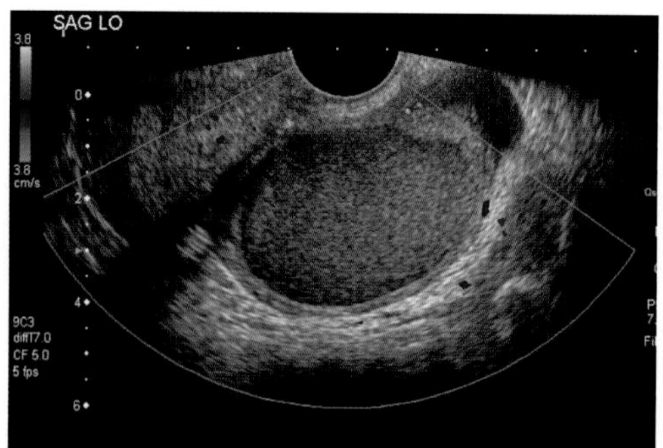

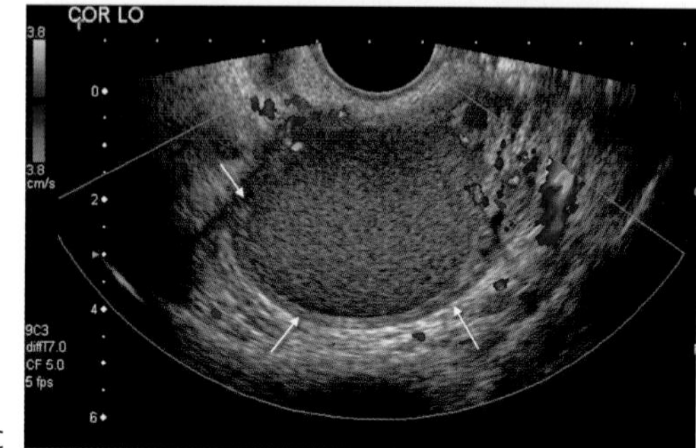

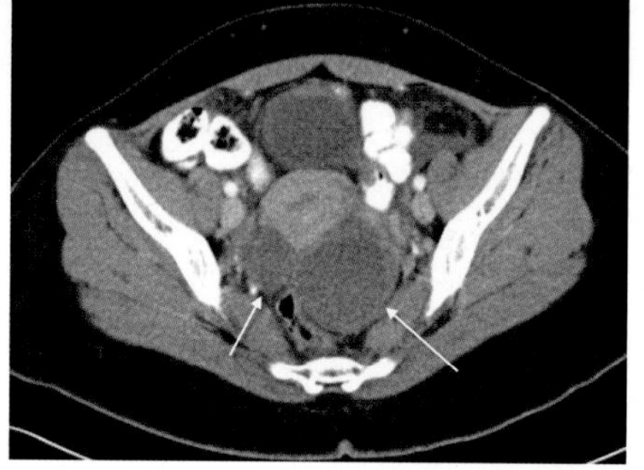

(A–C) Ultrasound (US) of the pelvis using transabdominal and transvaginal approach shows two large complex cystic lesions in the pelvis with low-level echoes (*white arrows*). The lesions appear paraovarian in location without evidence of flow. **(D)** Follow-up computed tomography (CT) scan of the pelvis obtained 3 months later shows the same cystic lesions in the pelvis without significant changes in size (*white arrows*).

Differential Diagnosis

- ***Endometrioma:*** The presence of diffuse low-level echoes in a cystic mass is suggestive of endometrioma.
- *Hemorrhagic ovarian cyst:* Fishnet or retracting blood clot is usually present. Fluid-fluid level could be seen. The lesions resolve on follow-up studies.
- *Pelvic abscess:* Appears as complex fluid collection with low-level echoes; no internal flow is seen on color images; peripheral flow occasionally can be seen.

Essential Facts

- Endometrioma is a pseudocyst formed by an accumulation of menstrual debris.
- Symptoms are dysmenorrhea, dyspareunia, premenstrual spotting, and vaginal bleeding.
- Increased risk of ovarian malignancy in patients with ovarian endometrioma.
- On US, it appears as a cystic mass with low-level echoes. Hyperechoic foci in the wall could be seen.
- Fluid-fluid levels are less common.
- Wall or internal calcifications could be seen.
- On magnetic resonance imaging, appears as cystic masses with high signal intensity on T1-weighted and low signal on T2-weighted images

✓ Pearls & × Pitfalls

✓ A cystic lesion in the pelvis with internal echoes is present in 95% of endometriomas.

× On rare occasions, a vascularized component arising from the wall could be seen and misdiagnosed as cystic neoplasm.

Case 32

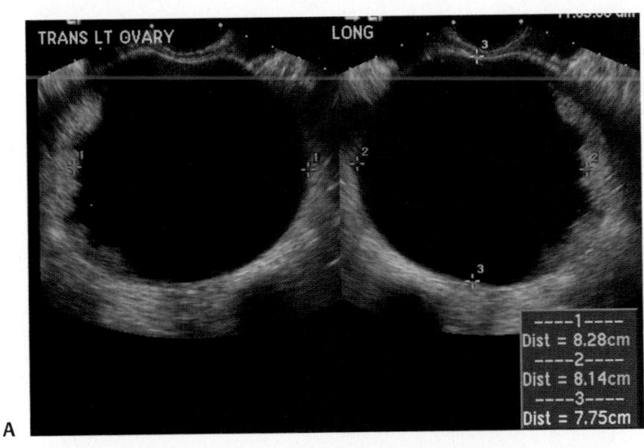

A

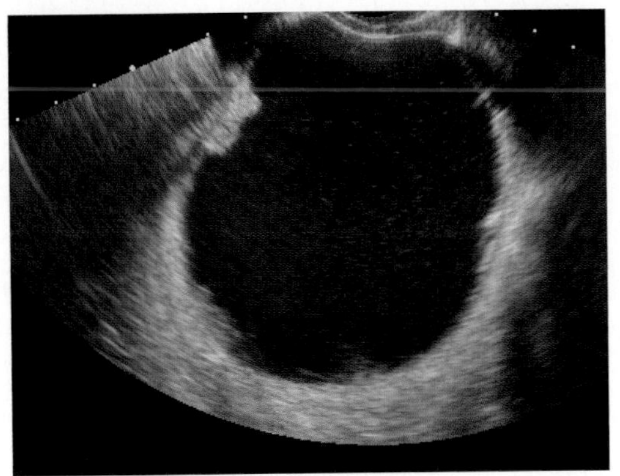

B

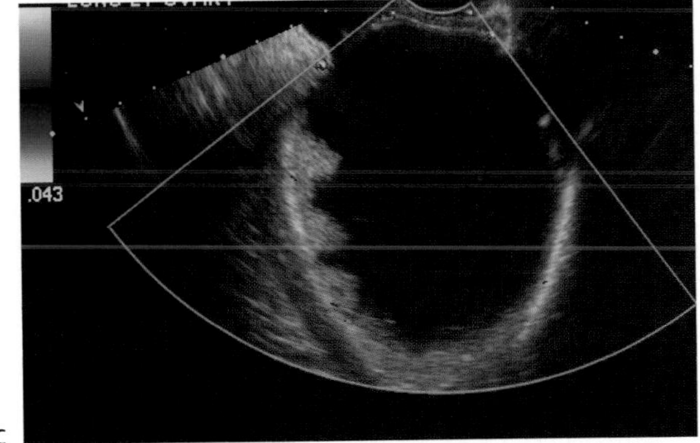

C

■ Clinical Presentation

A 34-year-old woman with left lower quadrant pain.

Imaging Findings

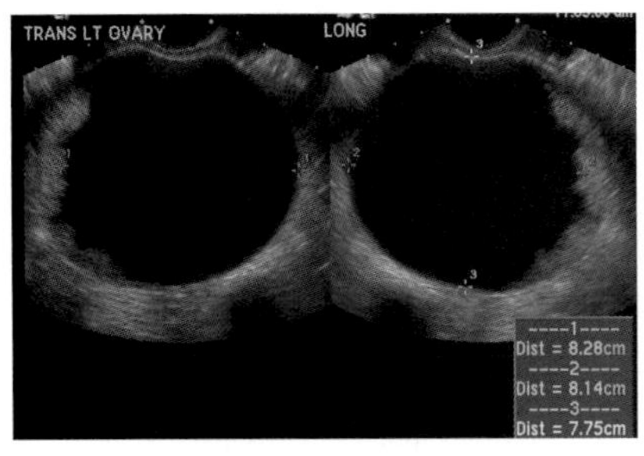

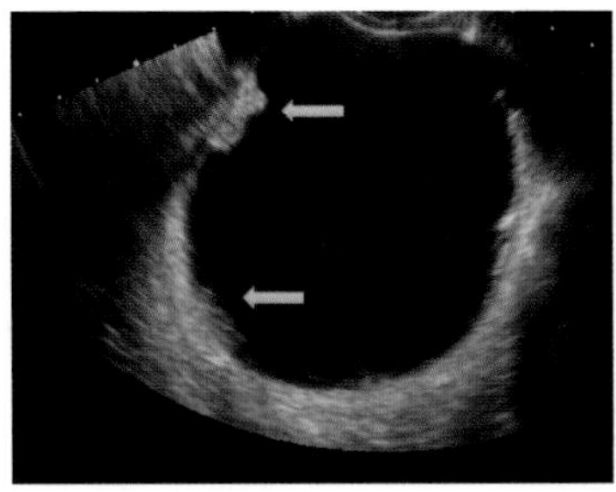
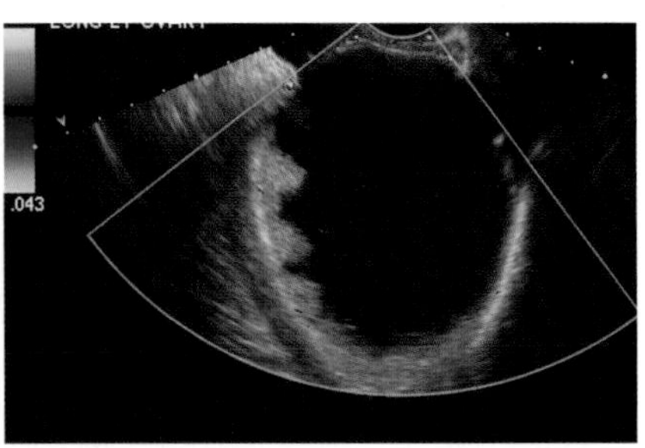

(A–C) Longitudinal and transverse images of the left ovary, which contains an 8-cm complex predominantly cystic lesion. Multiple small nodules are present in the periphery of the lesion (*arrows in B*). The nodules are isoechoic to hyperechoic. **(C)** With color Doppler imaging, no flow is identified within the nodules.

Differential Diagnosis

- ***Ovarian neoplasm with papillary excrescences:*** Papillary excrescences are small nodules grouped along the wall of a cystic neoplasm. Flow is often seen within papillary excrescences in malignant lesions.
- *Dermoid:* Demoids classically have echogenic nodules without vascularity. Dermoids may have calcifications or linear echogenic foci (hair). It would be difficult to distinguish this lesion (preoperatively) from a dermoid without additional imaging.
- *Atypical hemorrhagic cyst:* Hemorrhagic cysts may have clots mimicking solid elements. These are often geographic, larger, and less echogenic.

Essential Facts

- The terms *papillary excrescences, papillary vegetations, papillary projections* and *peripheral nodularity* are used interchangeably.
- They are small nodules grouped in the periphery of a cystic lesion. They are a sign of malignancy but can be seen in benign neoplastic lesions.
- Flow within papillary excrescences is a sign of malignancy and such lesions, regardless of size, should be removed.

Other Imaging Findings

- Small papillary excrescences may not be visible with computed tomography and may be better evaluated with magnetic resonance imaging. Many surgeons will operate based on the ultrasound findings and clinical scenario.

✓ Pearls & × Pitfalls

✓ The more solid elements a cystic ovarian lesion contains, the more likely it is to be malignant.
× Papillary excrescences can be seen in both benign and malignant lesions.
✓ Flow within papillary excrescences or other solid elements is a sign of malignancy.
✓ The sonographic morphology of an ovarian lesion is a more useful predictor of malignancy than its size.

Case 33

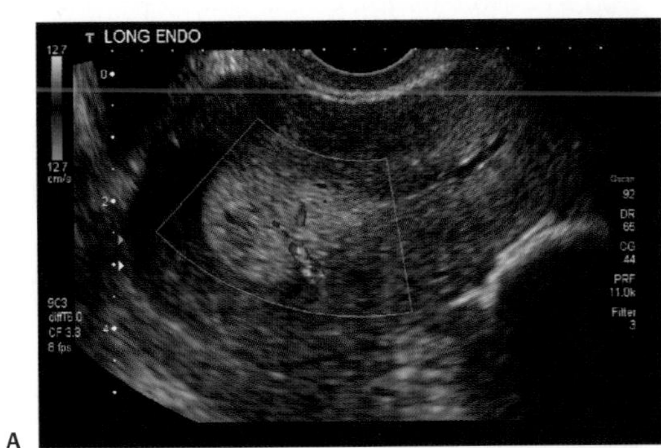

A

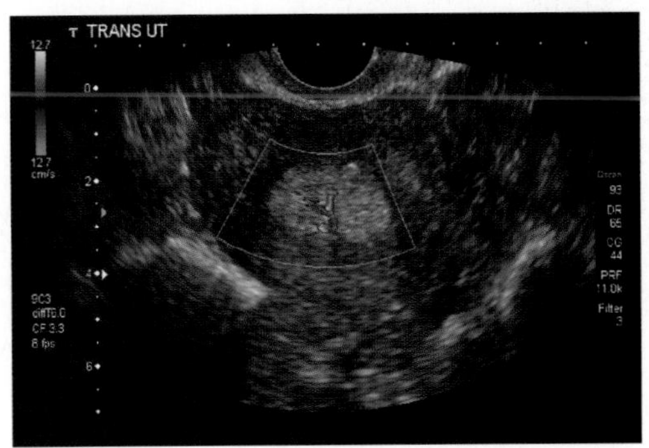

B

■ Clinical Presentation

A 70-year-old woman with history of breast cancer presents with a history of vaginal bleeding.

■ Further Work-up

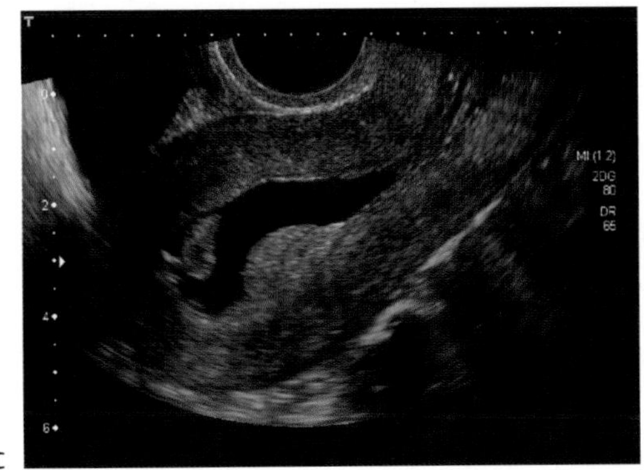

C

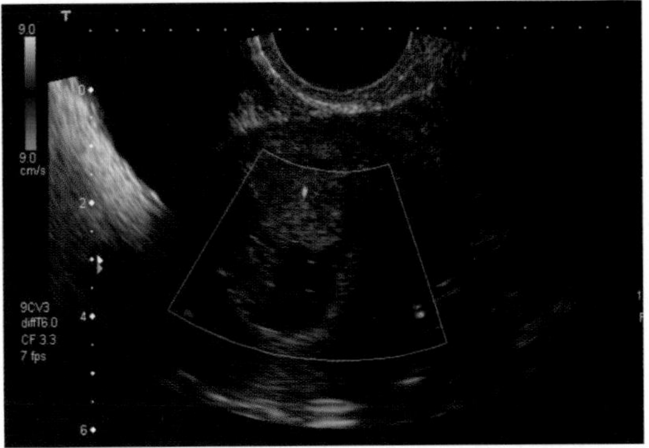

D

Imaging Findings

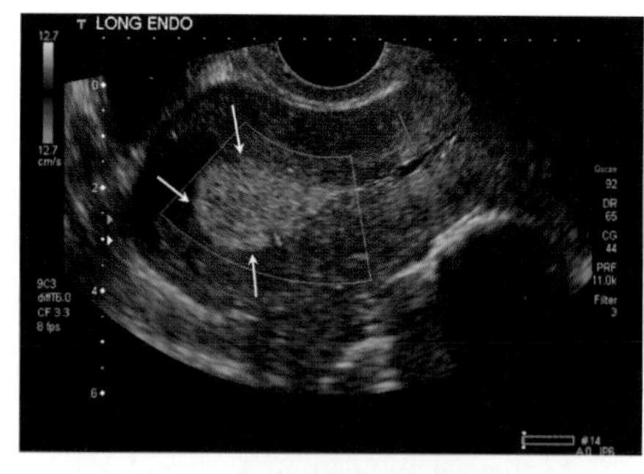

A

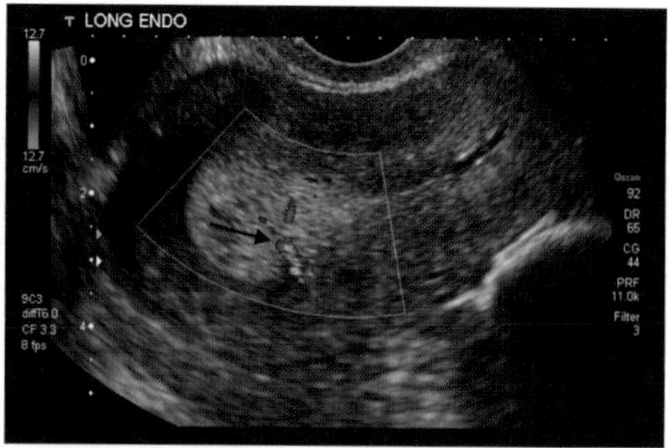

B

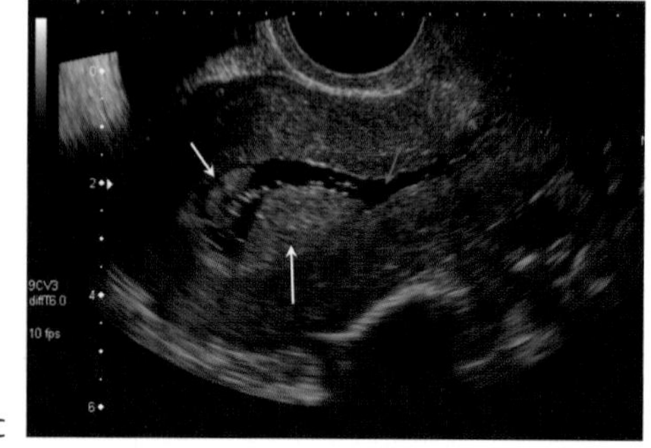

C

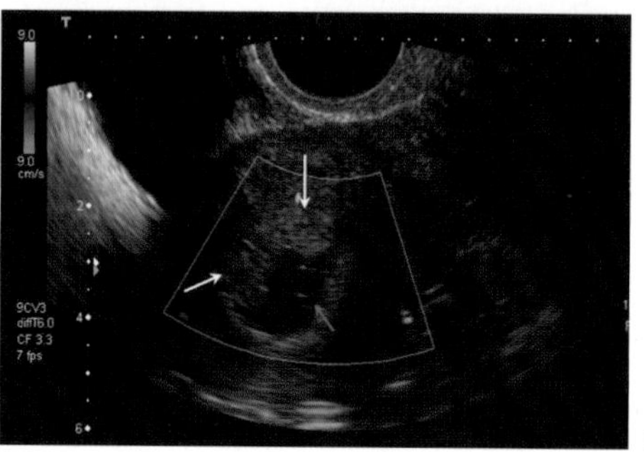

D

(A, B) Ultrasound (US) images of the endometrium show markedly thickened endometrium for a postmenopausal woman (*white arrows*). A feeding vascular flow noted on color Doppler (*black arrow*). Trace amount of endocervical fluid is present (*red arrow*) and is considered abnormal giving the patient's age. **(C, D)** Follow-up sonohysterogram demonstrate a total of three separate endometrial-based lesions (*two white arrows on the longitudinal view and the third lesion noted on the transverse view*). The largest is in the posterior wall.

Differential Diagnosis

- ***Endometrial polyps:*** Common; benign lesions frequently visualized in perimenopausal and postmenopausal women. Sonographically, polyps appear as nonspecific echogenic endometrial thickening, which could be diffuse and/or localized. An echogenic endometrial mass occasionally visualized. A flow within the stalk could be seen. Sonohysterogram is a study of choice for diagnosing endometrial polyps and extension.
- *Focal endometrial hyperplasia:* Endometrial hyperplasia is defined as a proliferation of glands of irregular size and shape associated with increase in gland/stroma ratio. The process is diffuse and less likely focal. Sonographically, the endometrium is thick and echogenic with well-defined margins. A small cyst may be seen in case of cystic hyperplasia.
- *Endometrial carcinoma:* The most common gynecology malignancy. It occurs in ~ 3% of women. Sonographically, a thickened endometrium is visualized in a postmenopausal woman. The thick endometrium may be well defined, echogenic, and indistinguishable from hyperplasia and/or polyps. Cancer is suspected when the endometrium has inhomogeneous echotexture with irregular or poorly defined margin.

Essential Facts

- Are common lesions frequently visualized in perimenopausal and postmenopausal women.
- The majority are asymptomatic; however, the patient could present with uterine bleeding.
- In menstruating women, patient presents with intermenstrual bleeding and/or menometrorrhagia; some patients present with infertility.
- Polyps represent overgrowth of endometrial tissue covered by epithelium.
- Polyps may be pedunculated and or broad-based.
- Twenty percent of endometrial polyps are multiple.
- Malignant degeneration is rare.
- Sonographically, polyps appear as nonspecific echogenic endometrial thickening, which could be diffuse and/or localized.
- Occasionally, an echogenic mass is visualized within the endometrial cavity.
- The diagnosis is easier when there is endometrial fluid and/or with sonohysterogram.
- Cystic areas may be seen within the polyp; a feeding artery through the pedicle could also be visualized on color Doppler.

✓ Pearls & × Pitfalls

✓ Sonohysterogram is valuable in differentiating endometrial polyps from submucosal fibroid; polyps usually visualized arising from the endometrium versus a submucosal fibroid are fully covered with the endometrium.

× Endometrial polyps may be missed on dilation and curettage (D & C), predominantly in cases of a polyp with long stalk. If abnormal bleeding persists after nondiagnostic D & C, hysteroscopy would be indicated.

Case 34

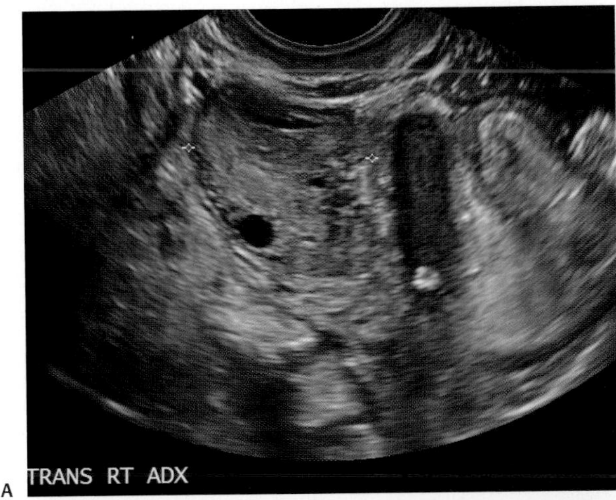

A

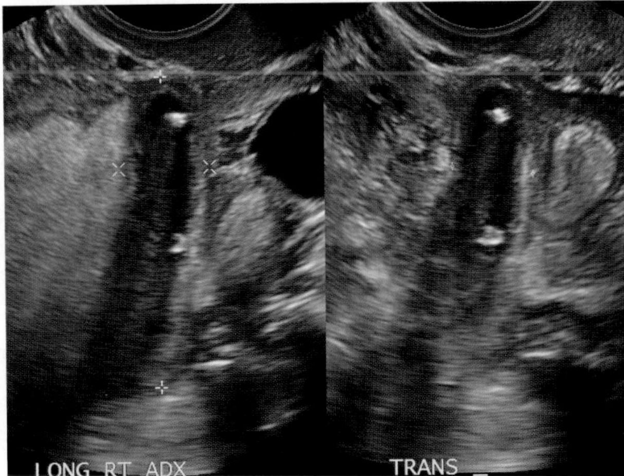

B

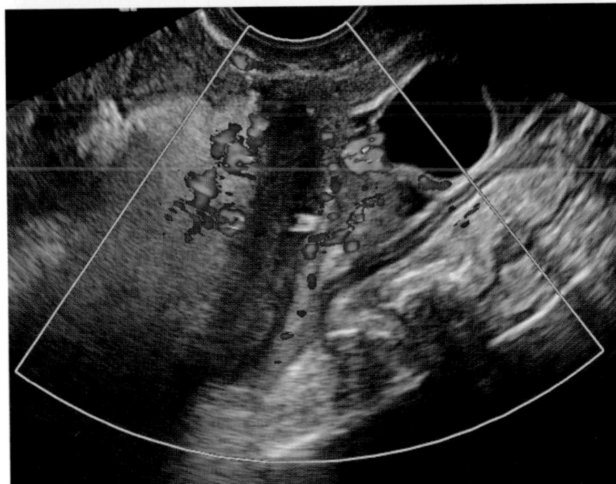
C

Clinical Presentation

A 25-year-old woman with right lower quadrant pain and fever, suspected tubo ovarian abscess (TOA).

Further Work-up

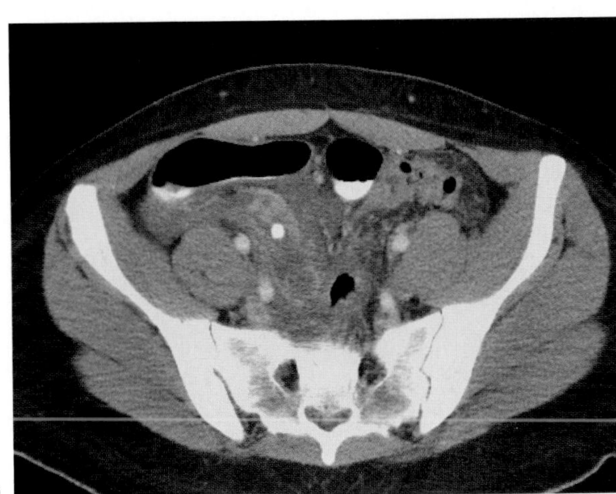
D

Imaging Findings

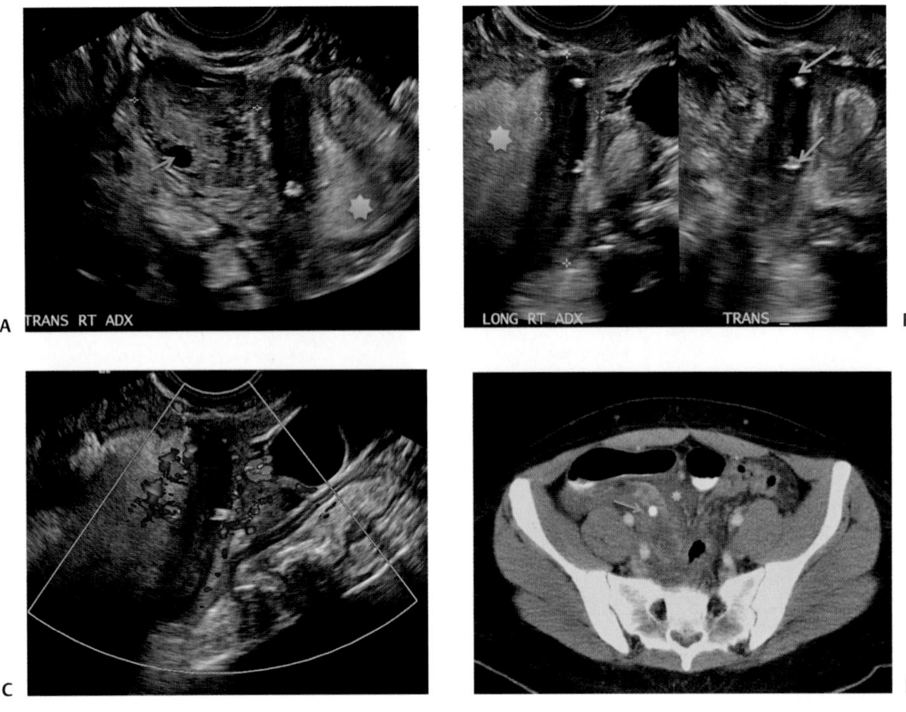

(A) Transverse image of the right ovary demonstrates a hypoechoic structure medial to a normal-appearing right ovary. Note the small follicle posterior in the ovary (*arrow*). Note the hyperechoic fat medially (*asterisk*). **(B)** Longitudinal and transverse images of the lesion defines a thick-walled tubular structure measuring 14 mm in diameter. It contains two punctate echogenic structures (*arrows*). Hyperechoic fat is seen cephalad (*asterisk*). **(C)** With color Doppler, imaging flow is present in the periphery of this lesion, indicating hyperemia. No flow is seen centrally. **(D)** Postcontrast axial computed tomography (CT) demonstrates a peripherally enhancing tubular structure draped over the right iliac artery and vein. It contains a calcification (*arrow*). Note the edema of the adjacent fat, particularly medially (*asterisk*).

Differential Diagnosis

- ***Acute appendicitis:*** A blind-ending hyperemic tubular structure in the right lower quadrant containing calcifications is consistent with a dilated inflamed appendix with appendicoliths.
- *Pyosalpinx:* The fallopian tube is more convoluted and would not contain stones. An inflamed tube can be nodular in contour, hence the term *cogwheel sign*.
- *Hemorrhagic corpus luteum:* A corpus luteum is intra-ovarian and is generally round, not elongated. Statistically it is the most common etiology for a complex adnexal lesion in a young patient.

Essential Facts

- The appendix, particularly an abnormal appendix, may be visible with transvaginal ultrasound (US) imaging of the pelvis.
- The diagnosis of acute appendicitis is difficult in women during the reproductive years, as the clinical presentation of acute appendicitis overlaps with gynecological disorders.
- Clinical mimickers of appendicitis include physiologic processes such as a ruptured ovarian cyst and pathological conditions, particularly pelvic inflammatory disease.
- Sonographic features of acute appendicitis include a dilated (> 7 mm), fluid-filled, blind-ending structure. Hyperemia is demonstrated with color or power Doppler as seen in our case. Appendicoliths may be visible.
- Inflamed periappendiceal fat is hyperechogenic as seen in our case (*asterisks*). It is a sign of inflammation.
- A ruptured or gangrenous appendix will have an atypical appearance.
- Patients will be tender when scanning near an abnormal appendix.

✓ Pearls & × Pitfalls

✓ A normal appendix should measure < 7 mm in diameter.

✓ Patients will be tender when the transvaginal probe is near an inflamed appendix.

× Free fluid in the pelvis can be physiologic in premenopausal women but can be due to inflammation from acute appendicitis.

× CT is more sensitive than US for the detection of acute appendicitis.

Case 35

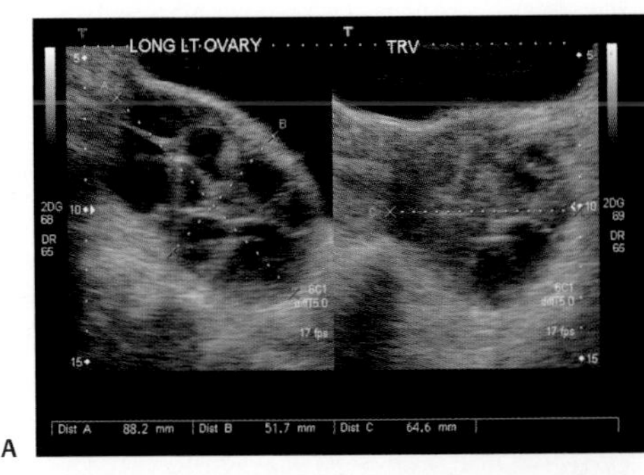

A

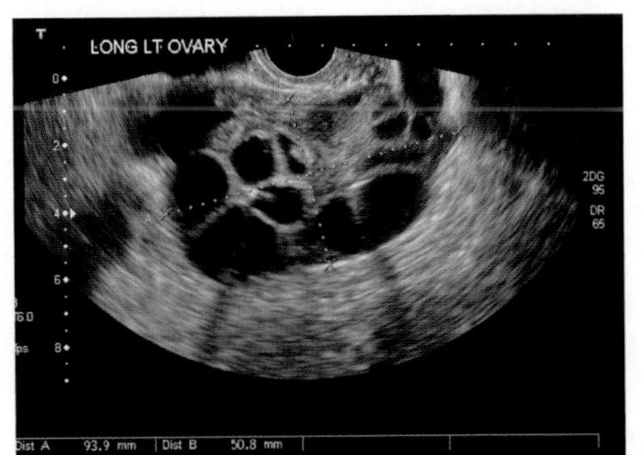

B

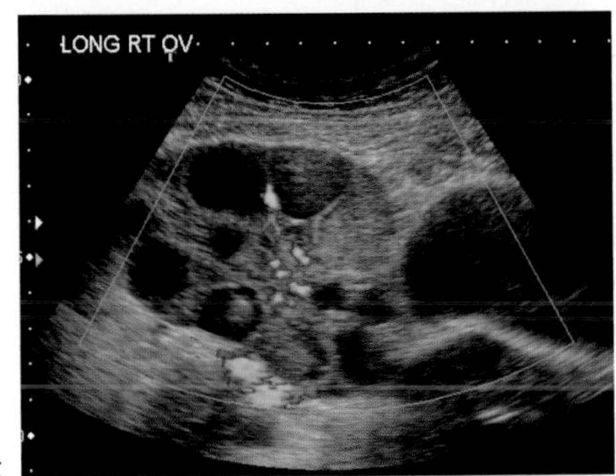

C

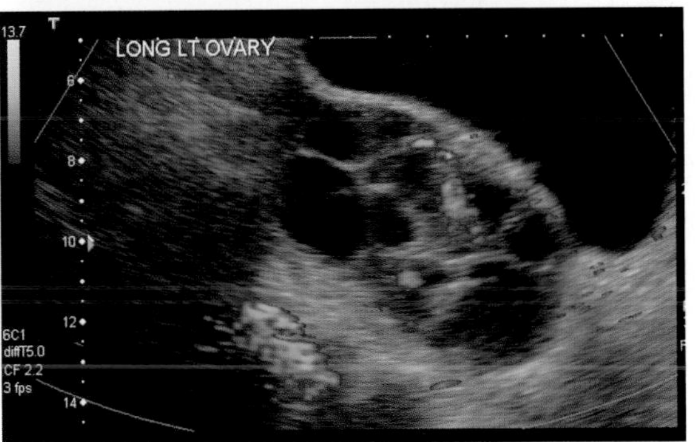

D

Clinical Presentation

A 32-year-old woman presents with abdominal pain and discomfort.

Further Work-up

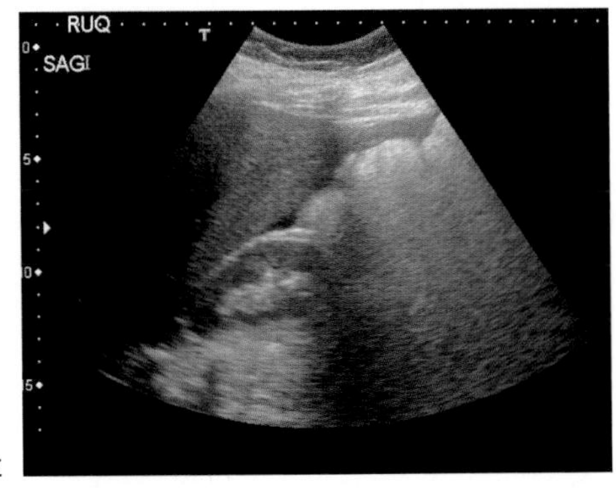

E

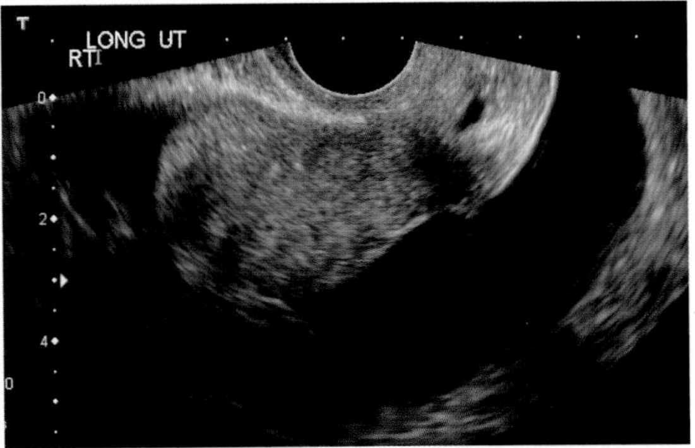

F

Imaging Findings

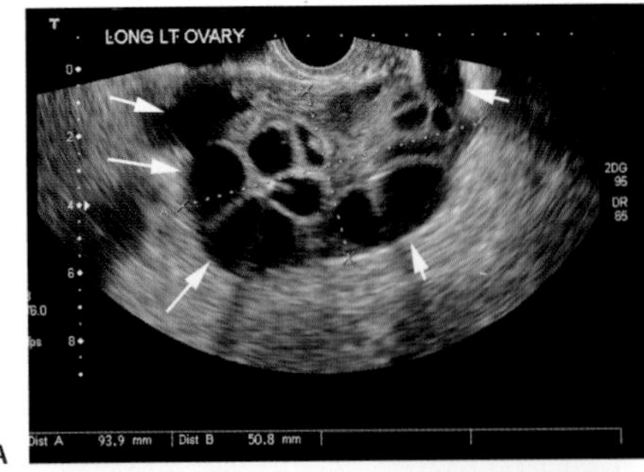

A

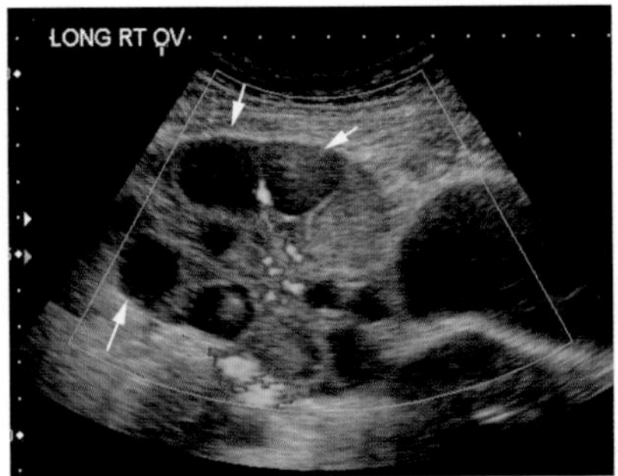

B

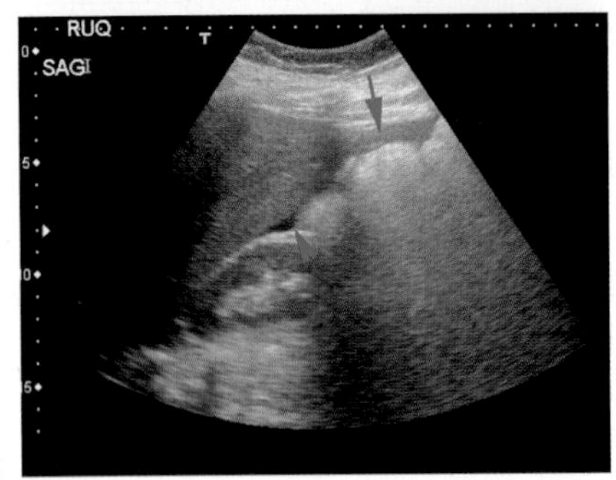

C

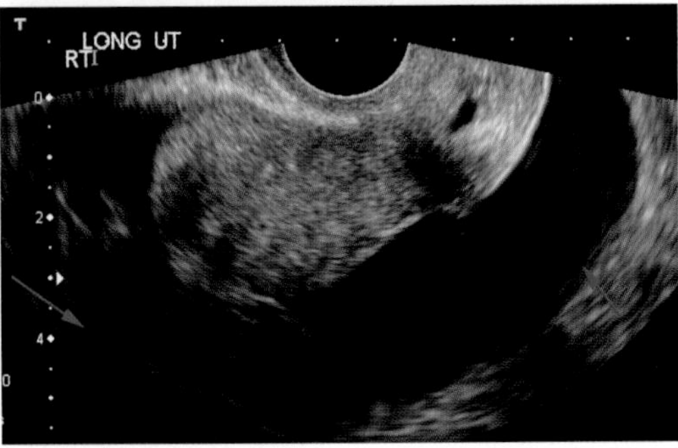

D

(A, B) Ultrasound (US) images of the pelvis using transabdominal and transvaginal scanning show enlarged ovaries with multiple large follicles (*white arrows*). Doppler flow in the ovaries is noted (*blue arrow*). **(C, D)** Further sonographic images show large amount of ascites in the pelvis extending to the right upper quadrant (*red arrows*).

Differential Diagnosis

- ***Ovarian hyperstimulation syndrome:*** Appears sonographically as enlarged ovaries with multiple large follicles. Ascites and/or effusion might be seen. The history of ovulation-induction therapy supports the diagnosis.
- *Polycystic ovarian disease:* Related to chronic anovulation with elevated luteinizing hormone/follicle-stimulating hormone ratio. Presents sonographically as enlarged ovaries containing small follicles. Increased stromal echogenicity is suggestive of the diagnosis. Unilateral involvement is rare.
- *Ovarian torsion:* Patient presents with sudden onset of abdominal pain. The sonographic findings depend on the duration of the process. Enlarged ovary and follicles secondary to edema usually present on US. The contralateral ovary is normal. The presence of arterial flow does not exclude the diagnosis of torsion.

Essential Facts

- Frequent complications seen in patients on ovulation-inducing drugs.
- Clinically could present as mild, moderate, or severe forms.
- In the mild form, the ovaries are enlarged, < 5 cm in diameter.
- In the severe form, the ovaries might exceed 10 cm diameter. The patient also complains of weight gain and abdominal distention.
- Sonographically, the ovaries are enlarged, containing large, thin-walled follicles.
- Ascites and pleural effusions are present in the moderate and severe forms.
- Intravascular fluid depletion and electrolyte imbalance could be seen in the severe form.

✓ Pearls & × Pitfalls

✓ Enlarged bilateral ovaries with multiple large follicles are suggestive of ovarian hyperstimulation syndrome in the proper clinical setting.

× Ovarian torsion could present as enlarged ovary with enlarged follicles. The finding could be misinterpreted as hyperstimulation syndrome. The presence of arterial flow does not exclude the diagnosis of torsion.

Case 36

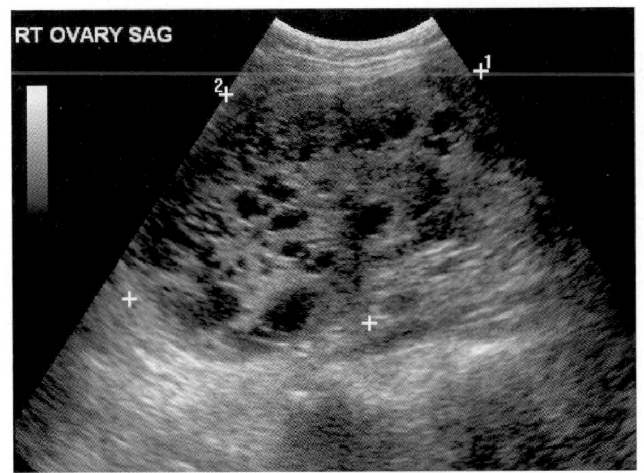

A

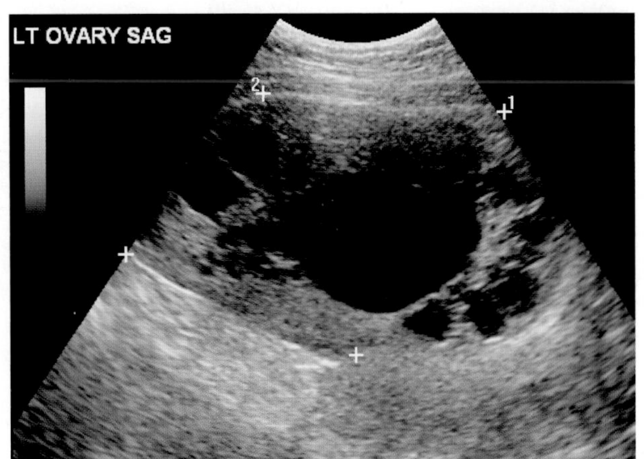

B

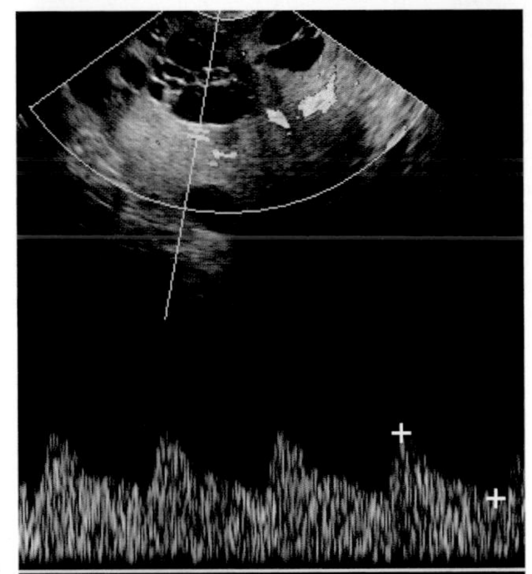
C

Clinical Presentation

A 32-year-old woman with abdominal bloating.

Further Work-up

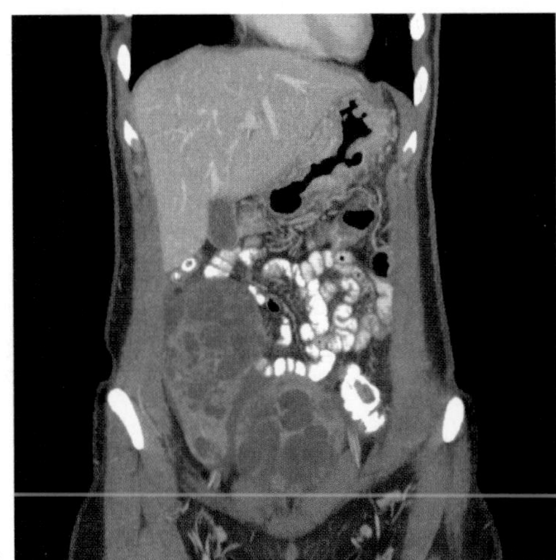
D

Imaging Findings

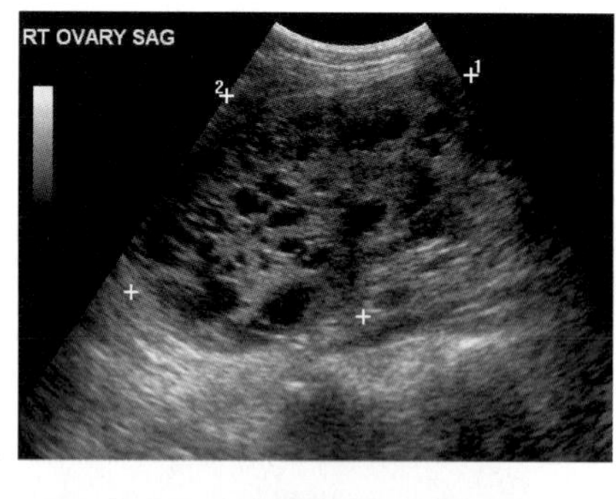

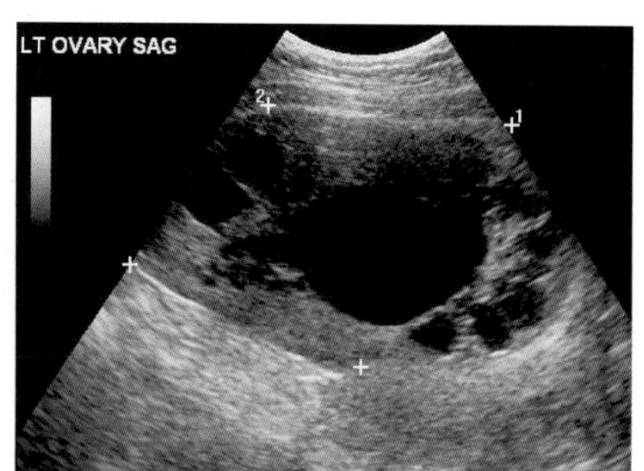

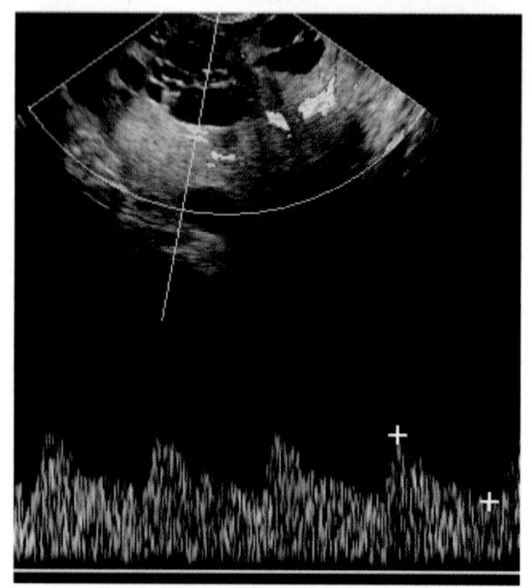

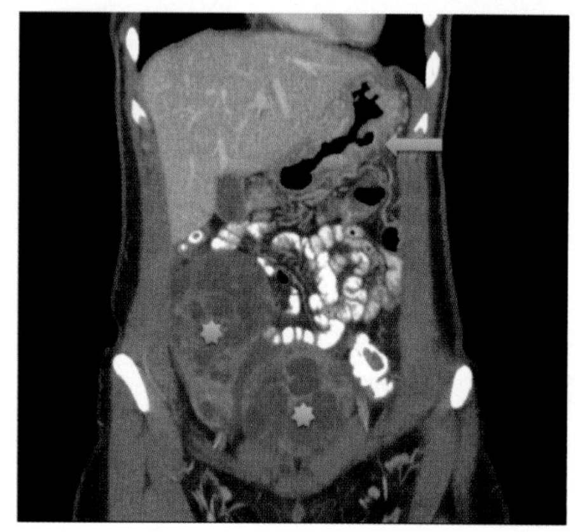

(A, B) Transabdominal images of the pelvis reveal right **(A)** and left **(B)**, partially cystic, partially solid adnexal masses presumably arising from the ovaries, as normal ovaries were not identified. **(C)** Spectral Doppler evaluation of the solid components reveals abundant low-resistance flow. **(D)** Coronal reformatted image confirms the bilateral cystic and solid adnexal lesions (*asterisks*). Note also the ulcerated mass along the greater curvature of the stomach (*arrow*).

Differential Diagnosis

- ***Krukenberg tumors metastatic from a gastric primary:*** Large bilateral ovarian masses with an ulcerating gastric mass, are most consistent with Krukenberg tumors.
- *Polycystic ovaries:* Polycystic ovaries would not be this large.
- *Bilateral epithelial ovarian malignancy:* Although epithelial ovarian cancer is much more common than Krukenberg tumors, they are usually more cystic, less often bilateral, and usually present in postmenopausal women.

Essential Facts

- Adenocarcinoma of the ovary with signet ring cells is known as Krukenberg tumors. They represent only 1 to 2% of ovarian cancers.
- They are usually metastatic from a gastrointestinal primary, most commonly gastric, carcinoma (70%).
- Signet ring cell adenocarcinomas of solid organs metastasize to the ovaries more commonly than other malignancies from the same organs. Spread is felt to be lymphatic.
- They are usually (80%) bilateral. They are complex but predominantly solid and can be very large.
- Krukenberg tumors can present with ascites and pleural effusions.
- The primary tumor can be occult. If the primary is occult, the prognosis is very poor. In general, Krukenberg tumors have a very low survival rate, 15% at 2 years.
- Average age at presentation is 45. Usually occurs in premenopausal women.

✓ Pearls & × Pitfalls

✓ Krukenberg tumors are generally more solid and more often bilateral than epithelial ovarian malignancies.

× The sonographic features of Krukenberg tumors overlap with the more common epithelial ovarian malignancies.

× The diagnosis of Krukenberg tumors is usually made at surgery.

✓ Krukenberg tumors present in younger women than ovarian cancer.

Case 37

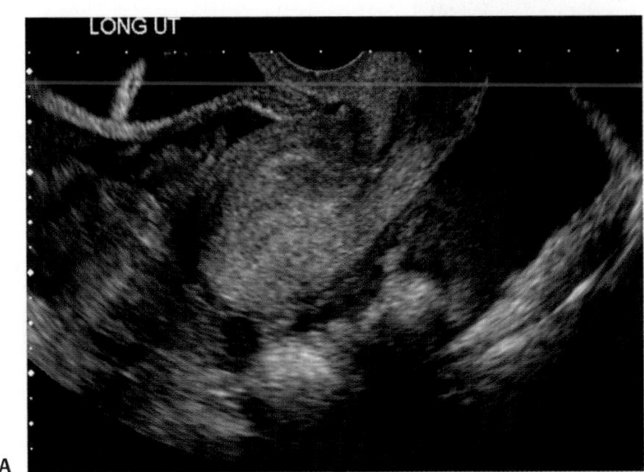

A

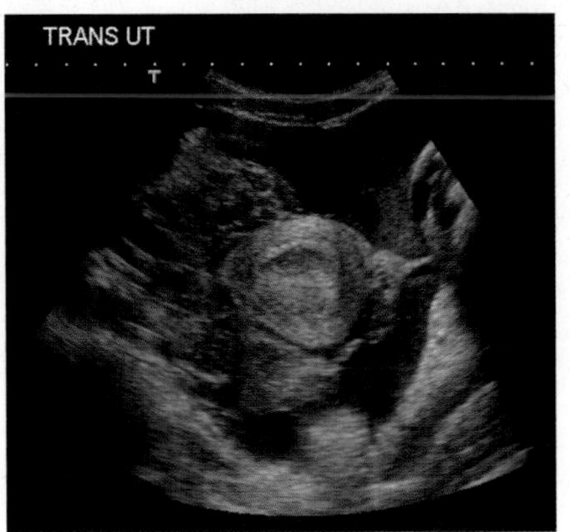

B

Clinical Presentation

A 19-year-old woman with positive pregnancy test presents with abdominal pain.

Further Work-up

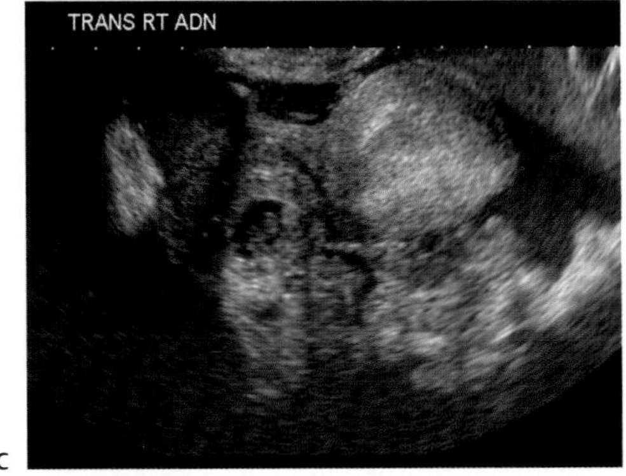

C

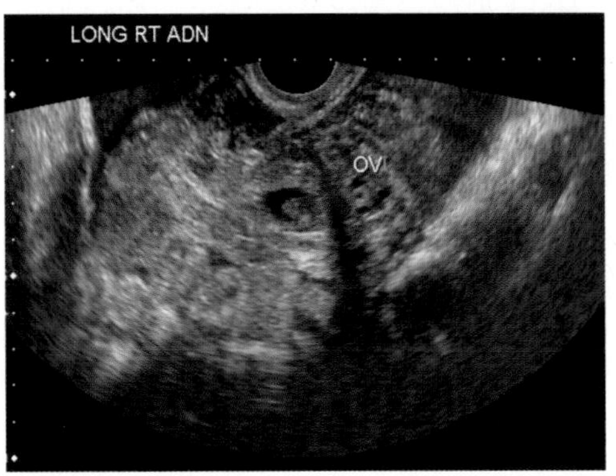

D

Imaging Finding

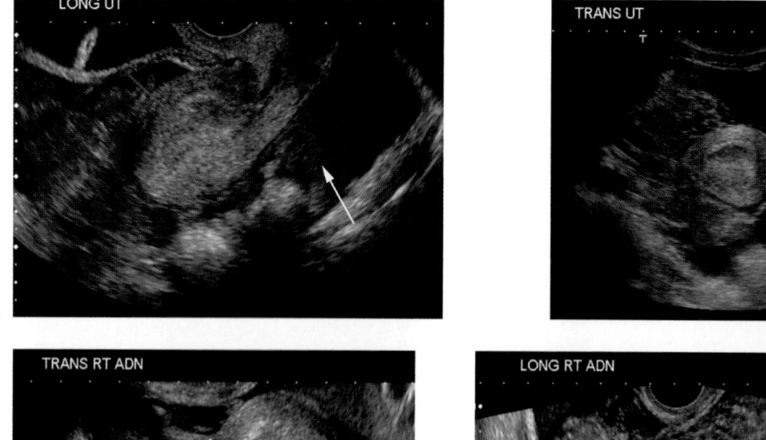

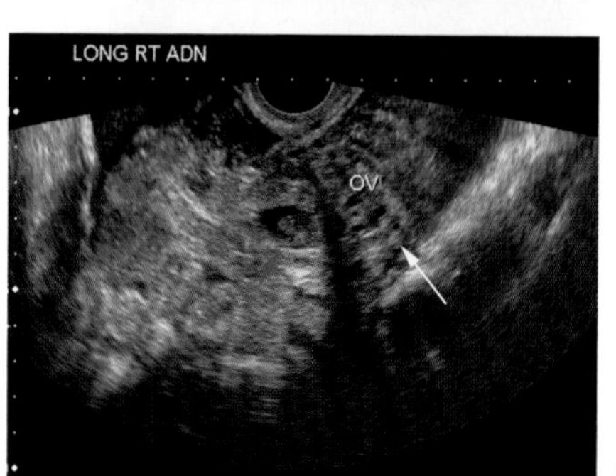

(A, B) Ultrasound (US) image of the pelvis with attention to the uterus shows no evidence of intrauterine gestation. The endometrial strip is thickened (*red arrow*). Large amount of complex fluid in the cul-de-sac is seen (*white arrow*). **(C)** Further imaging of the right adnexa demonstrates a complex paraovarian cystic mass (*white arrows*). A tubular structure is noted within the mass with sonographic appearance similar to a fetal pole (*red arrow*). **(D)** The described cystic lesion is paraovarian in location (*red arrow*) and is visualized adjacent to the ovary (*white arrow*) on the same image.

Differential Diagnosis

- ***Ectopic pregnancy:*** The presence of adnexal mass in a pregnant patient without visualization of intrauterine gestation is suggestive of the diagnosis. The presence of fetal pole or yolk sac is diagnostic of ectopic pregnancy. Visualization of large amount of blood in the cul-de-sac is suggestive of ruptured ectopic.
- *Tubo-ovarian abscess:* Appears as multiloculated adnexal mass with septations and irregular wall. The presence of low-level echo likely represents abscess formation. Elevated white blood cell count and cervical motion tenderness helps in narrowing the diagnosis. In chronic infection, paraovarian adhesions could form with subsequent formations of tubo-ovarian complex.
- *Tubal malignancy:* Adenocarcinoma is the most common type. Sonographically, it appears as a sausage-shaped solid or cystic mass with papillary projections.

Essential Facts

- Increased incidence of ectopic pregnancy with tubal abnormalities, previous ectopic pregnancy, pelvic inflammatory disease, intrauterine device, maternal age, and previous cesarean section.
- Clinical presentation of pain, vaginal bleeding, and adnexal mass.
- The presence of intrauterine pregnancy makes ectopic pregnancy unlikely.
- Intrauterine gestation usually seen on transvaginal US when B-hCG level is above 1,000 IU.
- Serial levels of human chorionic gonadotropin (B-hCG) will differentiate ectopic pregnancy, intrauterine pregnancy, and miscarriage.
- The presence of blood in the cul-de-sac in pregnant patients without visualization of intrauterine pregnancy is suggestive of possible ectopic pregnancy. The possibility of ruptured ectopic pregnancy needs to be considered when a large amount of blood is noted.
- Ninety-five percent of cases occur in the ampulla or isthmus; 2 to 3% are interstitial. Ovarian, cervical, and abdominal ectopic pregnancies are rare.
- The presence of ovarian lesions makes ectopic pregnancy less likely.

✓ Pearls & × Pitfalls

✓ The presence of intrauterine pregnancy almost excludes ectopic gestation secondary to extremely low incidence of heterotopic gestation (1 in 6,000).

× In patients undergoing ovulatory induction, the presence of intrauterine pregnancy does not exclude ectopic pregnancy despite the low incidence of heterotopic gestations. (Incidence of heterotopic gestation is 1%).

Case 38

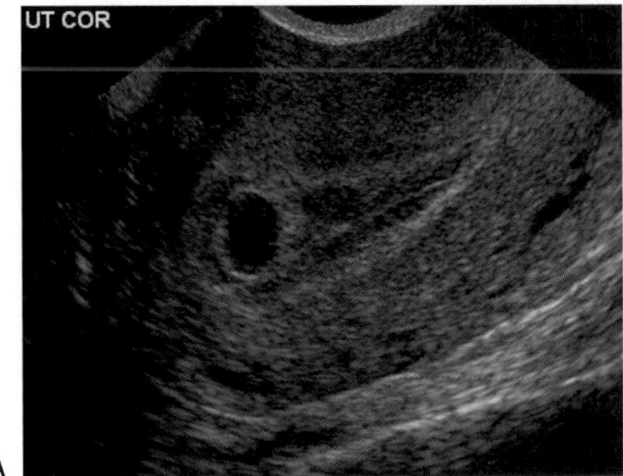

A

Clinical Presentation

A 21-year-old woman with irregular periods and positive pregnancy test.

Further Work-up

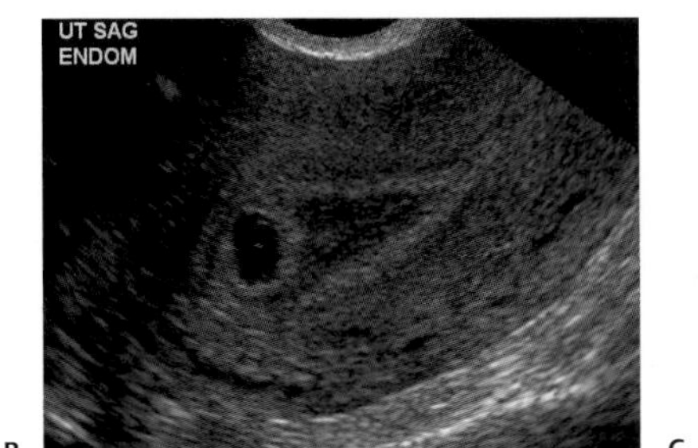

B

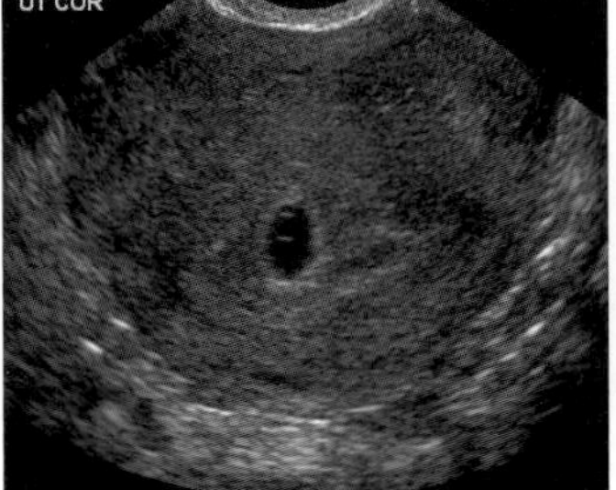

C

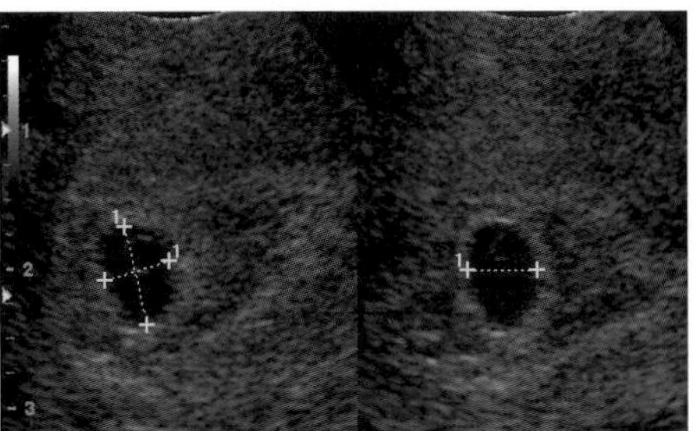

D

Imaging Findings

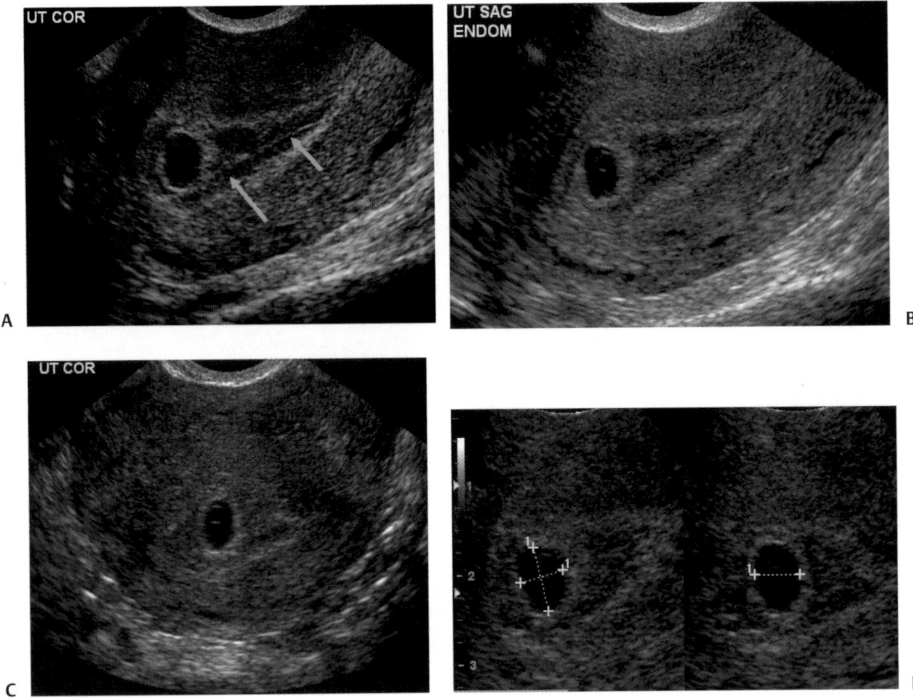

(A) Longitudinal transvaginal image of the uterus reveals a 1 cm rounded fluid collection near the fundus. Note its position in relation to the thin echogenic line (*arrows*) representing the two opposing layers of the endometrium **(B)** Higher-resolution images in a slightly different plane reveal a yolk sac. The presence of a yolk sac confirms that this is an intrauterine gestation. **(C)** The eccentric location of the gestational sac is also evident in this transverse image of the uterus. The gestational sac is eccentrically located due to implantation. **(D)** Sagittal and transverse transvaginal images demonstrate the proper way to measure a gestational sac. Even though the sac is composed of an echogenic peripheral rind, this is not included in the measurement. The central fluid collection is measured in three planes and divided by three for the mean sac diameter (MSD). In this case, the MSD is 5.9 mm and the yolk sac is already visible.

Differential Diagnosis

- ***Intrauterine gestation:*** An eccentrically located intrauterine fluid collection with a discreet echogenic rim separate from the echogenic endometrium is consistent with an early intrauterine gestation. It is usually round.
- *Pseudo sac:* A pseudo sac would be centrally located within the endometrial cavity. It is located between the two layers of the endometrium and would not demonstrate the echogenic rim seen with an intrauterine pregnancy. Pseudo sacs are often irregular in configuration.
- *Implantation bleeding:* The hypoechoic area surrounding the early gestational sac in this case represents the normal endometrium. Implantation bleeding would be more irregular.

Essential Facts

- The intradecidual sign demonstrated by this case consists of an intrauterine fluid collection with a discreet echogenic rim eccentrically positioned in the endometrium and separate from the distinct echogenic line (*arrows* in **A**) that represents the decidualized endometrium.
- The intradecidual sign distinguishes an early intrauterine pregnancy from a pseudo sac seen with ectopic pregnancy.
- The endometrium becomes decidualized with conception. The regions of the decidua are named in relation to the gestational sac. Decidua basalis (beneath the implanted embryo) decidua capsularis (covers the gestational or chorionic sac), decidua parietalis (DP) lines the remainder of the uterine cavity away from gestational sac. The DP is also referred to as the *decidua vera.*
- A yolk sac should be visible with a gestational sac > 8 mm. An embryo should be visible with a gestational sac > 16 mm.
- A failed pregnancy can be definitively diagnosed if no cardiac activity is present with an embryo ≥ 7 mm.
- A failed pregnancy can be definitively diagnosed in the setting of an intrauterine gestational sac measuring ≥ 25 mm without an embryo.
- The yolk sac should measure < 4 mm. It does not grow with time. It is visible into the early second trimester.
- Abnormalities of the yolk sac are associated with a poor prognosis. Abnormalities include a yolk sac that is large, irregularly shaped, thickened, or calcified.

✓ Pearls & × Pitfalls

✓ Abnormal size or shape of the yolk sac is associated with a poor outcome.

× Although a yolk sac should be visible with a sac size of 8 mm, technical factors should be taken into account as they may limit visualization of the yolk sac. In large patients, the yolk sac may not be visible until it is > 8 mm.

✓ The yolk sac is helpful in evaluation of twins in the first trimester. Two yolk sacs are seen with diamnionic twinning. A single yolk sac is seen with monoamnionic twins.

Case 39

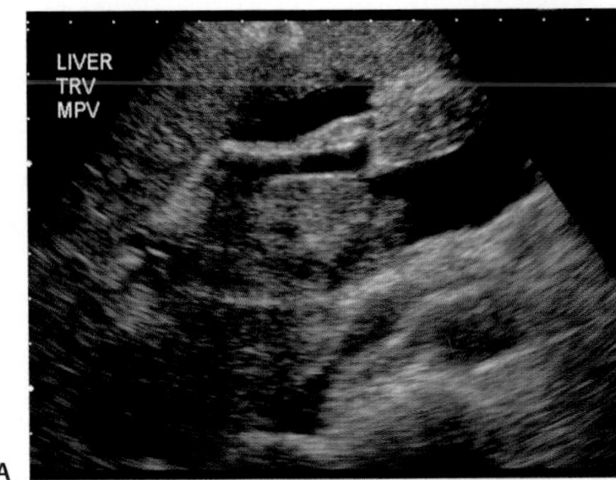

A

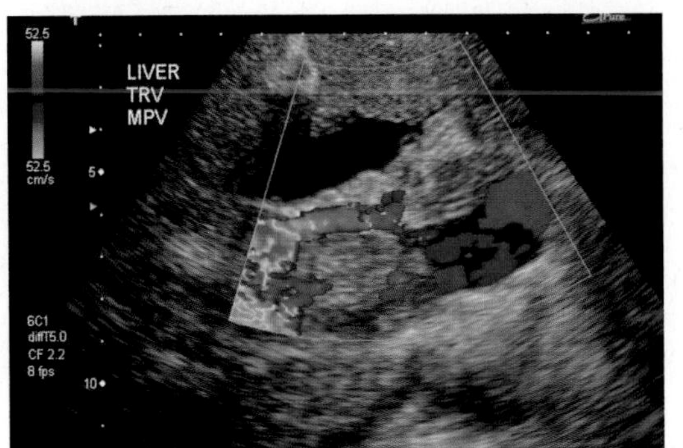

B

Clinical Presentation

A 58-year-old man with a history of hepatitis C presents with abdominal distention.

Further Work-up

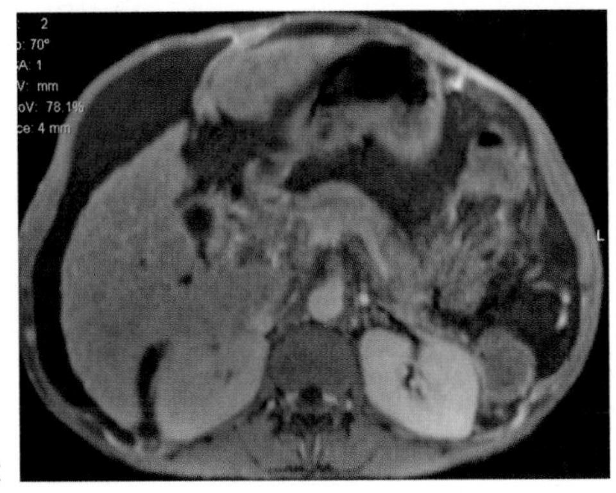

C

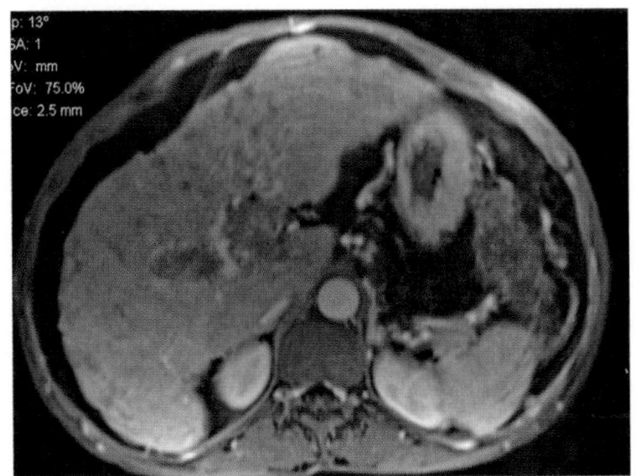

D

Imaging Findings

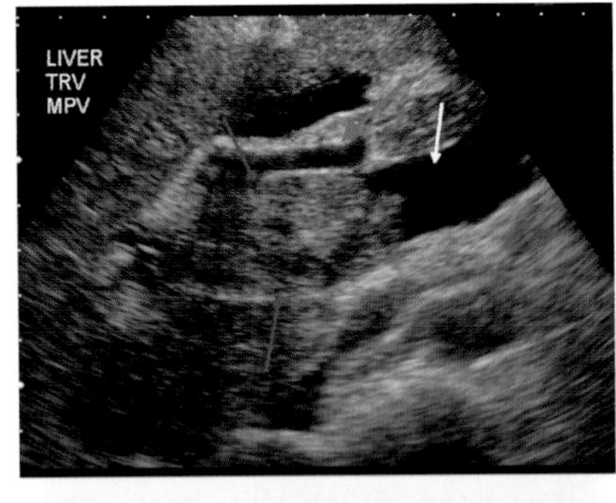

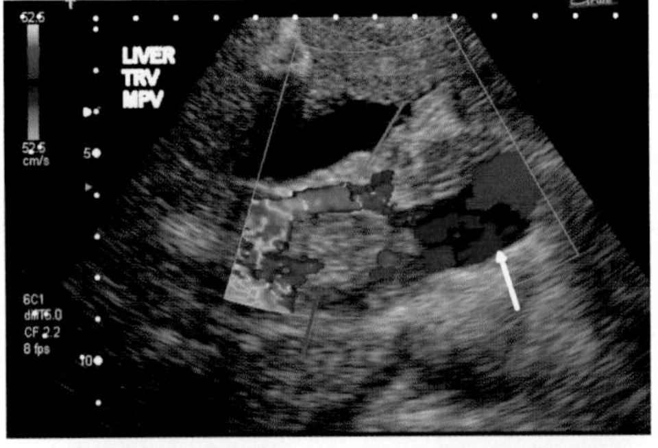

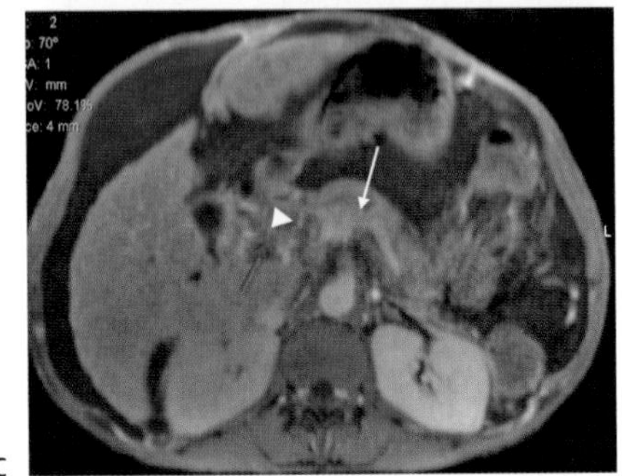

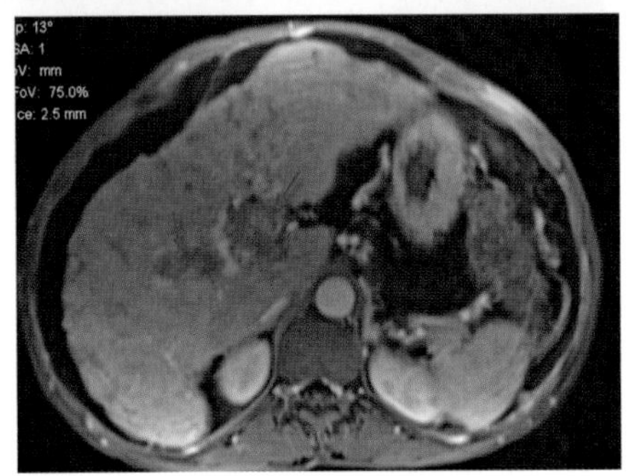

(A, B) Ultrasound (US) images of the liver in the region of the porta hepatis show echogenic filling defect in the portal vein (*red arrows*); minimal sluggish flow is noted in the portal vein (*white arrow*). A dominant hepatic artery is noted (*green arrow*). **(C, D)** Follow-up magnetic resonance imaging (MRI) imaging of the liver with contrast shows filling defect (*red arrows*) in the portal vein (*white arrow*). Flow within the filling defect is noted (*arrowhead*). Involvement of the intrahepatic branches is also noted.

Differential Diagnosis

- ***Tumor thrombus of the portal vein:*** Mostly seen in patients with hepatocellular carcinoma or pancreatic cancer. On US, it appears as echogenic filling defect in the portal vein. The presence of pulsatile flow in the portal vein/thrombus is suggestive of the diagnosis.
- *Bland thrombus of the portal vein:* Can be seen in patients with cirrhosis, hypercoagulable state, chronic pancreatitis, pregnancy, infectious or postsurgery (postsplenectomy). On US, it appears as a filling defect in the portal system without definite arterial flow. Continuous flow can be seen on Doppler US. Collateral and cavernous transformation of the portal vein usually noted in the chronic type.

Essential Facts

- The patient is usually asymptomatic; however, symptoms such as gastrointestinal bleeding, abdominal pain, varices, ascites, and splenomegaly might be seen.
- Complications such as portal hypertension and bowel ischemia could also be present.
- The presence of portal vein tumor thrombus is associated with poor prognosis.
- The common sonographic appearance is echogenic thrombus; hypoechoic thrombus is occasionally seen.
- Hepatofugal flow and varices also could be seen on US.
- The presence of pulsatile flow in the portal vein favors the diagnosis.
- The presence of pulsatile flow is 95% specific and 62% specific in diagnosing malignant thrombus of the portal vein.
- On contrast-enhanced imaging, tumor thrombus shows arterial enhancement with washout; bland thrombus usually follows the liver enhancement with mild retention of contrast similar to liver parenchyma.

✓ Pearls & × Pitfalls

✓ Cavernous transformation of the portal vein occurs over a prolonged period of time and is likely to associate with benign etiologies.

× Varices in the porta hepatis associated with portal hypertension could be misinterpreted as cavernous transformation of the portal vein secondary to chronic portal vein occlusion.

Case 40

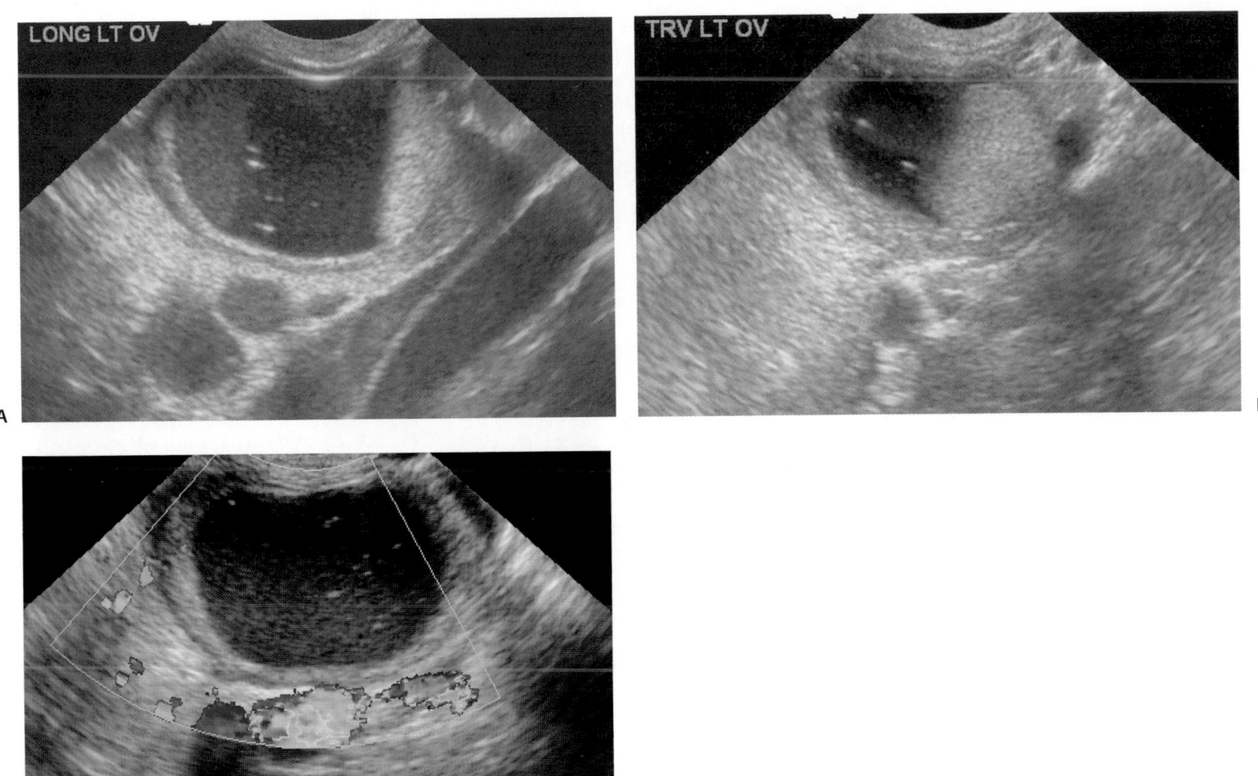

Clinical Presentation

A 27-year-old woman with left pelvic pain.

Further Work-up

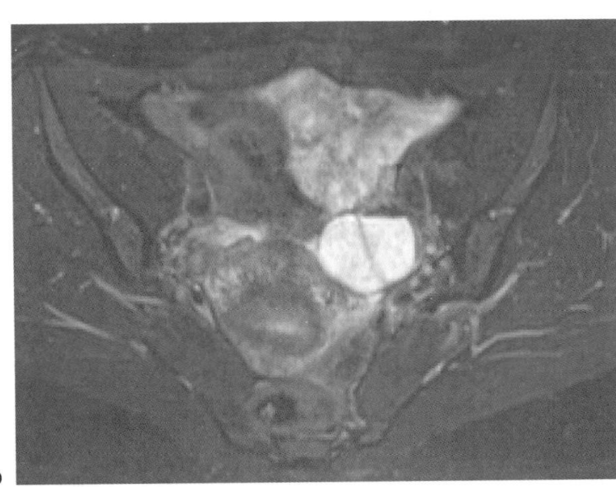

Imaging Findings

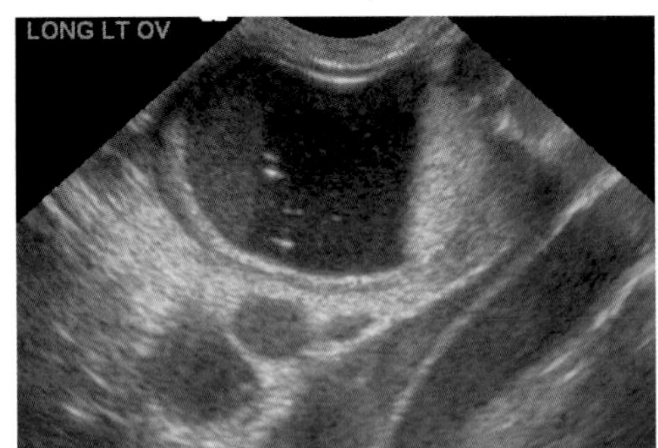

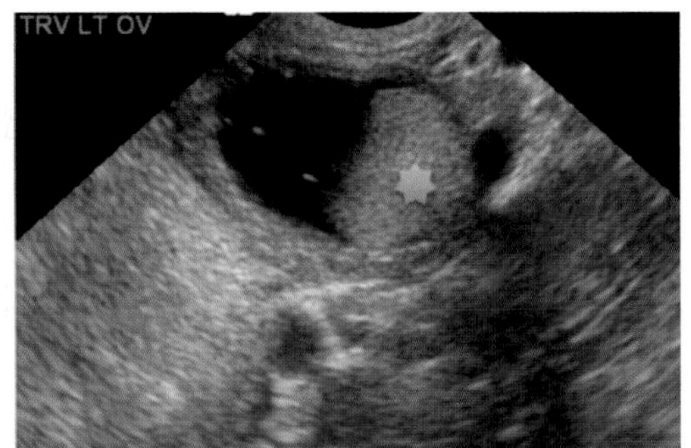

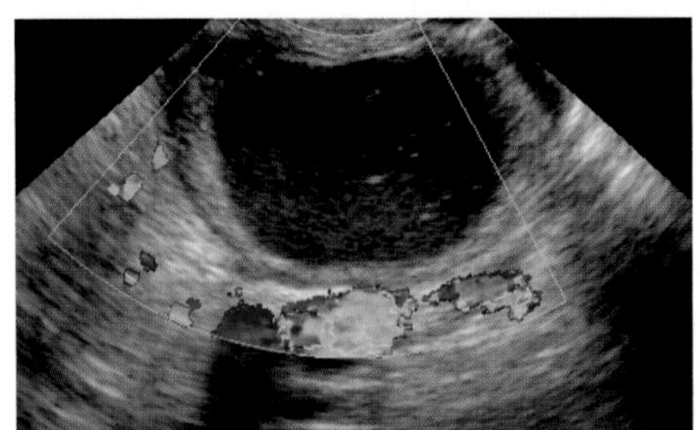

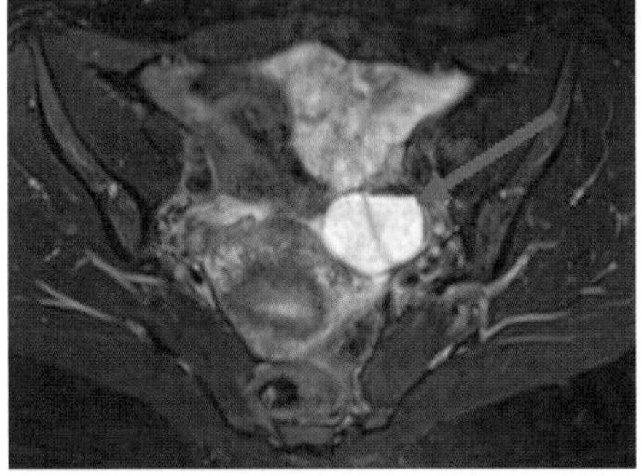

(A) Longitudinal view of the left ovary demonstrating a triple fluid layer. **(B)**, Transverse images through different layers of the lesion. There is a geographic area of hyperechogenicity that causes dirty shadowing (*asterisk*). **(C)** No flow is identified within the lesion with color Doppler. **(D)** Fat suppressed axial image reveals a fat fluid layer in the lesion anteriorly (*arrow*).

Differential Diagnosis

- ***Dermoid:*** Fluid-fluid layers with a geographic area of increased echogenicity that causes dirty shadowing are a classic finding of a dermoid.
- *Endometriomas:* The transverse image (C) contains homogeneous low-level echoes mimicking an endometrioma. Although endometriomas can contain small echogenic nodules in the periphery, they are usually smaller and would not be as echogenic nor cause acoustic shadowing.
- *Hemorrhagic cyst:* Occasionally, a hemorrhagic cyst will contain a fluid-fluid layer or retracting clot mimicking a fluid-fluid layer. It would not be as discrete and linear as the layers formed in a fat fluid interface of a dermoid.

Essential Facts

- Mature cystic teratomas, more commonly referred to as *dermoids*, are the most common ovarian neoplasm. They are almost always benign.
- Dermoids can have a variety of sonographic appearances. The triple-layer appearance above is likely due to a fat-fluid layer on top and a fluid-hair clump layer on the bottom.
- The classic sonographic feature of dermoids is a focal or diffuse echogenic component, hyperechoic lines and dots, areas of acoustic shadowing, and no internal flow.
- Most dermoids contain a clump of hair as in this case, which both absorbs and reflects sound at ultrasound (US) as seen above. The net effect is a focal hyperechogenic area that gradually attenuates sound and results in a gradual shadow.
- Absolutely no flow should be present in a dermoid.
- Dermoids warrant follow-up US even in the premenopausal patient.
- They are usually surgically removed because of the risk of rupture and the risk of torsion.
- There is a small risk of malignant transformation (< 2%). This tends to occur in women older than 50 years and in tumors larger than 10 cm.

Other Imaging Findings

- A T2 fat saturation magnetic resonance imaging image demonstrates a small fat-fluid layer in the lesion with fat density in the nondependent portion of the lesion anteriorly (*arrow*).
- Calcifications or fat are often detectable in dermoids on computed tomography.

✓ Pearls & × Pitfalls

✓ Lesions with features classic for a dermoid usually do not need other imaging modalities to establish the diagnosis.

✓ Dermoids should be followed with US annually to evaluate for malignant transformation.

✓ Signs of malignant transformation include solid elements with internal vascularity.

× Vascularity can be seen in the periphery of a dermoid and may represent surrounding ovarian stroma.

Case 41

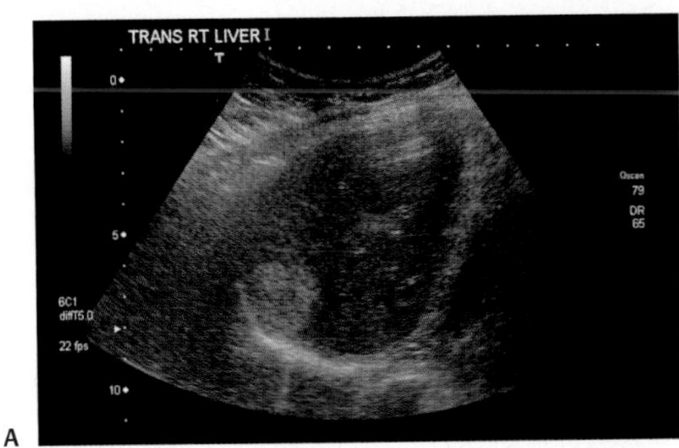

A

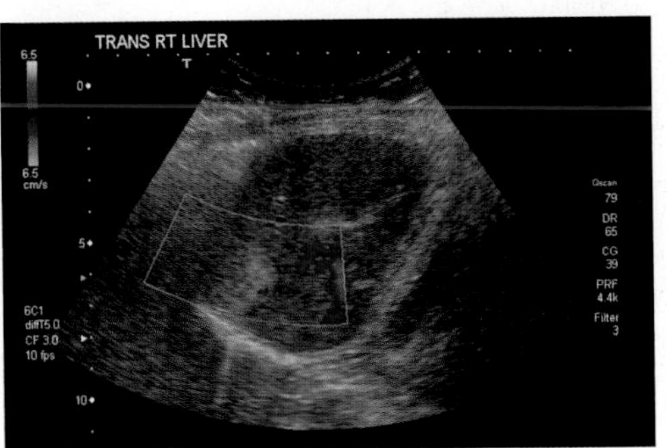

B

■ Clinical Presentation

A 52-year-old woman presents with a history of right upper quadrant pain for 6 months.

■ Further Work-up

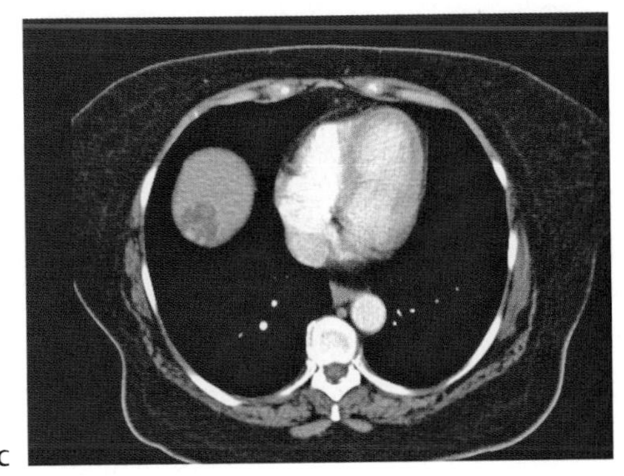
C

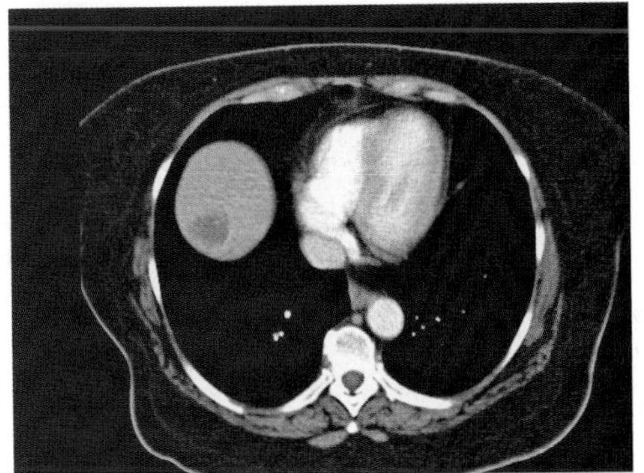
D

Imaging Findings

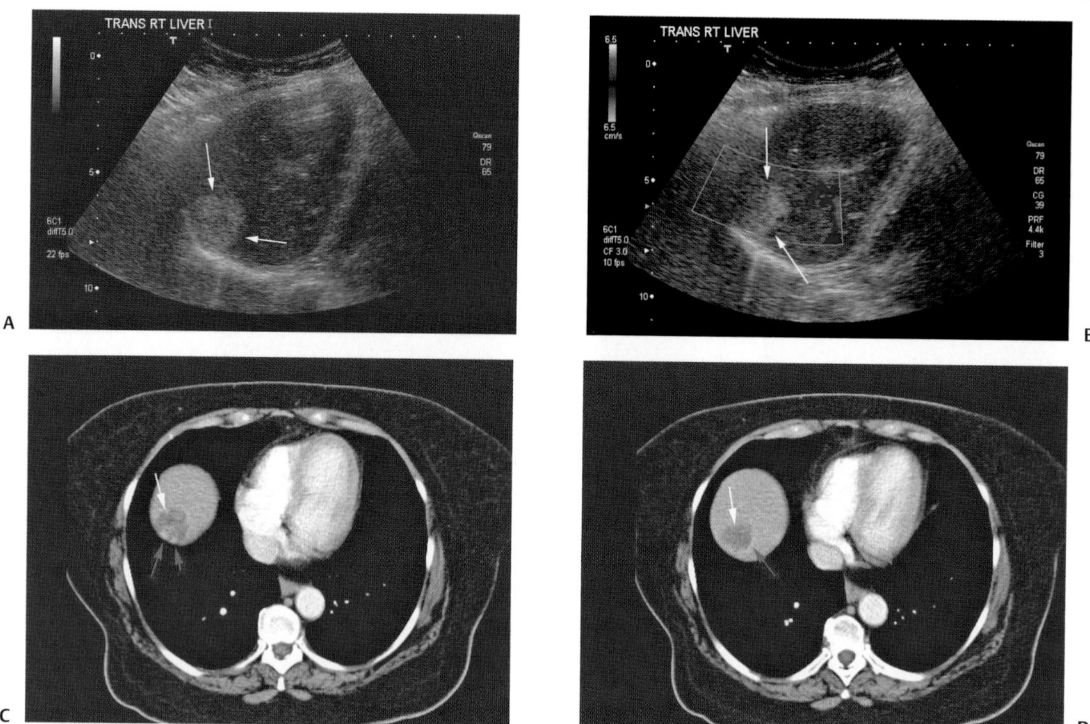

(A, B) Ultrasound (US) images of the liver demonstrate echogenic mass lesion in the dome of the liver in segment 8 (*white arrows*). Doppler color image shows no significant flow within the described lesion in the liver. **(C, D)** Follow-up computed tomography (CT) scan of the liver shows a hypodense lesion in the same location in segment 8 (*white arrow*). The lesion demonstrate peripheral, interrupted nodular enhancement (*red arrows*)

Differential Diagnosis

- ***Hepatic hemangioma:*** Most common benign hepatic tumor. The most common sonographic appearance is an echogenic mass with enhanced through transmission. Color or power Doppler flow usually shows no flow.
- *Hepatic adenoma:* Associated with oral contraceptive usage. Sonographically, the lesion could be echogenic, hypoechoic, isoechoic, or mixed echogenicity. In the presence of hemorrhage, a fluid component could be seen in or surrounding the lesion. The sonographic appearance of blood is variable.
- *Echogenic primary and metastatic malignancies:* Could be seen with gastrointestinal, islet cell, carcinoid, renal cell, hepatocellular, and vascular malignancies. The sonographic appearance overlaps with other lesions; however, the presence multiple lesions of different sizes and hypoechoic rim is suggestive of the diagnosis.

Essential Facts

- Most common benign liver tumor.
- More common in women with 5:1 ratio.
- Incidentally discovered; large lesions occasionally cause pain.
- Sixty-seven to 79% of hemangiomas are hyperechoic, the presence of enhanced transmission improves the diagnostic confidence.
- Large lesions are heterogeneous with central hypoechoic foci corresponding to central scar.
- The flow is extremely slow and usually not detected by color or power Doppler.
- Contrast-enhanced US shows early peripheral enhancement and sustained enhancement on the delayed images.
- Contrast-enhanced CT and magnetic resonance imaging and tagged red blood cell scintigraphy could be used to confirm the diagnosis.
- Transcutaneous biopsy could be performed for definite diagnosis when indicated.

✓ Pearls & × Pitfalls

✓ Echogenic liver metastasis could overlap with hemangioma on US.

✓ The presence of halo rim sign in the periphery of the lesion is suggestive of malignancy.

× Slow growth of hemangioma could be observed on a serial follow-up studies.

Case 42

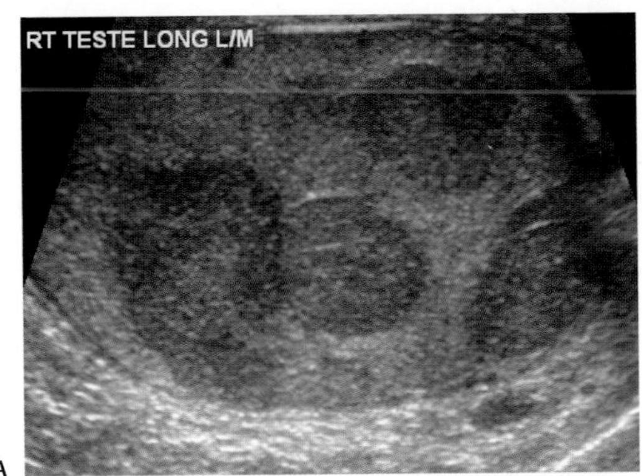

A

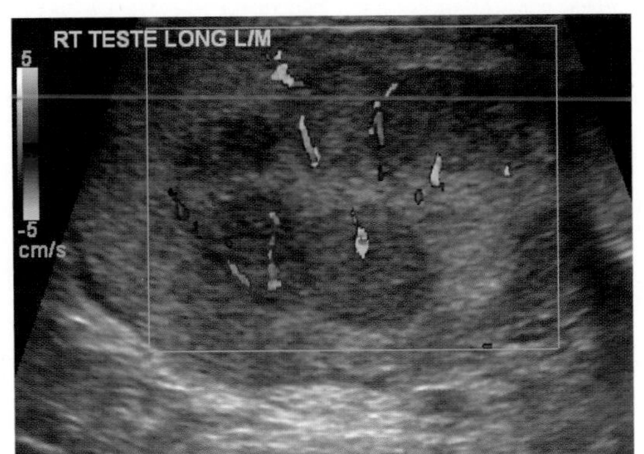

B

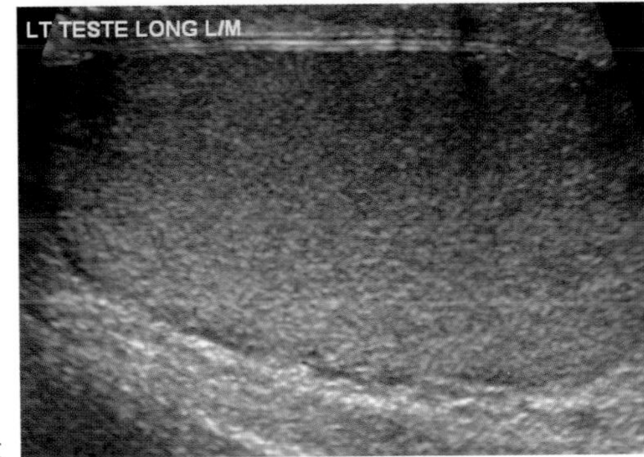

C

Clinical Presentation

A 36-year-old healthy man with right scrotal pain and enlargement.

Imaging Findings

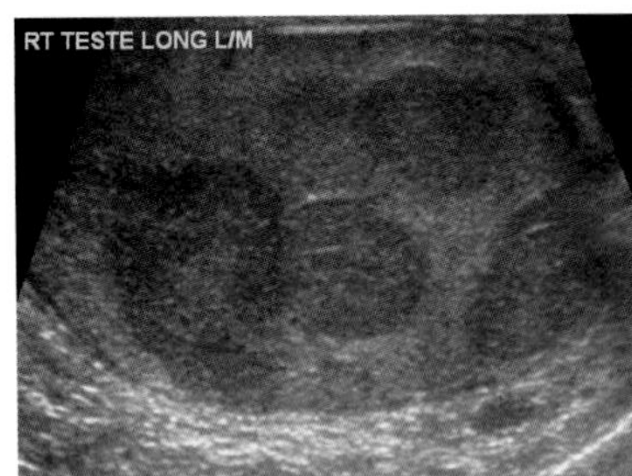

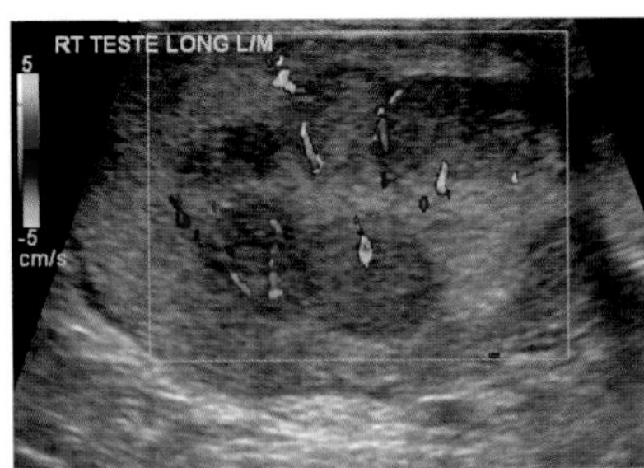

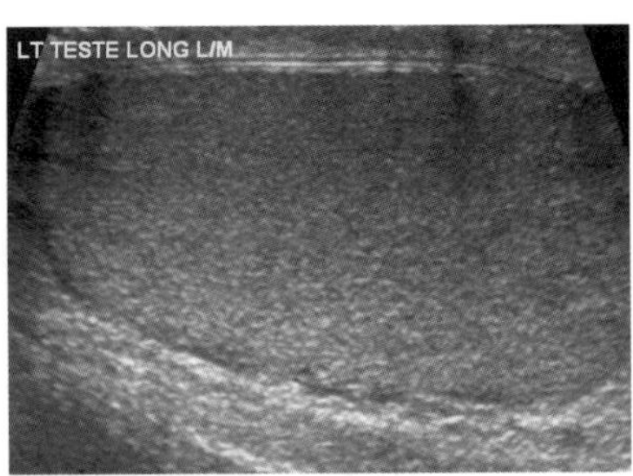

The right testicle **(A)** contains multiple round uniformly hypoechoic lesions that demonstrate internal vascularity with color Doppler imaging **(B)**. The right testicle measures larger than the left (measurements not shown). The left testicle **(C)** is homogeneous in echotexture without focal lesions.

Differential Diagnosis

- ***Multifocal seminoma:*** Homogenous, hypoechoic vascular masses in a single testicle are most consistent with multifocal seminoma.
- *Lymphoma:* Leukemic or lymphomatous involvement of the testicles is invariably bilateral. The testicles contain a barrier to chemotherapeutic agents that allows them to harbor leukemic or lymphomatous cells.
- *Metastases to the testes:* Metastases to the testes is usually bilateral and usually occurs in the setting of widespread metastatic disease.

Essential Facts

- Testicular carcinoma represents only 1% of all neoplasms in men but is the most common malignancy in the 15- to 34-year-old age group.
- The typical ultrasound (US) appearance of seminomas is a rounded, homogenous, well-circumscribed, intratesticular lesion that demonstrates flow with color Doppler ultrasound.
- Seminomas are the most common germ cell neoplasm (GCT). Other cell types include embryonal, yolk sac, choriocarcinoma, and teratoma.
- GCTs can be of a single cell type (pure) or mixed. Seminoma is the most common pure GCT. Pure seminomas account for 50% of all GCTs. Seminomas are the most common component of mixed GCTs.
- Seminomas are usually pure, which explains the classic homogenous hypoechoic appearance on US.
- Seminomas, in comparison with nonseminomatous GCTs, occur in a slightly older patient population, with the average age at presentation of 40.5 years.
- Because of the extreme sensitivity to radiation and chemotherapy, seminomas have the most favorable prognosis of the GCTs. Seventy-five percent of patients present with disease limited to the testes.
- Ninety-five percent of testicular tumors are malignant GCTs. The remaining types include stromal tumors (Sertoli cell and Leydig cell) and lymphoma or metastases.

✓ Pearls & × Pitfalls

✓ Seminomas can be lobulated in contour and rarely multifocal as in this patient. Bilateral seminomas are rare (< 2%) and are almost always asynchronous.

✓ Bilateral testicular masses are usually due to metastatic disease, lymphoma/leukemia, infection, and rare systemic diseases such as sarcoidosis.

✓ Seminomas are generally well-defined homogeneous lesions, whereas the nonseminomatous GCTs have a much more varied appearance.

× Seminomas can be atypical in appearance with cystic areas due to necrosis or tumor obstruction of the rete tubes with resultant cystic dilation. Larger tumors may be heterogeneous.

Case 43

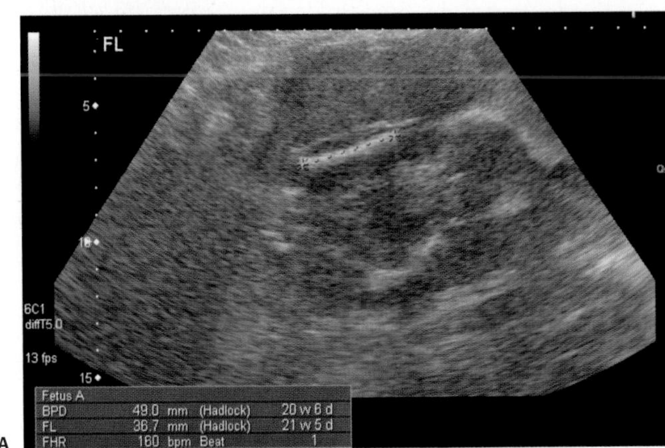

A

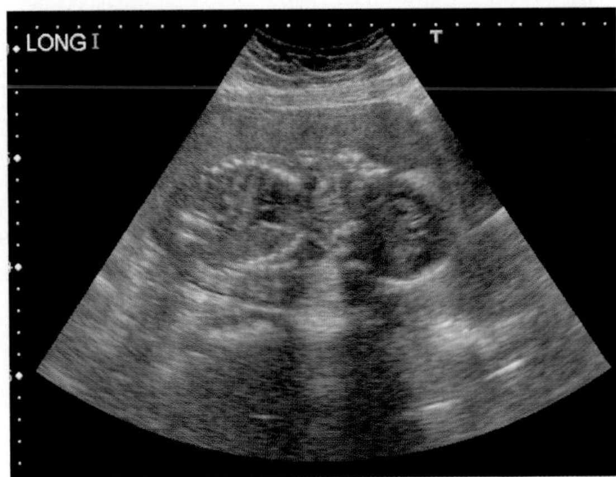

B

Clinical Presentation

A 25-year-old pregnant woman presents with abdominal pain.

Further Work-up

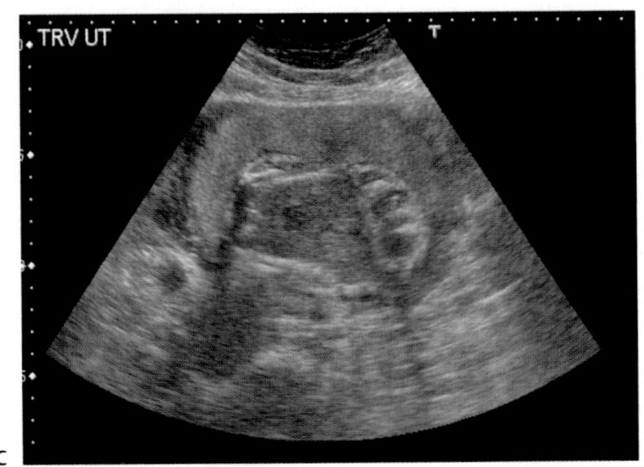

C

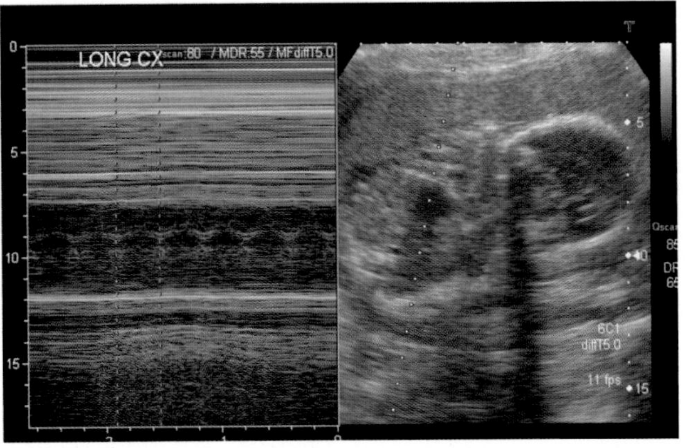

D

Imaging Findings

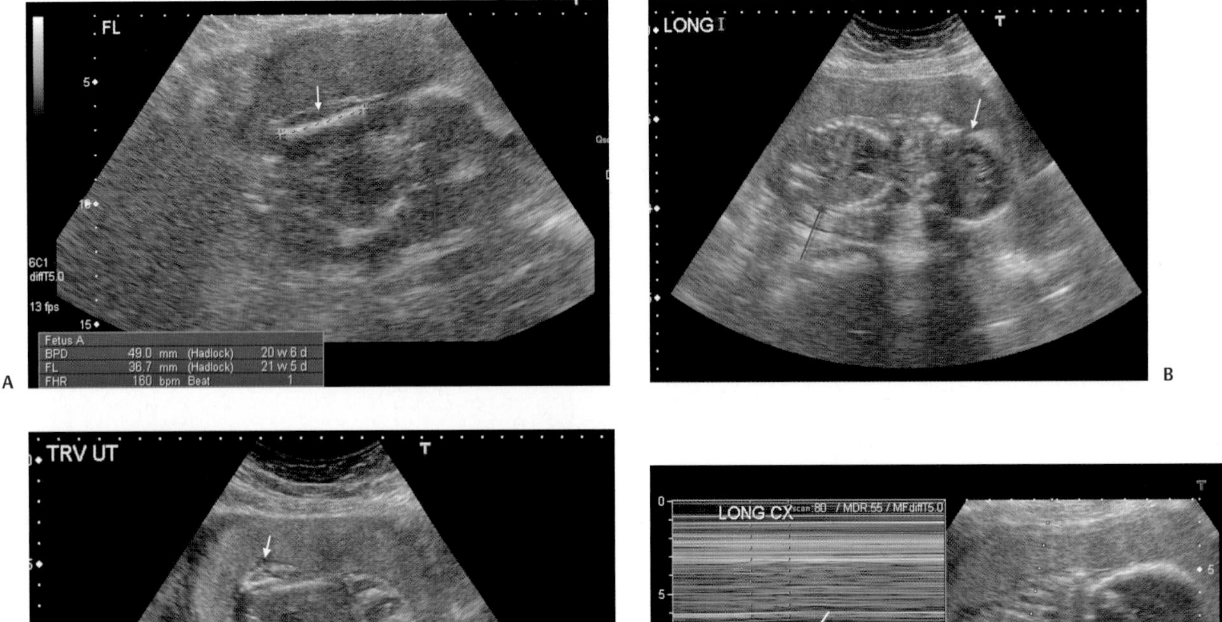

(A–C) Ultrasound (US) images of the pelvis using transabdominal approach show an intrauterine gestation at ~ 20 weeks and 6 days. Only a trace amount of amniotic fluid is noted around the fetus (*white arrow*). The fetal anatomy is ill defined due to the lack of amniotic fluid (*red arrow*). The placenta appears normal on gray scale image. **(D)** Cardiac activity is present on M-mode image, suggesting viability (*white arrow*).

Differential Diagnosis

- ***Anhydramnios secondary to premature rupture of membrane:*** Occasionally could be transient. Sonographic and physical assessment of the cervix could be helpful for the diagnosis. Occasionally, cases are associated with amniocentesis and/or uterine rupture.
- *Anhydramnios secondary to poor production of amniotic fluid:* Usually related to poor or nonfunctioning kidneys in the second trimester and is associated with poor prognosis. Evaluation of both kidneys and signs of lower urinary tract obstruction is critical for accurate diagnosis.
- *Oligohydramnios:* Defined as amniotic fluid index < 2 standard deviations for the gestation age. It could be related to intrauterine growth restriction, postterm pregnancy, or rupture of membrane and fetal anomalies.

Essential Facts

- Perinatal morbidity and mortality significantly higher
- Successful management requires accurate detection of etiology.
- Prolonged oligohydramnios/anhydramnios can result in pulmonary hypoplasia and fetal compression syndrome.
- Detailed assessment of fetal anomaly is critical.
- The presence of normal-appearing kidneys and lack of lower urinary tract obstruction should be documented.
- Assessment of maintained cervix, closed os, and lack of signs of premature rupture of membrane.
- Sonographic assessment of the gray scale placenta and Doppler might be helpful.

✓ Pearls & × Pitfalls

✓ The presence of anhydramnios in the second trimester with no signs for premature rupture of membranes indicates urinary tract abnormality.

× The umbilical cord coiled in a quadrant could be misinterpreted as a pocket of fluid; Doppler is critical in clarification.

Case 44

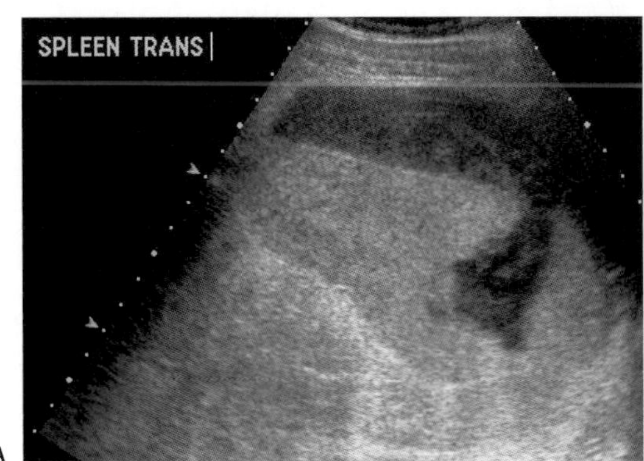

A

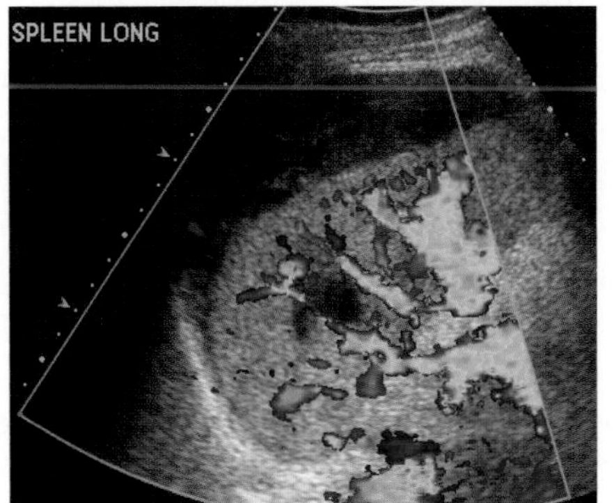

B

Clinical Presentation

A 25-year-old patient, recently diagnosed with mononucleosis, presents with abdominal and left shoulder pain.

Further Work-up

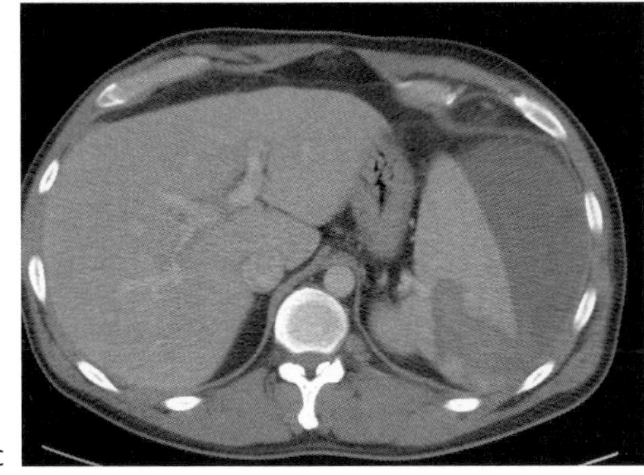
C

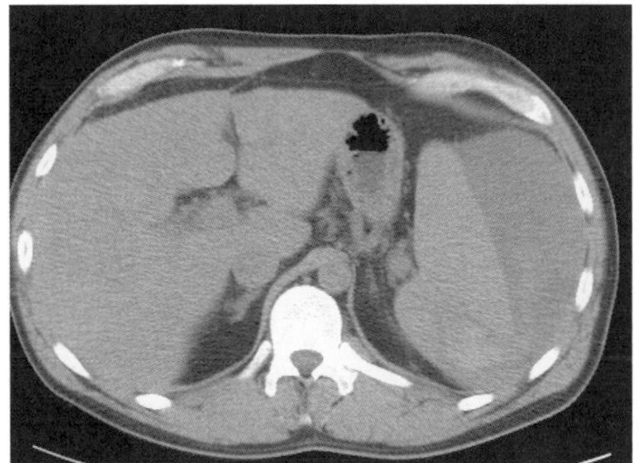
D

Imaging Findings

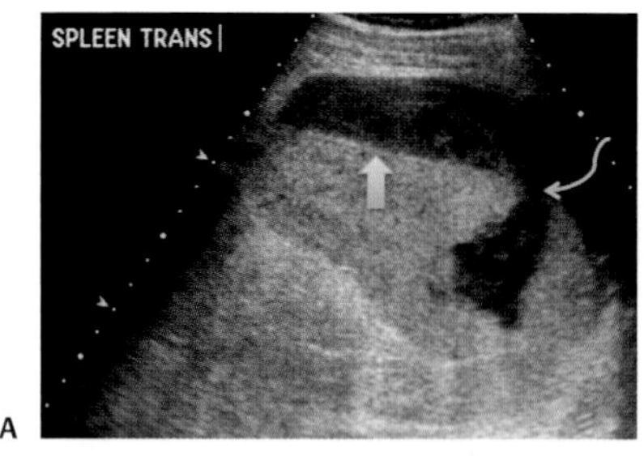

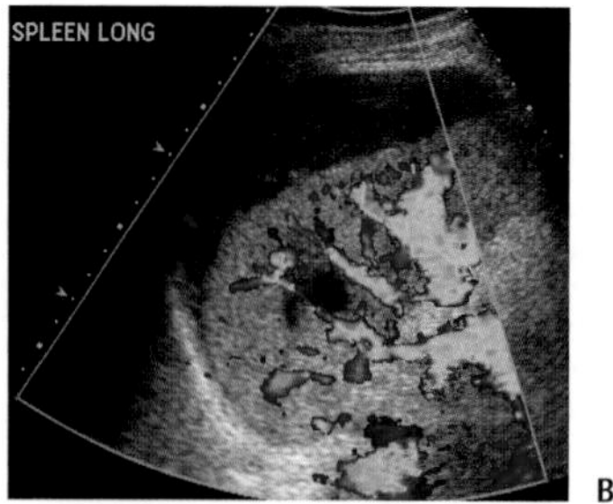

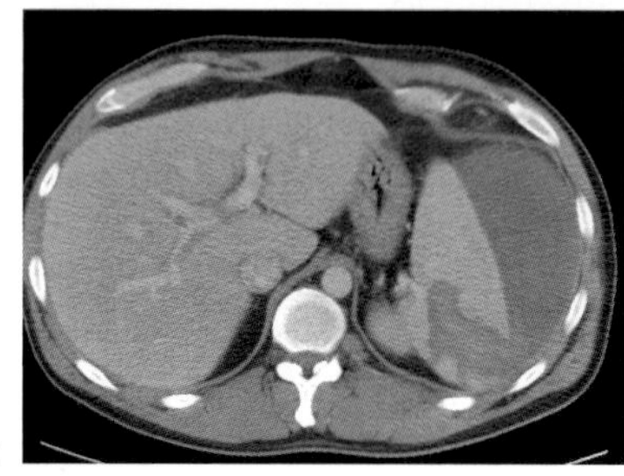

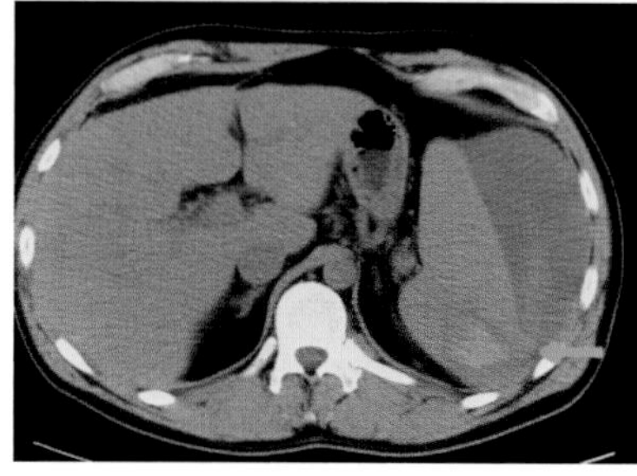

(A) Transverse gray scale image through the spleen reveals a large defect in the spleen laterally (*curved arrow*). Note the heterogeneous hypoechoic collection lateral to the spleen. Flattening of the splenic contour (*arrow*) indicates a subcapsular location. **(B)** Color Doppler imaging revealed a large area without obvious vascularity. **(C)** Postcontrast computed tomography (CT) reveals a large area of nonenhancement of the spleen posteriorly. Capsular disruption is better seen with contrast. **(D)** Noncontrast CT reveals a large high-density subcapsular collection causing mass effect on the spleen. Note the area of increased density within the splenic parenchyma posteriorly and disruption of the splenic capsule posterolaterally (*arrow*). High-density free fluid is also seen in the pelvis.

Differential Diagnosis

- ***Spontaneous splenic rupture related to mononucleosis:*** Disruption of the capsule, subcapsular hematoma, and hemoperitoneum are consistent with splenic rupture. In the setting of mononucleosis, this is related to splenomegaly.
- *Posttraumatic splenic rupture:* Because there was no history of trauma these findings would indicate spontaneous rupture of the spleen. The ultrasound (US) findings of splenic rupture are the same regardless of etiology.
- *Lymphoma:* Lymphomatous involvement of the spleen can have a variety of appearances but would not be expected to have a subcapsular collection or capsular disruption.

Essential Facts

- Splenic rupture is usually posttraumatic. Less frequently it is spontaneous.
- Spontaneous rupture usually occurs with an enlarged or abnormal spleen. The classic spontaneous rupture is in the setting of splenomegaly with mononucleosis.
- The spleen is the most frequently injured abdominal organ in the setting of trauma.
- US criteria for splenic rupture include hemoperitoneum, subcapsular hematoma, intraparenchymal bleeding, and fragmentation of the spleen with capsular disruption.
- Surgical versus conservative treatment of splenic rupture is determined by the grade injury (and patient status).
  - Grade 0: Perisplenic blood.
  - Grade 1: < 3 cm subcapsular hematoma and/or laceration.
  - Grade 2: > 3 cm subcapsular hematoma and/or laceration.
  - Grade 3: Capsular disruption.

✓ Pearls & × Pitfalls

✓ US is very sensitive for detection of free intra-abdominal fluid but not as sensitive for detection of acute splenic parenchymal lacerations or hematoma.

✓ Subcapsular collections will cause mass effect and a flattened contour.

× Acute hematomas can be echogenic and difficult to distinguish from the spleen.

✓ Kehr sign (left shoulder pain) occurs in ~ 50% of splenic ruptures and is due to irritation of the diaphragm.

✓ Color Doppler evaluation of the spleen should be performed in the setting of trauma to evaluate for devitalized tissue.

Case 45

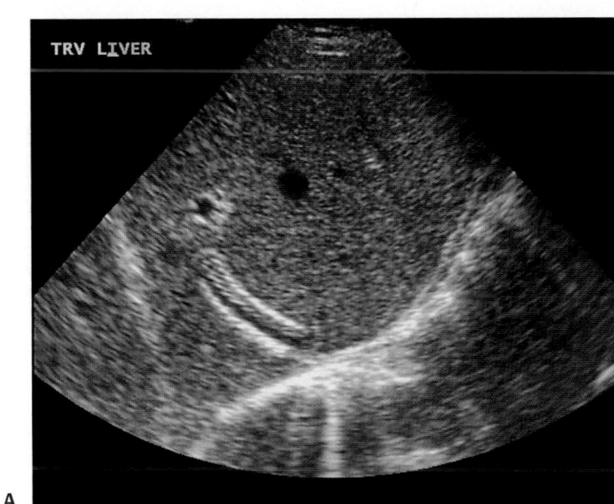

A

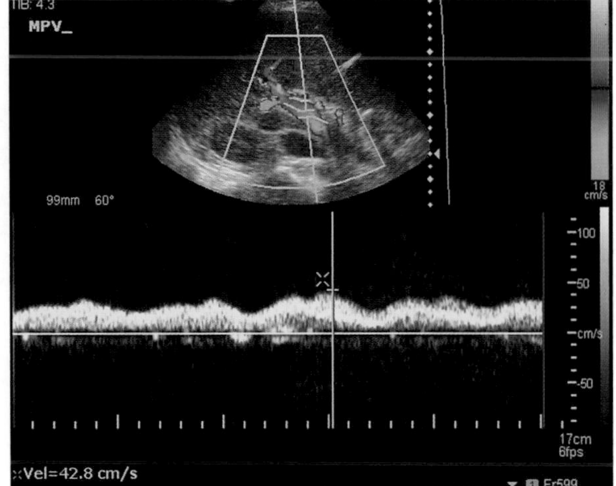

B

Clinical Presentation

A 55-year-old man presents for assessment of TIPS (transjugular intrahepatic portosystemic shunts) patency.

Further Work-up

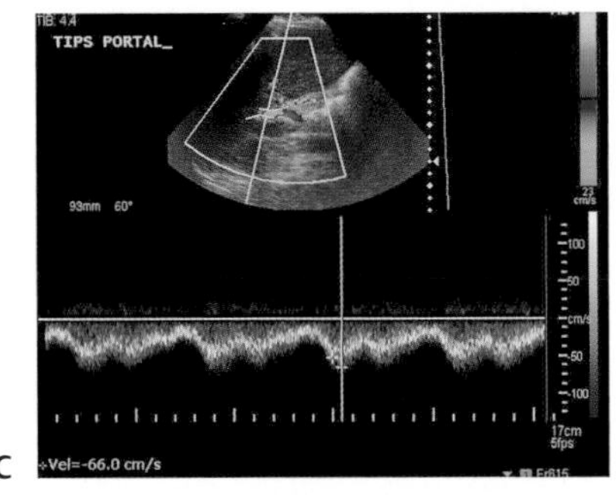

C

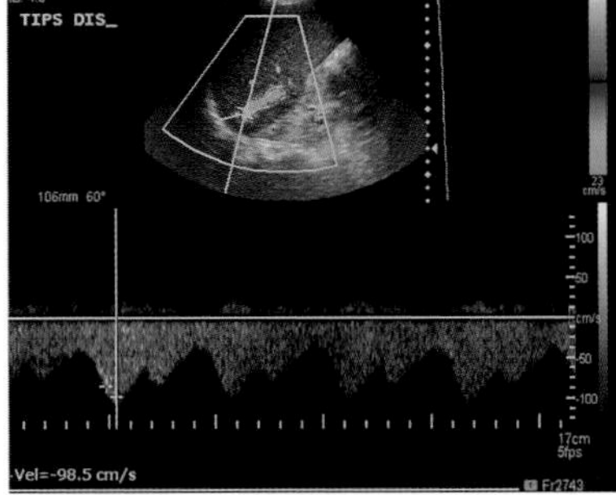

D

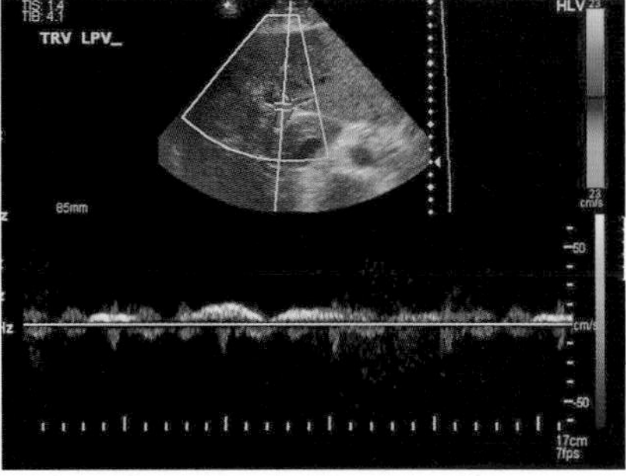

E

Imaging Findings

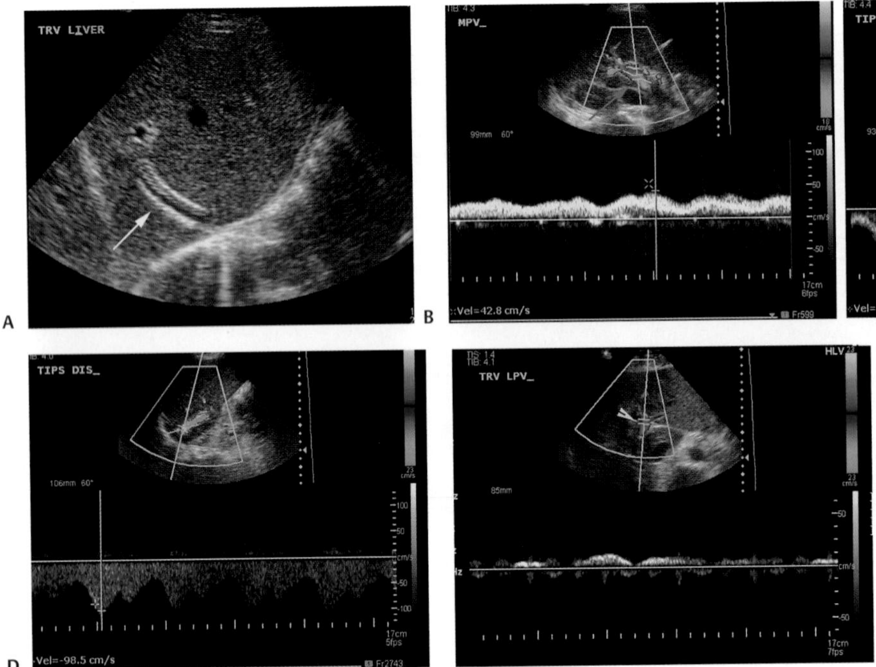

(A–E) A gray scale image shows a TIPS extending from the right portal vein to the right hepatic vein (*white arrow*). Doppler assessment of the portal vein shows antegrade flow (*green arrow*). The velocities in the proximal TIPS (*red arrow*) and distal TIPS (*red arrowhead*) are borderline. Flow in the left portal vein is antegrade (*white arrowhead*).

Differential Diagnosis

- ***Early TIPS malfunction:*** The sonographic appearance of early TIPS malfunction is nonspecific and could include abnormal direction of flow intrahepatically distal to the TIPS and slight increased velocity and gradient within the TIPS. The presence of secondary signs of TIPS malfunction is a late manifestation.
- *Normal TIPS Doppler:* The typical sonographic appearance includes normal direction of flow within the main portal vein, normal waveform and velocity within the TIPS, and reversal of flow within the intrahepatic portal vein distal to the TIPS. The velocities and gradient should be assessed in the proximal, mid, and distal segments of the TIPS.
- *Normal TIPS Doppler with recanalized para-umbilical vein:* In case of recanalized para-umbilical vein, flow within the left portal vein could remain antegrade despite the presence of TIPS. An antegrade flow within the left portal vein in the presence of recanalized paraumbilical vein does not imply the presence of an early TIPS malfunction.

Essential Facts

- The most common cause of TIPS malfunction is stenosis and/or intimal hyperplasia.
- Clinical monitoring of TIPS patency is relatively insensitive for early detection.
- Stenosis is more common on the hepatic vein side.
- The sonographic appearance is nonspecific; however, early detection could be critical in maintaining functional TIPS.
- The sonographic Doppler findings include changes in direction of flow within the intrahepatic branches, decreased pulsatility of the main portal vein, velocity gradient > 50 cm/sec through the TIPS, and increased and/or decreased velocity within the TIPS (normal velocities are 50 to 200 cm/sec).
- The presence of focal narrowing on gray scale images is suggestive of significant stenosis.
- The presence of color aliasing also requires further assessment.

✓ Pearls & × Pitfalls

✓ Any changes from baseline imaging should be considered as potential early TIPS malfunction; further assessment would be critical in maintaining functional TIPS.

× The left portal vein could remain antegrade in the presence of the recanalized paraumbilical vein; this should not be considered TIPS malfunction.

Case 46

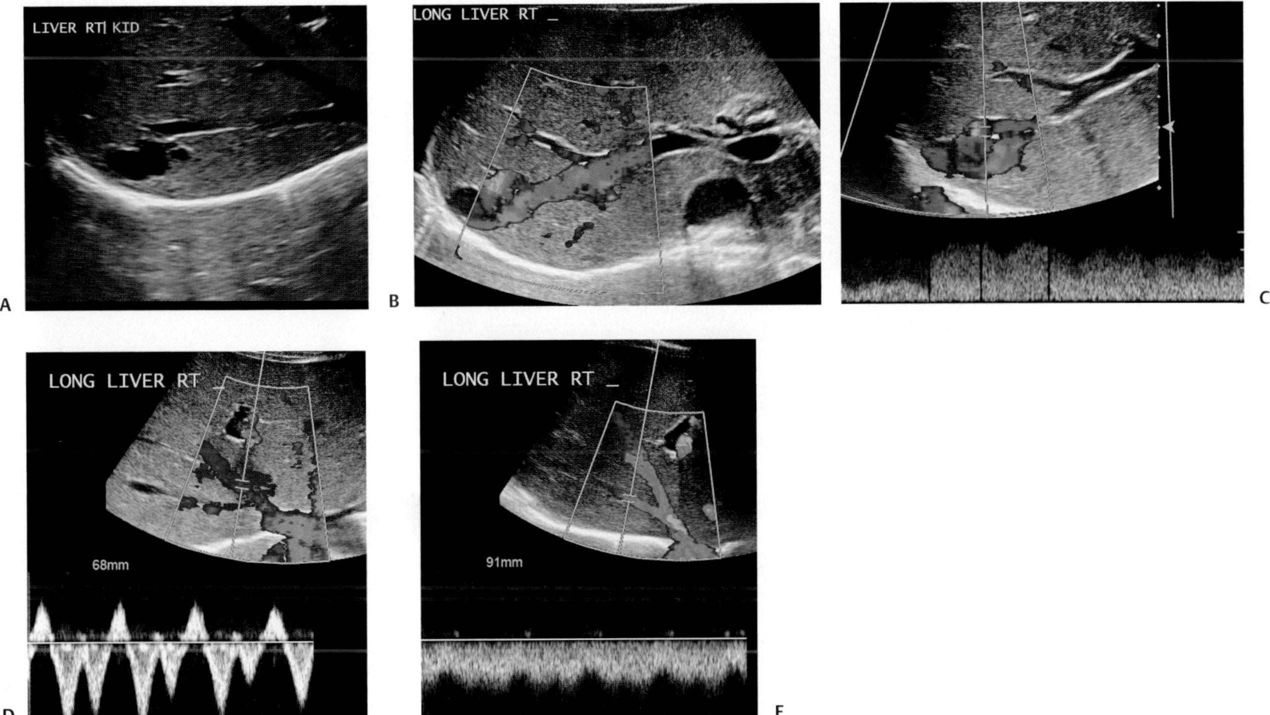

Clinical Presentation

A 35-year-old patient with hypertension referred for ultrasound (US) evaluation for renal artery stenosis (RAS). An incidental liver lesion was seen at US.

Imaging Findings

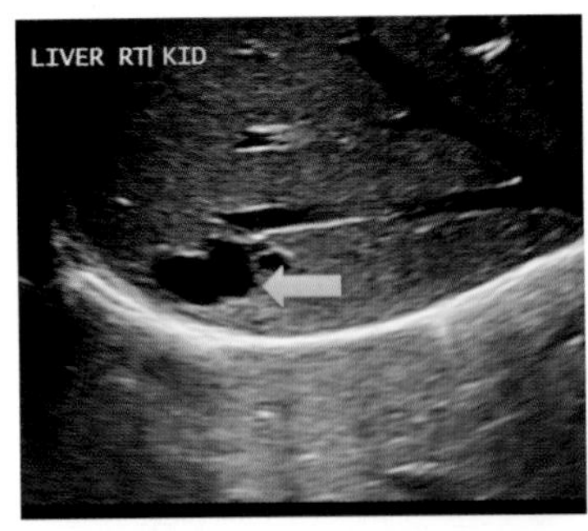

A

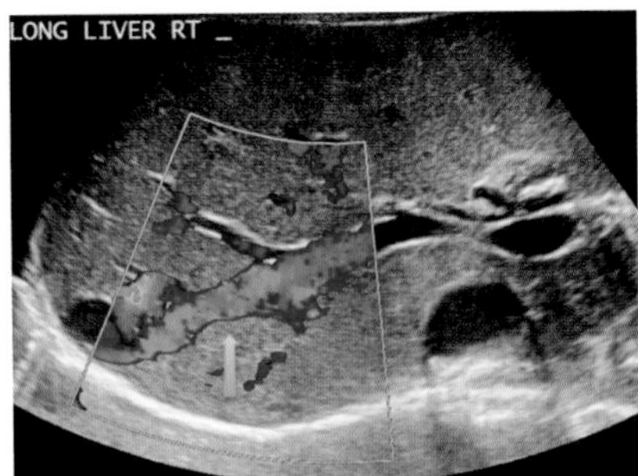

B

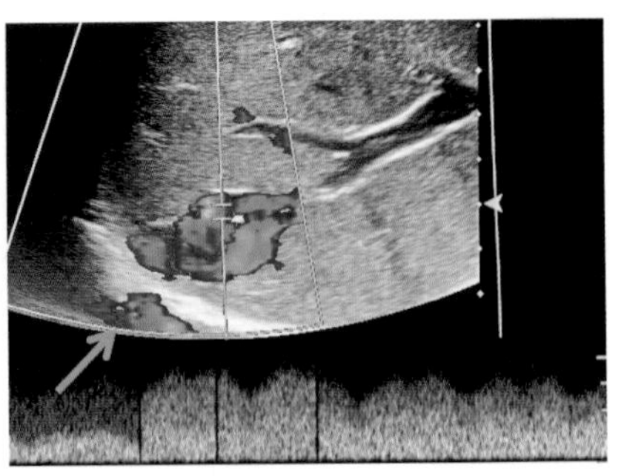

C

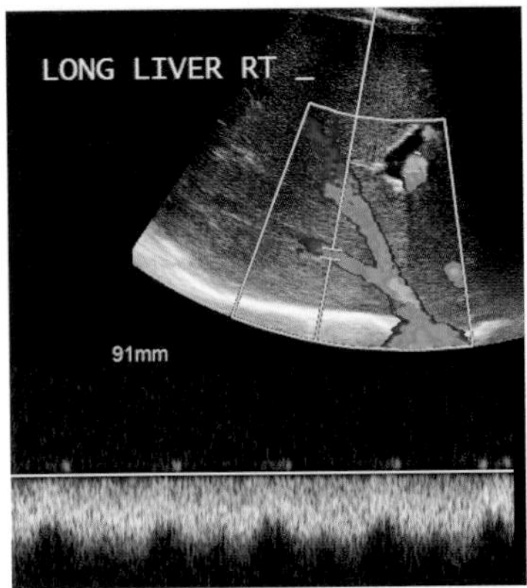

D

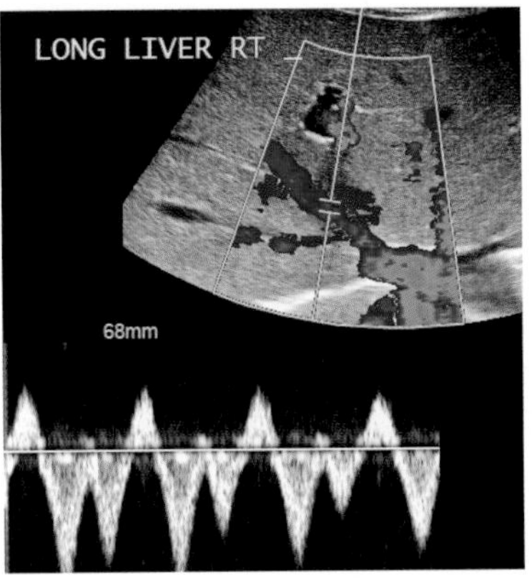

E

(A) Gray scale transverse image demonstrates a lobulated cystic lesion (*arrow*) in the periphery of the liver posterior to a branch of the right portal vein. **(B)** With color Doppler imaging, the lesion is an aneurysmal vascular structure connected to the right portal vein (*arrow*). Note that a mirror image artifact occurs with both color (arrow in C) and gray scale. **(C)** Turbulent high-velocity flow is present within the lesion. The hepatic vein that drains the lesion demonstrates turbulent flow **(D)** compared with the adjacent hepatic vein **(E)**, which demonstrates a normal hepatic venous waveform.

Differential Diagnosis

- ***Congenital intrahepatic portosystemic shunt:*** An aneurysmal vascular structure directly supplied by the portal vein and drained by the hepatic vein is consistent with a congenital portosystemic shunt.
- *Abernethy malformation:* Eponym for a congenital extrahepatic portosystemic shunt. This shunt occurs in the portal vein prior to the liver.
- *Arteriovenous fistula (AVF) following biopsy:* AVF formation is a known complication of liver biopsy. AVF is a hepatic artery to hepatic or portal vein connection. This patient had not had a biopsy or trauma.

Essential Facts

- Congenital intrahepatic portosystemic venous shunts are uncommon hepatic vascular anomalies that are often seen in a normal liver, as in this case.
- Intrahepatic shunts are connections within the liver between branches of the portal vein (PV) and the systemic veins, usually hepatic veins. These are most commonly seen with cirrhosis. They can be created (transjugular intrahepatic portosystemic shunts [TIPS]) or posttraumatic (biopsy). Less commonly they are congenital, as seen in this case.
- Portosystemic shunts can be intrahepatic or extrahepatic. Extrahepatic shunts occur central to the bifurcation of the PV. Both types most commonly develop as a result of portal hypertension. Rarely, they are congenital.

✓ Pearls & ✗ Pitfalls

✓ Cirrhosis is the most common cause for portal-to-systemic venous shunting.

✓ Congenital portosystemic shunts can be an incidental finding in normal livers. With increased use of imaging studies, these lesions are likely to be increasingly encountered.

✓ Color and spectral Doppler are critical to make the diagnosis of a vascular shunt.

✓ Vascular shunting results in turbulence and increased velocities.

✗ Abernethy malformation is an eponym for congenital extrahepatic portosystemic shunts but is used generically to describe any portosystemic shunts.

Case 47

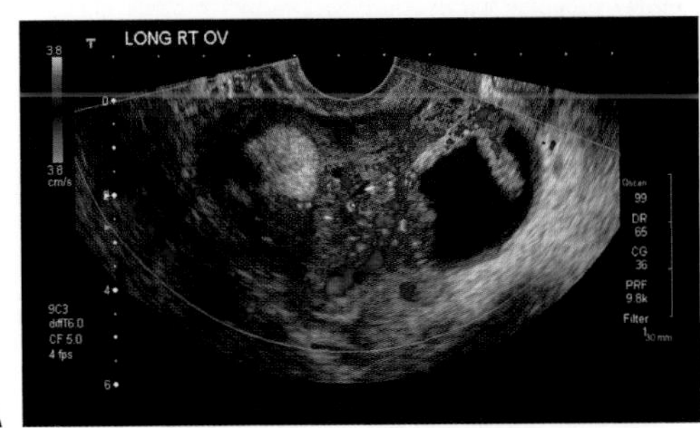

A

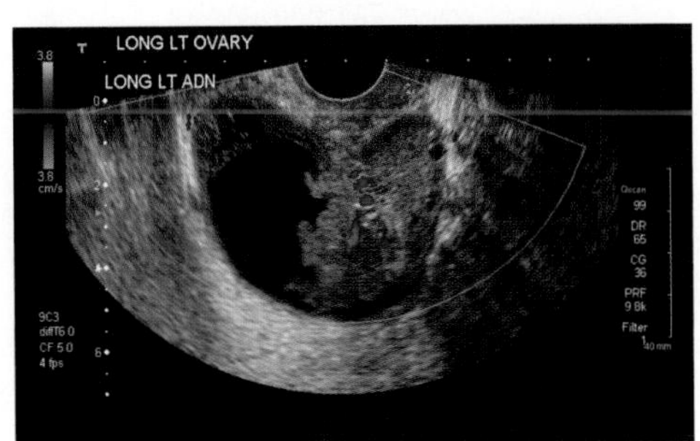

B

Clinical Presentation

An 18-year-old woman with chronic pelvic discomfort presents with acute exacerbation of pain.

Further Work-up

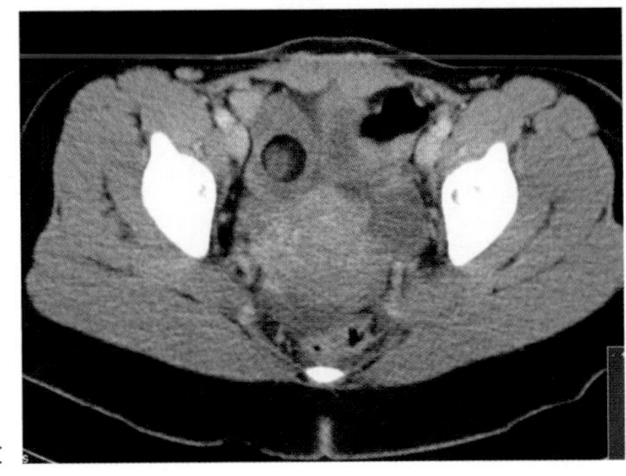

C

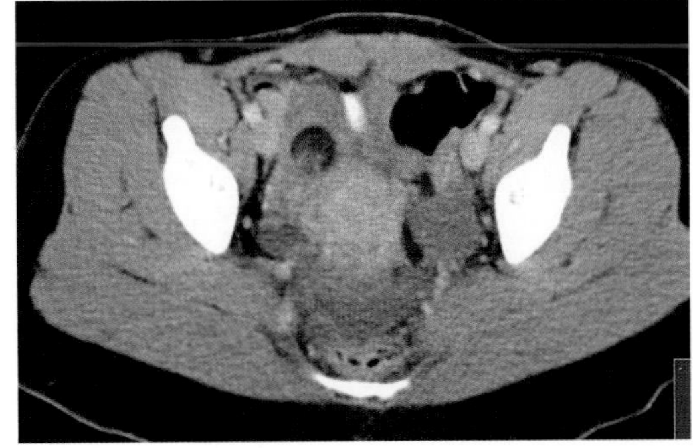

D

Imaging Findings

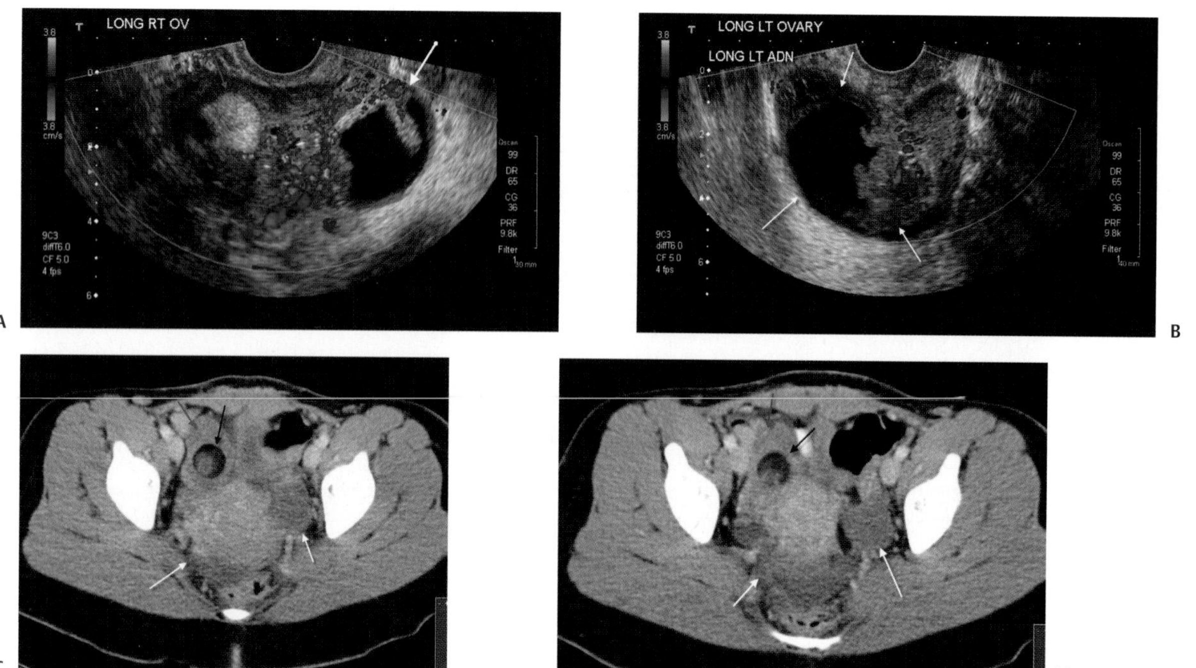

(A, B) Ultrasound images of the adnexa bilaterally show poorly defined ovarian (*red arrow*) margins bilaterally with complex bilateral tubular structures (*white arrows*), demonstrating irregular thickened walls and low-level echoes. An echogenic mass in the right ovary is also seen (*red arrow*). **(C, D)** Computed tomography scan images of the pelvis show dilated fluid-filled tubular structures in the pelvis with poorly defined adnexa (*white arrows*). Fat-containing lesion (*black arrow*) in the right ovary (*red arrow*) is also present.

Differential Diagnosis

- ***Tubo-ovarian complex:*** Occurs secondary to chronic inflammation in the pelvis. Sonographically, it appears as a complex ill-defined soft tissue mass in the adnexa. Acute onset of pain in the adnexa and local tenderness to physical examination are common presentations. Right ovarian dermoid is also noted.
- *Tubal carcinoma:* Rare and occurs in postmenopausal women. A sausage-shaped solid or cystic mass usually noted on ultrasound. The presence of thick papillary projections suggests tubal origin of the mass. Right ovarian dermoid is also noted.
- *Ovarian vein thrombosis:* Patients usually presents with fever, abdominal pain, and palpable mass. Ultrasound demonstrates inflammatory mass in the adnexa. The ovarian vein can be seen as tubular distended structure containing echogenic clot. Right ovarian dermoid is also noted.

Essential Facts

- Annually, there are ~ 1 million cases of pelvic inflammatory diseases in the United States.
- Complications of pelvic inflammatory diseases and tubo-ovarian abscess include infertility, increased risk of ectopic pregnancy, and chronic pelvic pain.
- In chronic infection, fibrosis and adhesions will form, obscuring the margins of the adnexa.
- The patients could present with acute onset of pain.
- The typical sonographic appearance of a tubo-ovarian complex is an adnexal mass, with ill-defined margins. The ovaries are not well separated from the mass.
- A tubo-ovarian abscess appears as a complex multiloculated complex mass with internal echoes.
- Ultrasound-guided transvaginal aspiration with antibiotics treatment is effective and safe for management of tubo-ovarian abscess.

✓ Pearls & × Pitfalls

✓ The appearance of benign and malignant adnexal masses could overlap on ultrasound; clinical correlation is important in narrowing the differential diagnosis.

× Ovarian vein thrombosis presenting with pelvic pain and fever could be misinterpreted as pelvic inflammatory disease with subsequent delay in the diagnosis.

Case 48

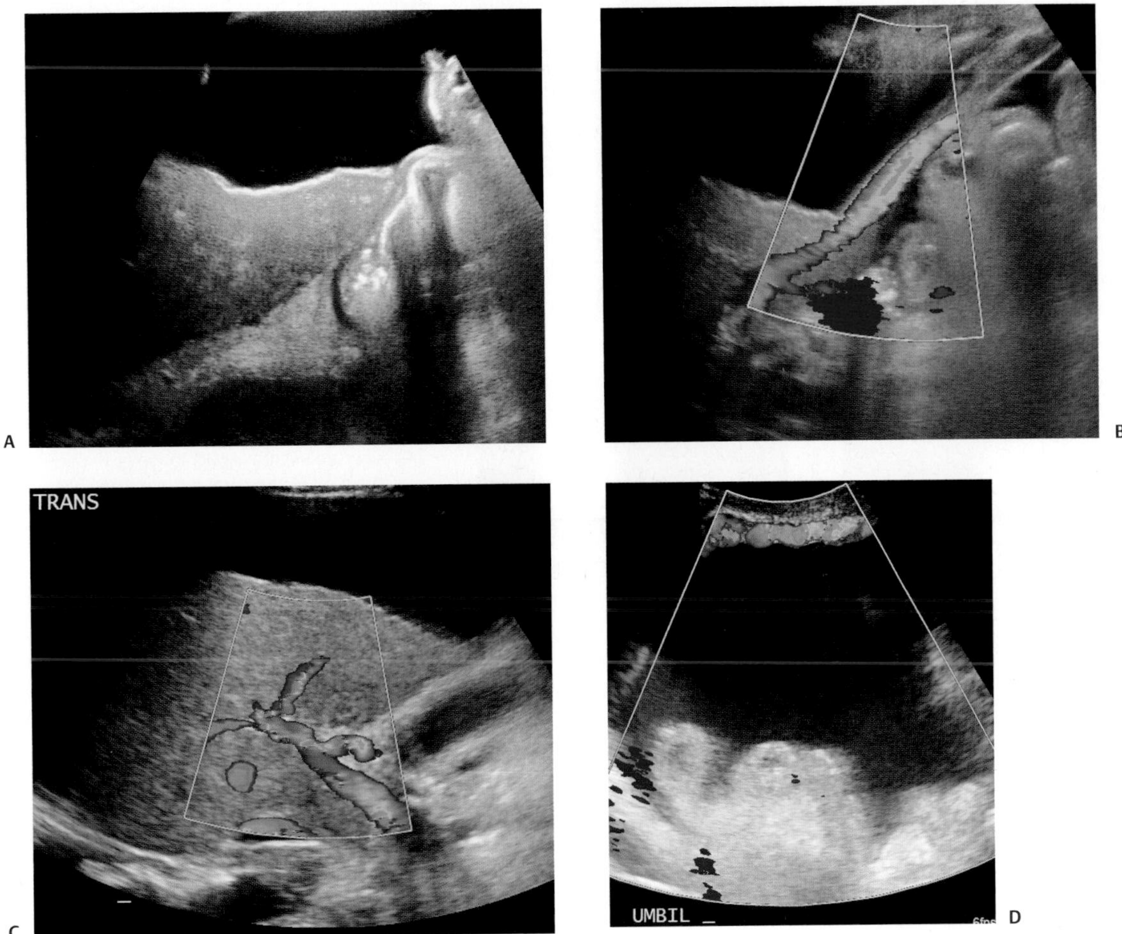

Clinical Presentation

A 53-year-old woman presents with increasing abdominal girth.

Imaging Findings

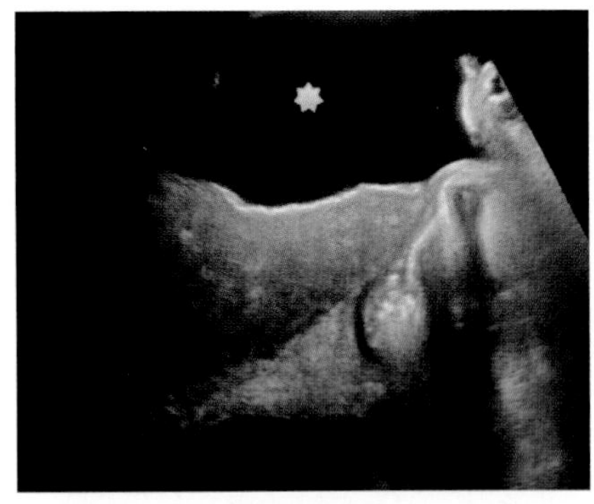

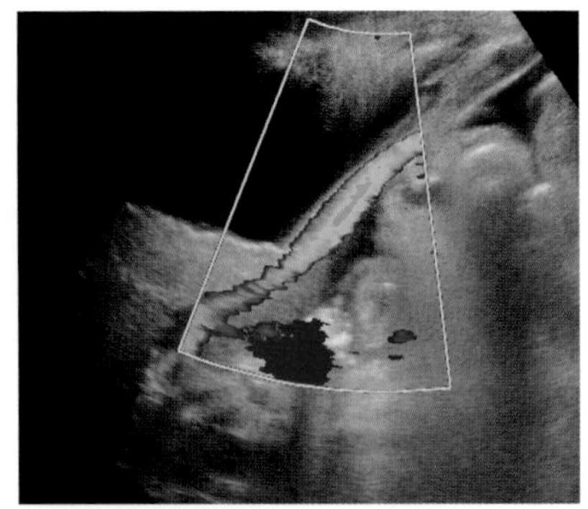

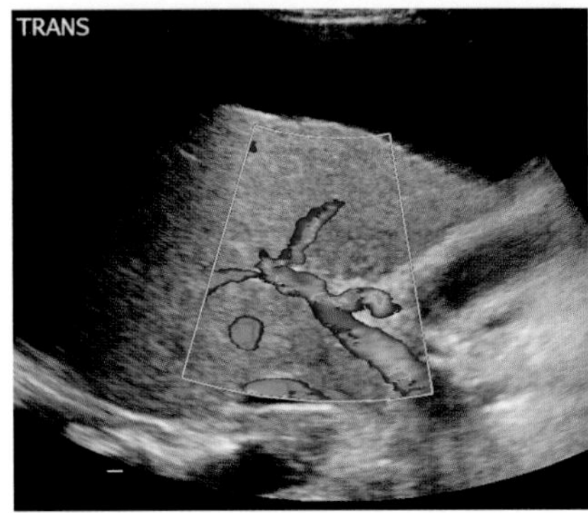

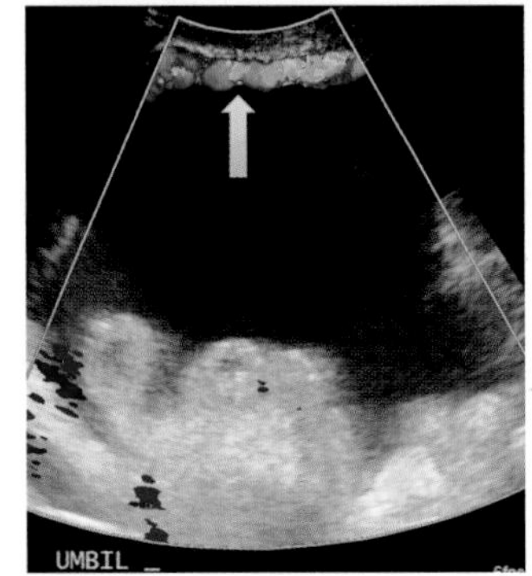

(A) Longitudinal gray scale image of the right upper quadrant demonstrates a shrunken liver with a very nodular anterior surface. Note the large amount of ascites (*asterisk*). **(B)** A large vessel is extending from the left lobe of the liver anteriorly. The direction of flow is away from the liver (red) or hepatofugal toward the anterior abdominal wall. **(C)** The main portal vein is patent with hepatopedal flow. **(D)** Color Doppler ultrasound reveals tortuous vessels along the anterior abdominal wall (*arrow*).

Differential Diagnosis

- ***Cirrhosis with a patent paraumbilical vein (PUV):*** A vessel extending anteriorly from the left lobe of a cirrhotic liver is consistent with a patent paraumbilical vein.
- *Cirrhosis with hepatofugal flow in the main portal vein:* This structure could be confused for the main portal vein (MPV) with hepatofugal flow. However, the MPV is identified separate from it.
- *Cirrhosis with a transjugular intrahepatic portosystemic shunt (TIPS):* TIPS are between a branch of the portal vein and a hepatic vein. They are located within the parenchyma of the liver.

Essential Facts

- A patent PUV is a spontaneous intrahepatic portosystemic shunt that occurs in the setting of portal hypertension usually due to cirrhosis. It results from recanalization of the left PUV.
- A patent PUV courses in the falciform ligament and forms collaterals with the superficial veins of the anterior abdominal wall called *caput medusa*.
- Blood travels from the left portal vein to the PUV bypassing the liver parenchyma. The larger the PUV and resultant shunt volume, the greater the risk for hepatic encephalopathy.
- Most extrahepatic portosystemic shunts due to portal hypertension are via the coronary vein, esophageal varices, or retroperitoneal collaterals.
- Congenital extrahepatic portosystemic shunts occur between the portomesenteric and systemic veins, bypassing the liver through a complete or partial shunt. They may be diagnosed in infancy and associated with other congenital anomalies including congenital heart defects.
- Abernethy malformation (sometime incorrectly spelled "Abernathy" with two a's instead of two e's) is an eponym for congenital extrahepatic portosystemic shunts but is often used to describe any portosystemic shunt.

✓ Pearls & × Pitfalls

✓ The presence of a PUV indicates portal hypertension.
× PUVs are frequently missed by US. Due to their anterior location, they are often overlooked.
✓ Flow in a PUV is away from the liver (hepatofugal).
✓ The presence of ascites increases the chances of identifying a PUV.
× Esophageal and gastric varices are difficult to visualize with US but clearly imaged with computed tomography.
× Treated liver mets can cause a nodular surface of the liver mimicking cirrhosis.

Case 49

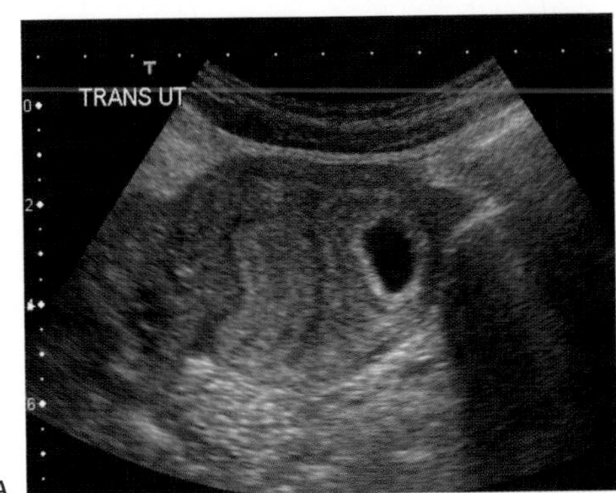

A

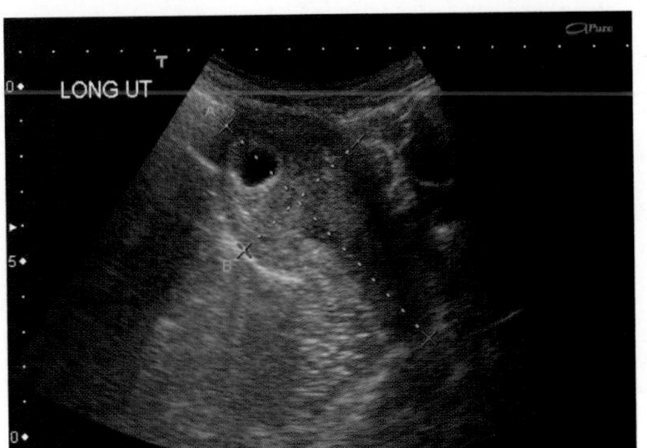

B

Clinical Presentation

A 21-year-old woman with positive pregnancy test presents for fetal age evaluation.

Further Work-up

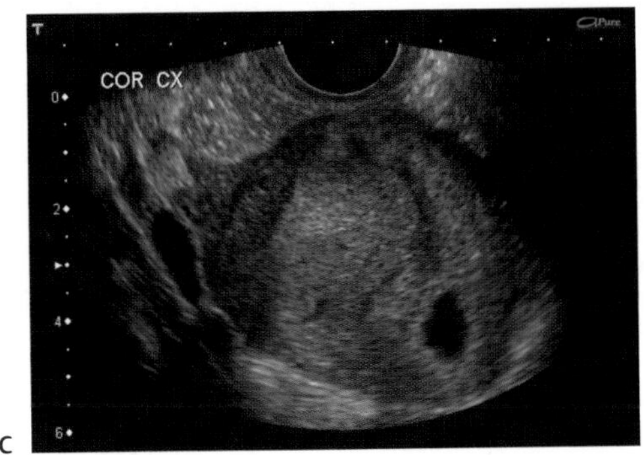

C

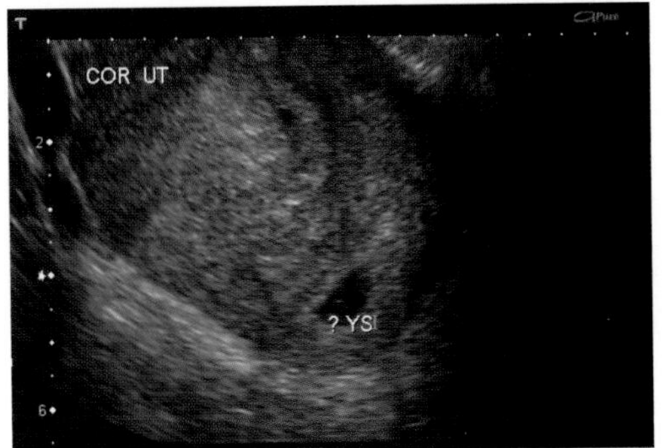

D

Imaging Findings

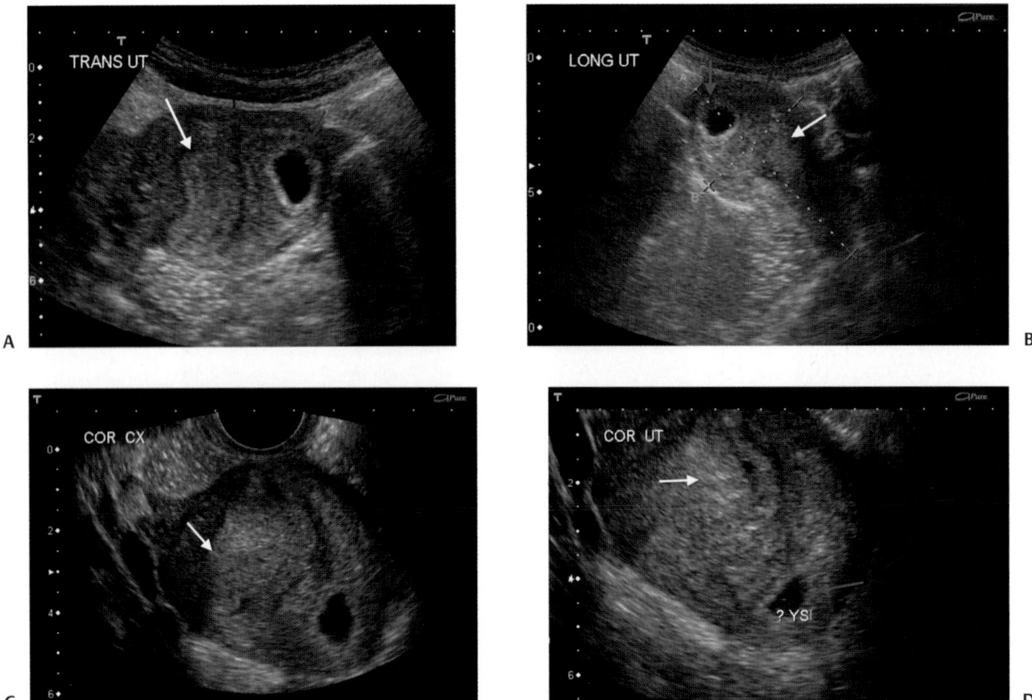

(A, B) Transabdominal ultrasound (US) images of the pelvis demonstrate intrauterine gestational sac (*red arrow*). A separate endometrium (*white arrow*) is noted. The two endometria are separated with thin hypoechoic line of tissue (*blue arrow*). **(C, D)** Transvaginal evaluation demonstrates similar findings of intrauterine gestational sac with yolk sac (*red arrow*). An additional endometrium with trace amount of endometrial fluid (*white arrow*) is also noted. The two endometria appear to be separated with a thin hypoechoic line (*blue arrow*). The fundus appears to be normal in contour.

Differential Diagnosis

- ***An intrauterine pregnancy in a septated uterus:*** The typical sonographic appearance includes the presence of two separate endometria and one cervix. The two endometria are separated by thin fibrotic tissue. The two endometria are close, with < 90-degree angle. The uterine fundus is normal in contour.
- *An intrauterine pregnancy in a bicornuate uterus:* An indentation on the uterine fundus is noted on transabdominal and transvaginal ultrasounds of the uterus. The two endometria are separated by a thick hypoechoic line of tissue. The angle between the two endometria exceeds 90 degrees. Only one cervix is visualized on the transvaginal evaluation.
- *An intrauterine pregnancy within a didelphys uterus:* Sonographic appearance usually resembles bicornuate uterus; however, duplication of the cervix is noted on transvaginal ultrasound as well as physical examination.

Essential Facts

- The uterus has a normal outline
- The two endometrial cavities are closer together.
- The two endometria are separated by thin fibrous septa.
- The septum has poor blood supply on Doppler.
- The septa could be partial or complete.
- Three-dimensional (3-D) US and hysterosalpingography provide accurate diagnosis.
- Septated uterus is treated by hysteroscopic incision of the fibrous septum.
- Increased incidence of urinary system anomalies.
- Early miscarriage is common within the septated uterus, likely secondary to poor blood flow in the septum.
- Late miscarriage likely related to space restriction.
- Higher incidence of other pregnancy-related complications.
- A full-term pregnancy in septated uterus is estimated at 10%.

✓ Pearls & × Pitfalls

✓ 3-D ultrasound images of the pelvis are helpful in accurately characterizing uterine anomalies.

× The sonographic appearance of partial septated uterus and arcuate uterus could overlap; adding volume sonography and hysterosalpingography would improve the diagnostic accuracy.

Case 50

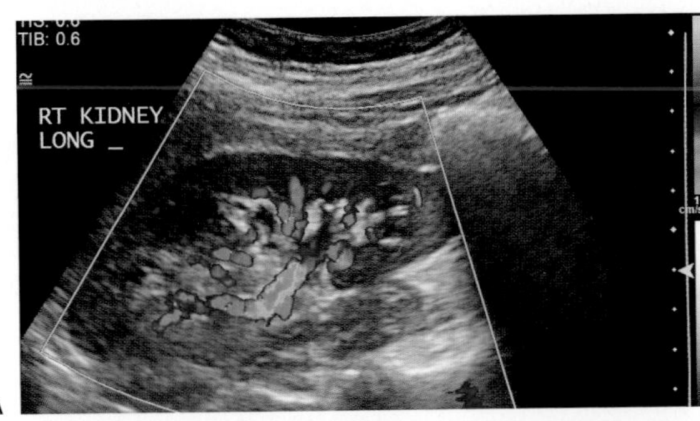

A

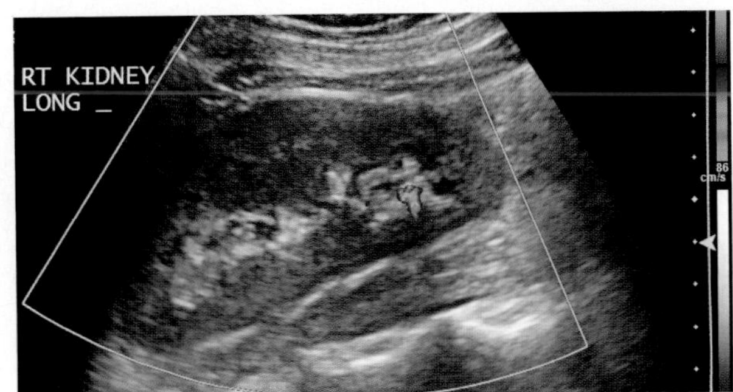

B

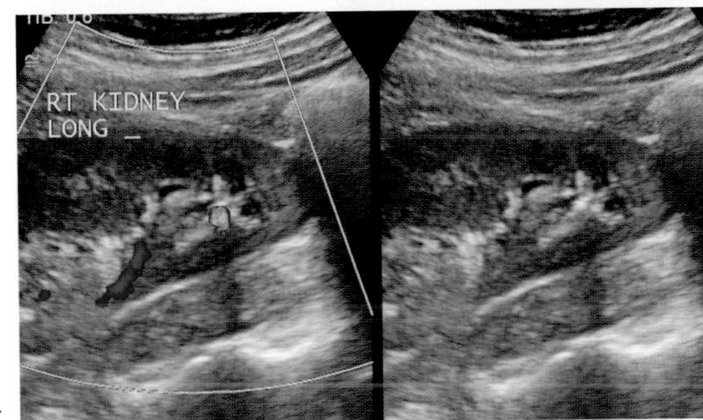

C

■ Clinical Presentation

A 30-year-old patient with right flank pain and hematuria.

■ Further Work-up

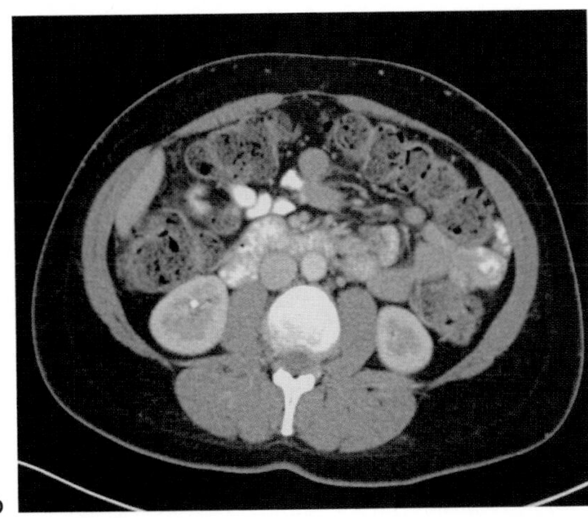

D

Imaging Findings

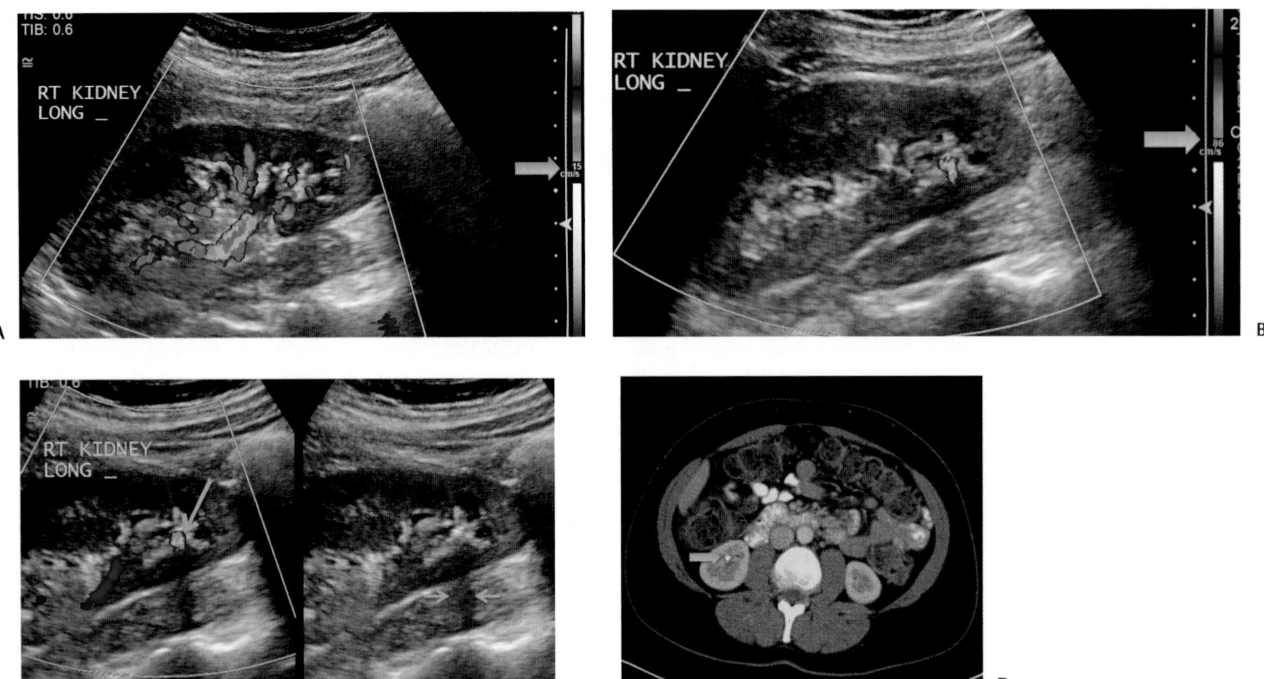

(A) Color Doppler longitudinal image of the right kidney demonstrates abundant hilar and intrarenal vessels. Note the color settings (scale 15 cm/sec) (*arrow*). **(B)** With color settings (*arrow*) for very fast flow (PRF 86 cm/sec), the normal intrarenal vessels no longer fill in with color. Note the focal color aliasing in a lower pole calyx. **(C)** A split-screen image with color on the left and gray scale on the right in longitudinal planes. An echogenic focus is present in a lower pole calyx in the area of color aliasing (*arrow*). Questionable shadowing is present (*arrows*). Twinkling occurs within only one of the many echogenic foci seen centrally in the kidney. **(D)** Post contrast CT of the abdomen reveals a 4 mm nonobstructing stone (*arrow*) in the lower pole of the right kidney.

Differential Diagnosis

- ***Nonobstructing stone in a lower pole calyx with twinkle artifact:*** An echogenic focus that causes color aliasing with a fast-flow velocity color scale is consistent with a stone. The stone is too small to cause obvious shadowing.
- *Small pseudoaneurysm or arteriovenous fistula (AVF) status post biopsy:* High flow is present in an AVF or pseudo aneurysm (PSA). However, these vascular structures would be anechoic on the gray scale images.
- *Small vascular renal mass:* It would be difficult to detect flow in a lesion of this size. Detecting flow in a lesion requires a much slower color scale or power Doppler.

Essential Facts

- Twinkling or the twinkle artifact was first described in 1996. It is an artifact that occurs with color Doppler ultrasound and improves detection of genitourinary calculi.
- Because small renal stones may not cause shadowing with ultrasound, the twinkle artifact is particularly helpful in this setting.
- The twinkling artifact appears as a rapidly alternating color Doppler signal that imitates turbulent flow. It occurs at or beyond the stone.
- The twinkle artifact becomes evident with color scales set for fast-flow velocities (high pulse repetition frequency, i.e., > 60 cm/sec). Increased PRF has the added benefit of reducing the detectable color flow seen normally in the kidney.
- Twinkle artifact occurs with noncalcified biliary calculi and any material with an irregular, rough, or reflective surface.
- Newer generation ultrasound machines using digital processing technology perceive the twinkle artifact more frequently than older generation scanners, which used analogue technology.
- The artifact is likely due to a form of intrinsic noise known as phase (or clock) jitter within the Doppler circuitry of the ultrasound machine.

✓ Pearls & ✗ Pitfalls

✓ The twinkle artifact has a high positive predictive value (PPV) for detecting renal and urinary tract calculi.

✗ The twinkle artifact is evident only with appropriate color scale.

✗ The twinkle artifact can be seen with parenchymal calcifications, mimicking renal stones.

✓ A spectral Doppler tracing placed on a twinkle artifact reveals noise. No arterial or venous tracing will be evident.

✗ Computed tomography remains the gold standard for detection of renal calculi.

Case 51

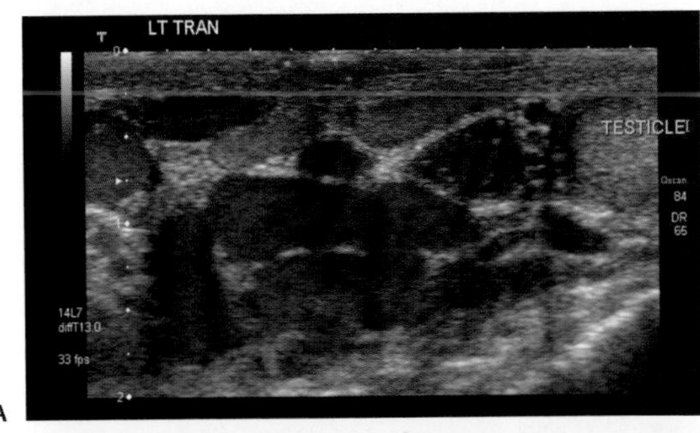

A

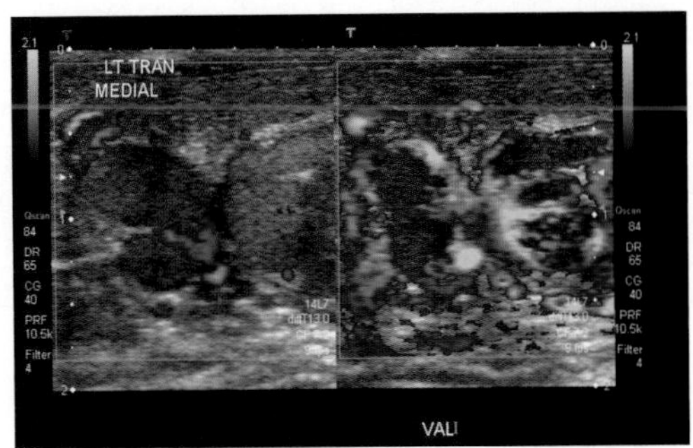

B

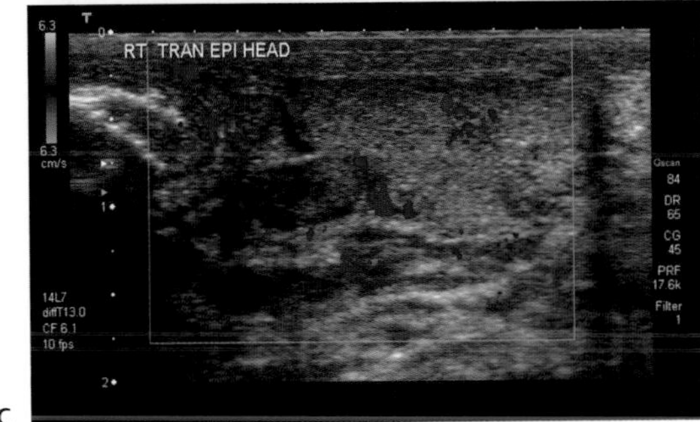

C

■ Clinical Presentation

An 86-year-old man presents with newly diagnosed left-sided palpable scrotal lesion.

■ Further Work-up

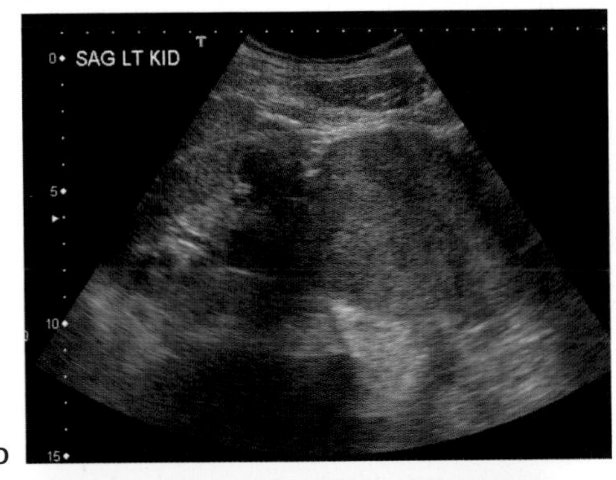

D

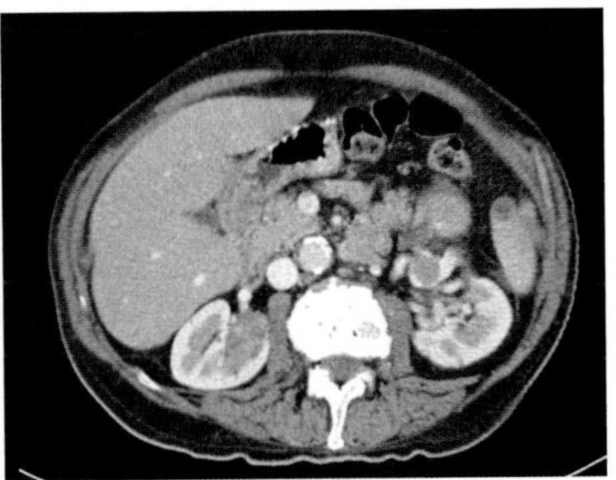
E

F

Imaging Findings

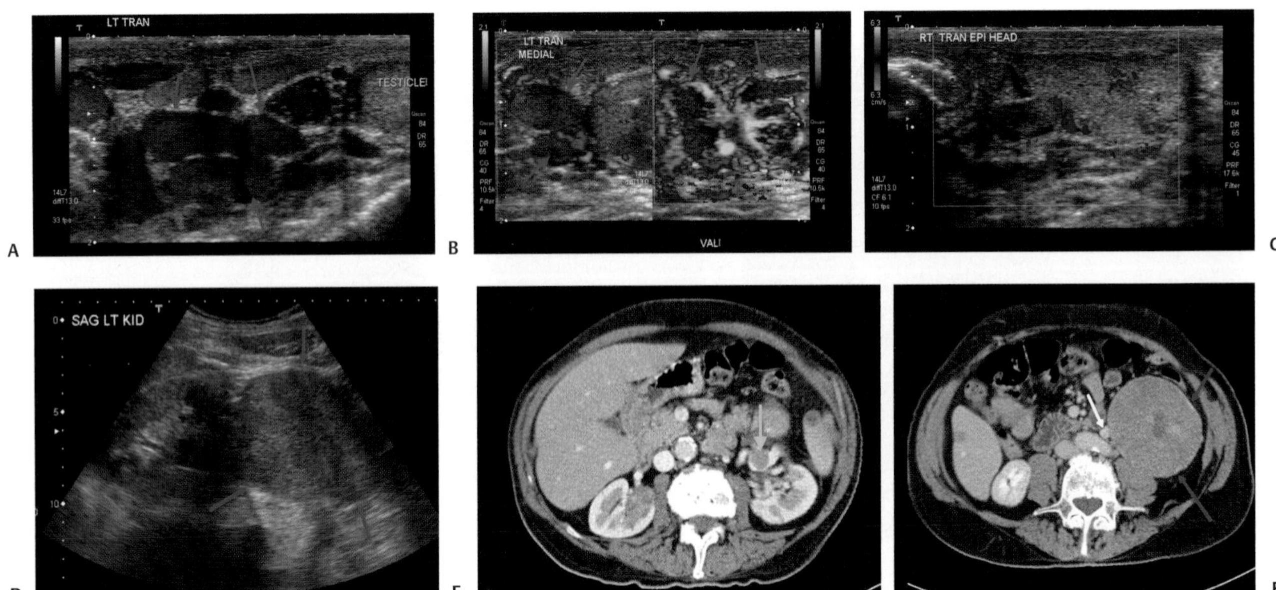

(A–C) Ultrasound (US) images of the right and left scrotum demonstrate a predominant cluster of dilated tubular structures with low-level echoes in the region of the left scrotum (*blue arrows*). This appears to be extratesticular in location. The tubular structures demonstrate flow on Doppler imaging. There was no significant change in size of the presumed dilated vessels with Valsalva maneuver. The right testicle appears normal. **(D–F)** Further US images of the left retroperitoneum demonstrate large retroperitoneal mass (*red arrows*), likely originating from the lower pole of the left kidney. Vascular flow within the mass is also present. The finding on US was confirmed with computed tomography (CT) of the abdomen. Dilatation of the gonadal vein on the left is noted on CT (*white arrow*). Filling defect in the renal vein is also noted (*yellow arrow*).

Differential Diagnosis

- ***Secondary varicoceles:*** Usually related to increased pressure in the spermatic vein. A search for neoplastic obstruction of the gonadal venous system must be undertaken in cases of right-sided noncompressible or newly diagnosed varicocele in patients older than 40 years old.
- *Primary varicoceles:* Usually related to incompetent valves in the internal spermatic vein. It is a common cause of male infertility, usually located on the left side and detected before age 25. It is bilateral in 70% of cases. The size of primary varicoceles usually changes with Valsalva maneuver.
- *Complex hydrocele:* Could be secondary to hematocele or pyocele. It appears sonographically as a complex collection with low-level echoes, loculation, and septations. The scrotal wall usually is thickened and might be hyperemic.

Essential Facts

- The clinical presentation includes scrotal pain, heaviness, and scrotal mass.
- Usually related to increased pressure in the spermatic vein, secondary to hydronephrosis, enlarged liver, and abdominal and/or retroperitoneal mass. Venous thrombosis in the gonadal vein or inferior vena cava (IVC) is a rare etiology.
- It is also visualized in nutcracker syndrome, compression of the left renal vein by the superior mesenteric artery.
- Usually occurs in patients older than 40 years.
- The presence of unilateral varicocele on the right side requires further assessment of the retroperitoneum to exclude obstructive process.
- The typical sonographic appearance is multiple serpentine anechoic structures > 2 mm in diameter, creating the appearance of tortuous multicystic collection.
- The veins follow the course of the spermatic cord into the inguinal canal.
- Varicoceles also could be intratesticular.
- Secondary varicoceles demonstrate no change in size during Valsalva maneuver.

✓ Pearls & × Pitfalls

✓ The presence of right-sided varicocele and/or recently diagnosed varicoceles in patients over 40 requires further assessment to exclude retroperitoneal pathology.

× Occasionally, varicoceles could be misinterpreted as complex septated hydrocele. The presence of Doppler flow, as well as visualization of the varicoceles along the spermatic cord, improves the sonographic accuracy.

Case 52

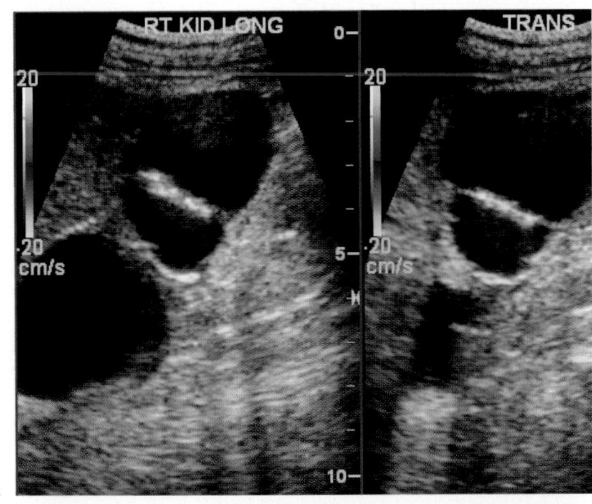

A

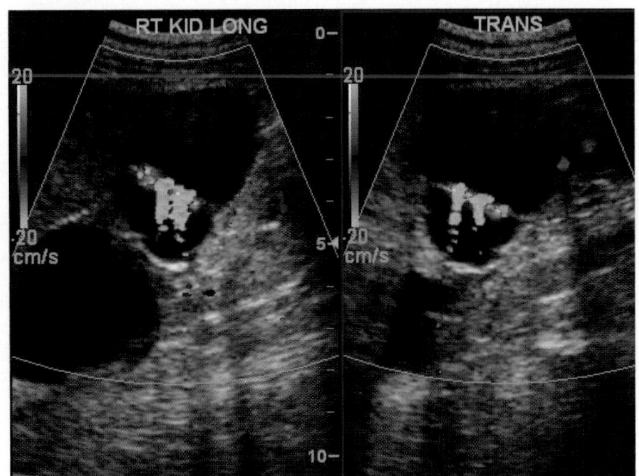

B

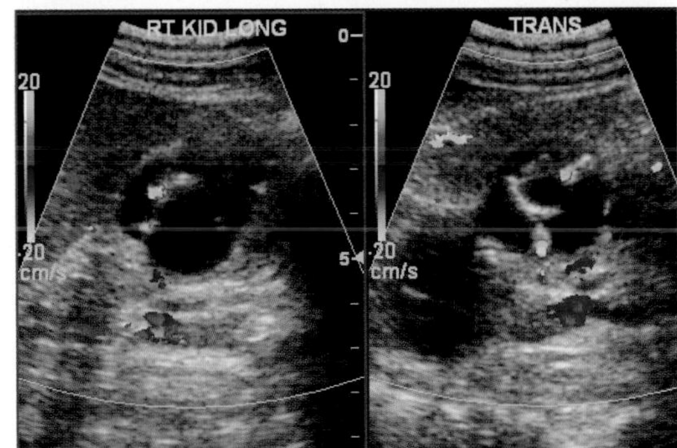

C

Clinical Presentation

A 60-year-old woman with hematuria. Images of the right kidney.

Further Work-up

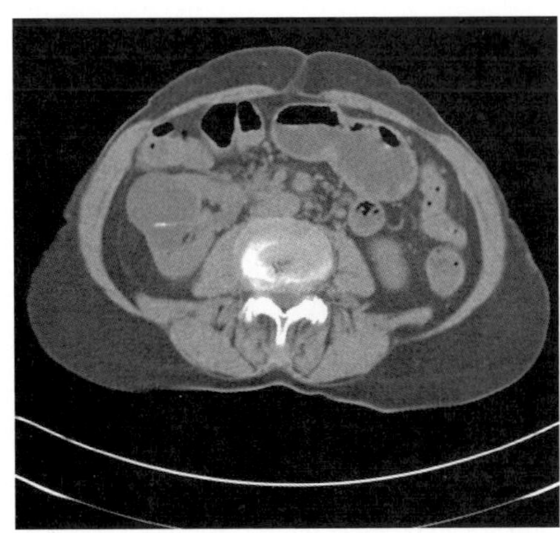
D

Imaging Findings

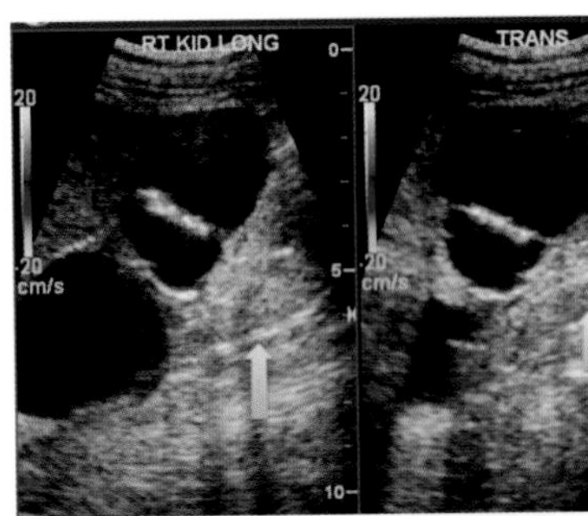

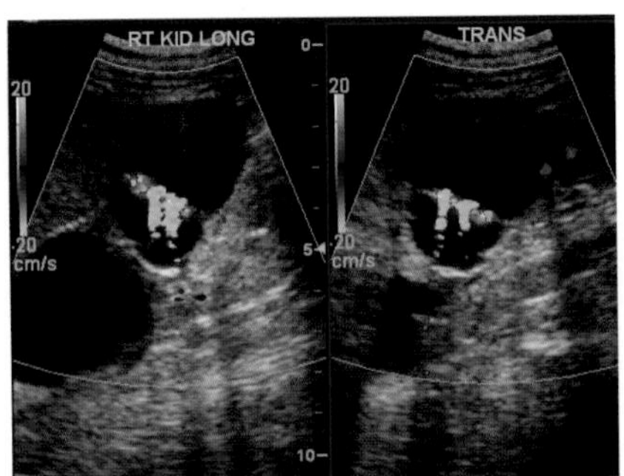

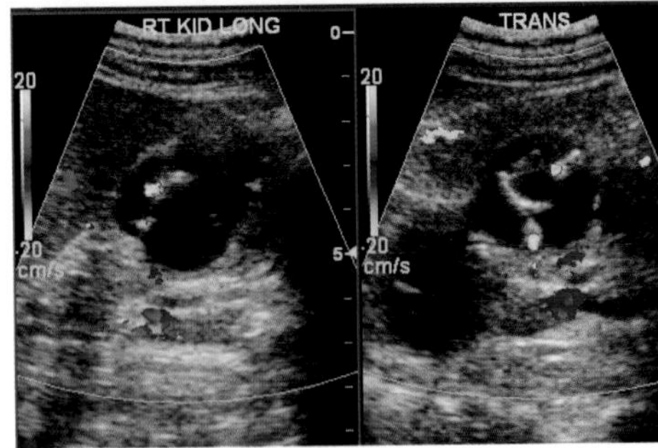

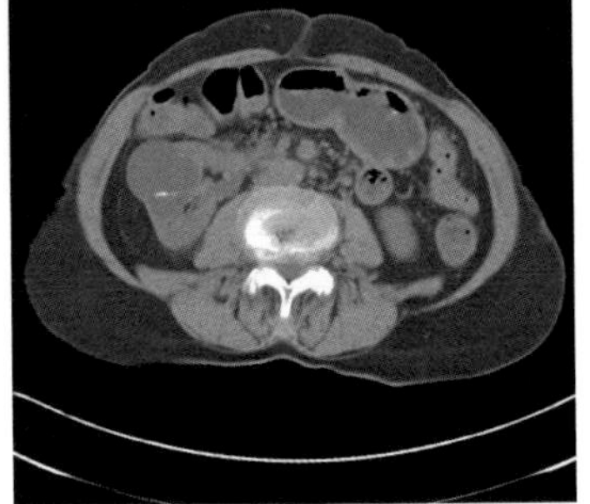

(A) Longitudinal and transverse images of the right kidney are focused on a cystic lesion in the anterior interpolar region. Renal cortex is seen posteriorly (*arrows*). The cyst contains an echogenic septation. **(B)** Longitudinal and transverse images of the lesion demonstrate color aliasing on and well beyond the septations. **(C)** Longitudinal and transverse images through a different plane of the lesion. Additional septations are seen. **(D)** Noncontrast computed tomography (CT) reveals a calcified septations within a right renal cyst.

Differential Diagnosis

- ***Calcified right renal cyst:*** A cyst with very echogenic septations that demonstrate twinkle artifact is consistent with calcified septations in a renal cyst. CT confirmed the presence of calcification. This is probably a Bosniak IIF lesion.
- *Multilocular cystic nephroma:* Would have multiple loculations, peripheral and curvilinear calcifications, and irregular borders. The classic feature of this lesion is extension into the central sinus and renal pelvis.
- *Cystic neoplasm with flow in septations:* Flow within septations would not extend beyond the septations, as is seen with the twinkle artifact in this case.

Essential Facts

- Simple renal cysts are commonly observed in normal kidneys, with an increasing incidence with age, typically after age 20 to 30.
- Renal cysts can be complex. Occasionally, renal neoplasms are cystic or have a cystic component or necrosis.
- Cysts may manifest complex features as a result of hemorrhage, infection, or inflammation.
- Bosniak classification for renal cysts was devised in 1986 for CT evaluation but is frequently used in ultrasound (US) and magnetic resonance imaging.
  - Class I: Malignant risk < 1%; no follow-up required
    - Simple cysts: anechoic, imperceptible walls, rounded
  - Class II: Malignant risk < 3%, no follow-up required
    - Minimally complex, may contain thin septations (< 1 mm), thin calcifications, or internal echoes. Hyperdense on CT. Less than 3 cm in size.
  - Class IIF: Malignant risk 5 to 10%; follow-up recommended
    - Increased number of septa, minimally thickened septa or wall. Thick calcification. Intrarenal, > 3 cm. No contrast enhancement.
  - Class III: Malignant risk 40 to 60%; surgical excision recommended
  - Thick or multiple septations, mural nodule. Enhances or demonstrates internal vascularity with US.
  - Class IV: Malignant risk > 80%; surgical excision recommended.
    - Solid mass with cystic or necrotic component. Enhances or demonstrates internal vascularity with US.

✓ Pearls & × Pitfalls

✓ Category IIF identifies lesions that are more complicated but not necessarily suspicious enough to warrant surgical exploration.

✓ US is more sensitive than CT in determining minimal complexity of a cyst.

✓ High-density cysts seen on CT can appear anechoic on US.

✓ The natural history of renal cysts is to increase in size over time.

× Further evaluation with CT or magnetic resonance imaging is often performed for renal lesions detected with US.

✓ Benign lesions tend to be more exophytic. Malignant lesions tend to be more endophytic.

✓ Nodular and septal enhancement is the most sensitive finding to discriminate cystic renal cell carcinoma (RCC) from complex benign lesions.

Case 53

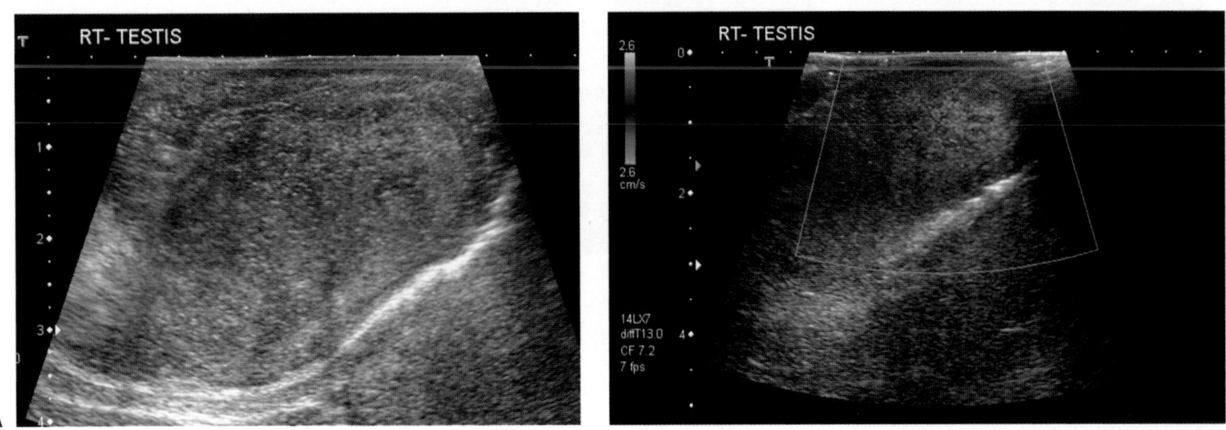

Clinical Presentation

A 61-year-old man, known case of Fournier gangrene that was treated with debridement, presents with right-sided testicular pain.

Further Work-up

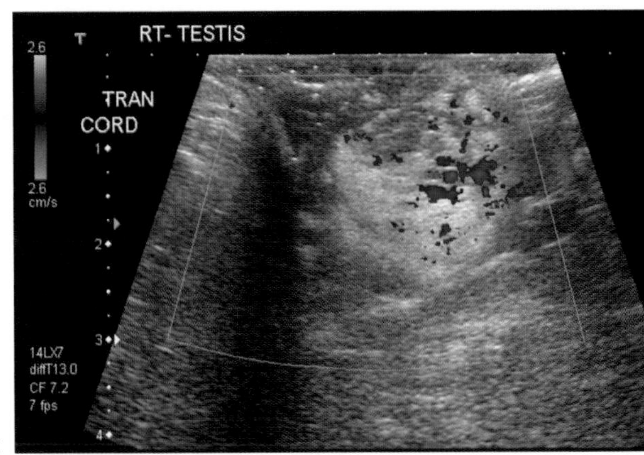

Imaging Findings

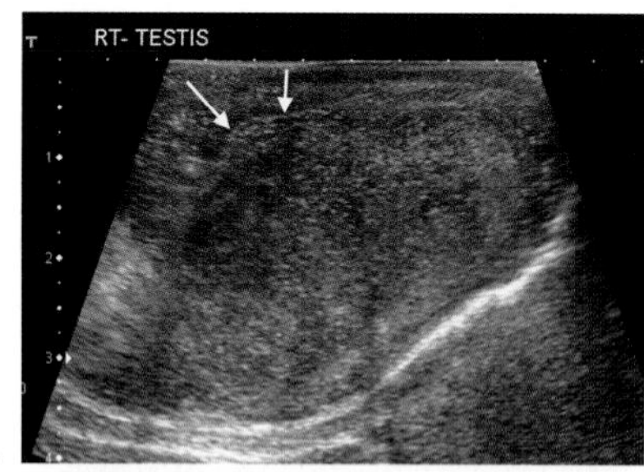

A

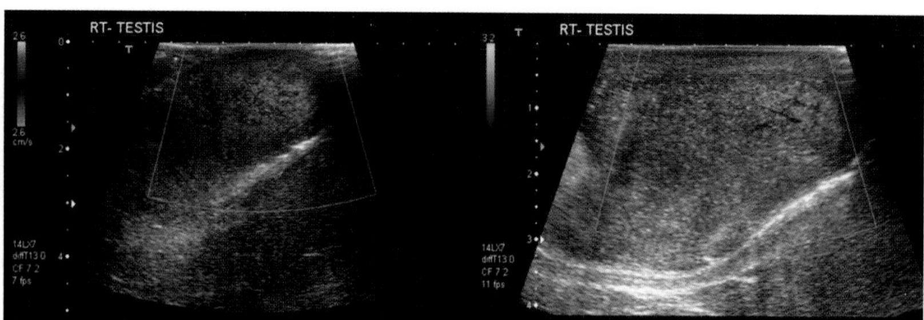

B

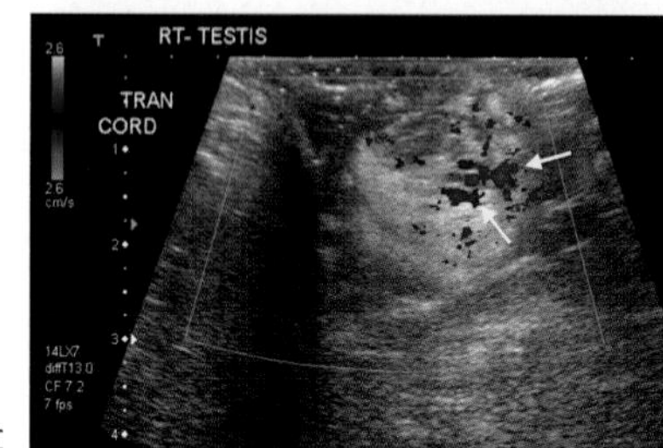

C

(A) Ultrasound (US) images show a diffusely heterogeneous testicle. The superior pole is more hypoechoic and ill defined (*white arrows*). **(B)** No flow is identified within the testicle on color or power images. **(C)** Flow is present along the course of the spermatic cord confirmed on color Doppler (*white arrows*).

Differential Diagnosis

- ***Testicular torsion:*** Patients present with acute onset of pain. US finding in testicular torsion varies depending on the length of time since the onset of symptoms. Gray scale US examination may be normal, especially early after onset; however, it may also demonstrate inhomogeneous echotexture with areas of hypoechogenicity and disruption of the architecture. On color Doppler, there is unilateral absent or decrease in flow.
- *Severe epididymitis/orchitis:* The patients present with more prolonged pain and occasionally fever. On gray scale images, swelling, edema, or occasionally small abscess is noted. In case of severe epididymitis/orchitis, testicular blood supply might be compromised. US demonstrates enlarged epididymis/testicles, significant thickening or effusion, decreased echogenicity with increased flow on color Doppler images; however, in severe cases, there will be decreased flow.
- *Testicular atrophy and infarction:* Combined axis measurements of the two sides differs by 10 mm or more and/or testicular size $< 4.0 \times 2.0$ cm. The atrophied testicle will demonstrate increased echogenicity secondary to fibrosis. If ischemia still exists, uniform hypoechogenicity will be observed (which is a marker for poor prognosis and outcome). Undescended atrophic testis will demonstrate hypoplastic vessels.

Essential Facts

- The most common causes of acute scrotal pain are testicular torsion and severe epididymitis or orchitis. Other causes are postinguinal hernia repair and posttrauma.
- Color Doppler is the most useful modality demonstrating decrease or no flow in the testicle.
- Tc 99m-pertechnetate scanning can help differentiate between torsion and inflammatory causes. Tc 99m scanning demonstrates decrease in testicular perfusion with torsion and increase with inflammatory causes.
- Ischemia, if not treated, may end up in testicular atrophy or infarction in which the size will decrease and echogenicity will increase because of fibrosis.

✓ Pearls & × Pitfalls

✓ Doppler and gray scale US of the scrotum represents the most common and useful imaging modality used to diagnose acute scrotum and scrotal ischemia.

× Color Doppler US may be falsely negative when there is incomplete torsion of the spermatic cord. In these situations, the systolic value is still recorded while the diastolic one is absent or reduced, and reactive hyperemia of the tunica vaginalis is wrongly interpreted as blood flow into the capsular arteries.

Case 54

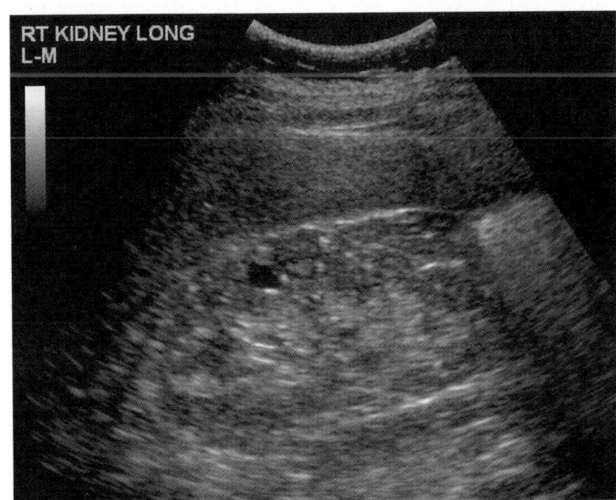

A

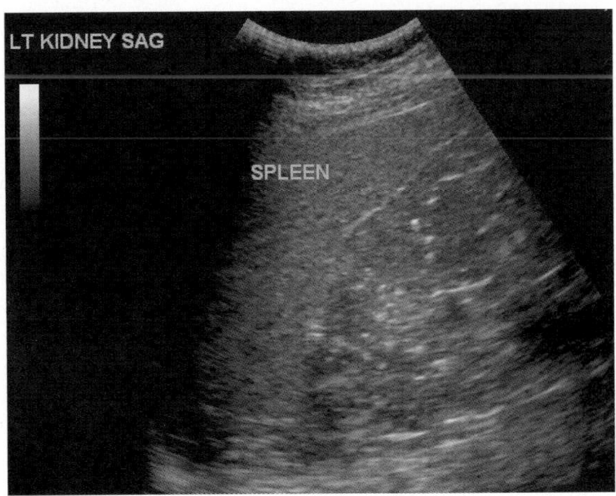

B

■ Clinical Presentation

A 60-year-old woman with long-standing bipolar disorder treated with lithium presents with elevated blood urea nitrogen and creatinine.

■ Further Work-up

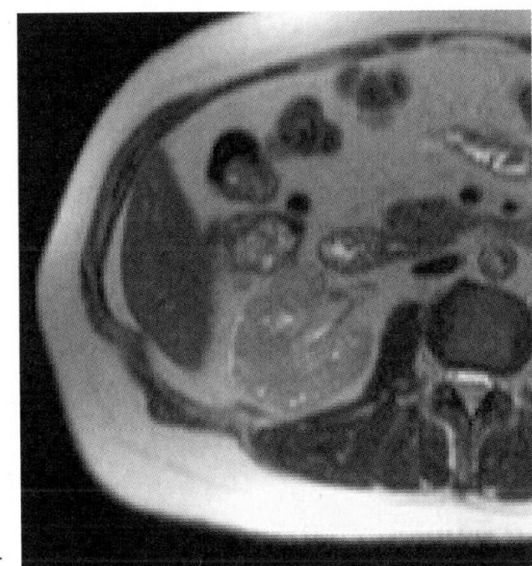

C

Imaging Findings

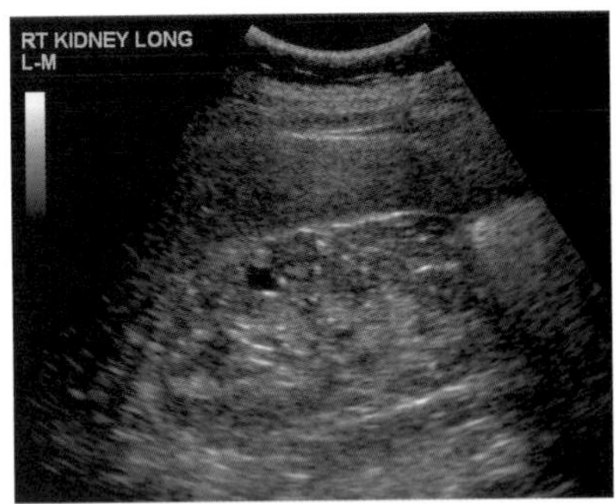

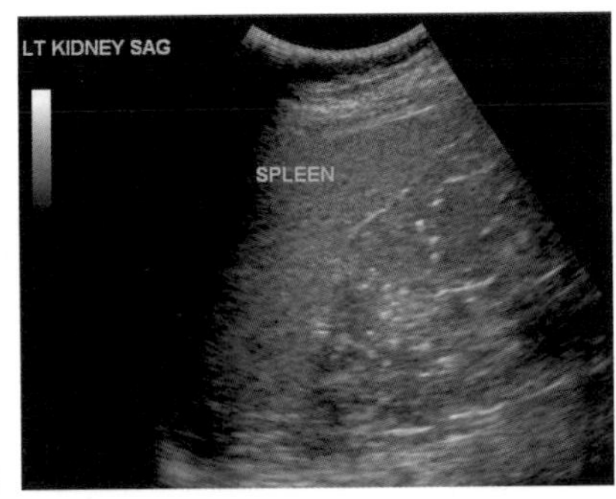

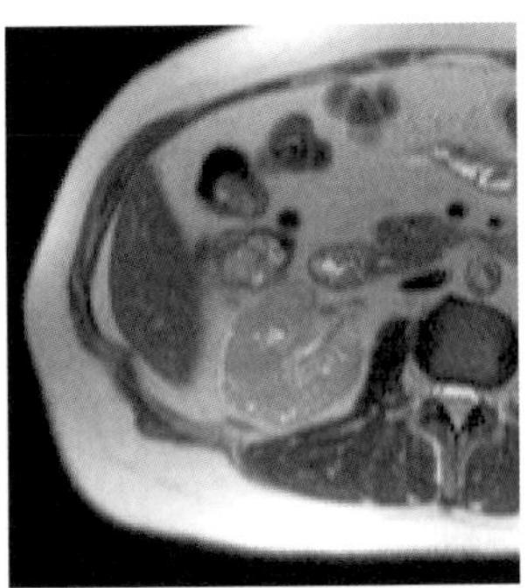

(A, B) Longitudinal gray scale images of both kidneys reveal innumerable echogenic foci scattered throughout the cortex and medullary portions of the kidneys. A 1 cm cyst is present in the upper pole of the right kidney in **(A)**. Note that the spleen is normal without echogenic foci. **(C)** Magnified T2-weighted transverse image of the right kidney demonstrates tiny hyperintense foci throughout the kidney.

Differential Diagnosis

- ***Lithium-induced microcysts:*** Numerous tiny echogenic foci in the kidneys that are T2 hyperintense on MRI correspond to microcysts and represent lithium-induced microcysts.
- *Extrapulmonary* Pneumocystis carinii *infection:* Aerosolized pentamidine use can result in systemic *P. carinii* infection with innumerable calcifications in the kidneys. Similar findings would be present in the liver and spleen.
- *Acquired cystic kidney disease:* Cysts would be larger and vary in size.

Essential Facts

- Lithium-associated microcysts are tiny (1 to 2 mm) cysts that appear echogenic on ultrasound. They occur in 30 to 60% of patients on chronic lithium therapy.
- These microcysts are abundantly and symmetrically distributed in both the cortex and the medulla of normal-sized kidneys.
- The findings of lithium-induced microcysts persist following cessation of treatment.
- When this finding is seen in the kidneys, a history of lithium use should be sought as a cause of nephropathy.

✓ Pearls & × Pitfalls

× The US appearance of lithium-induced microcysts is very similar to tiny calcifications.

✓ Lithium-induced microcysts may be too small to visualize on computed tomography. They are best seen on US and MRI.

✓ Larger cysts (> 3 mm) can be seen in addition to microcysts in lithium nephropathy.

✓ Kidney size is usually normal in the setting of lithium nephropathy.

Case 55

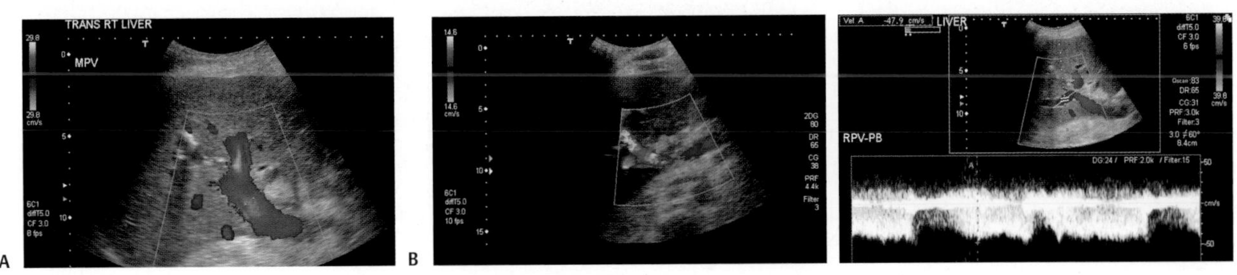

Clinical Presentation

A 65-year-old man 24 hours postliver transplant presents with abnormal liver function tests.

Further Work-up

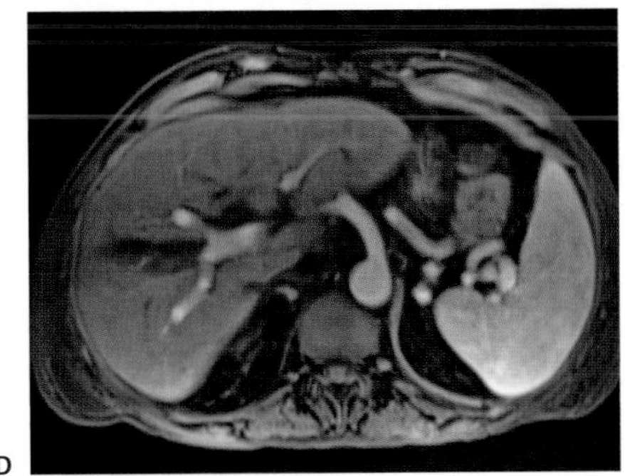

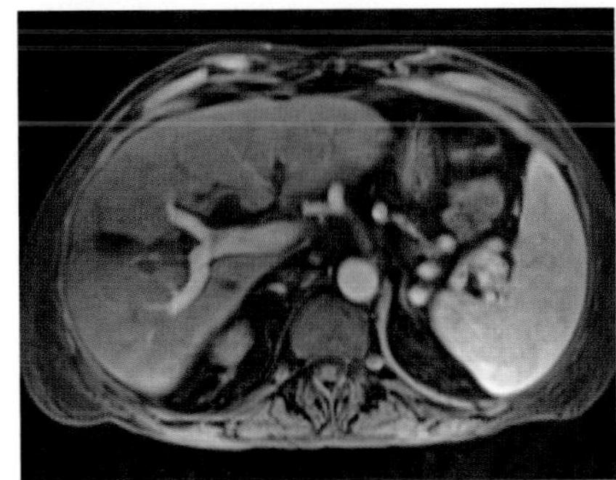

Imaging Findings

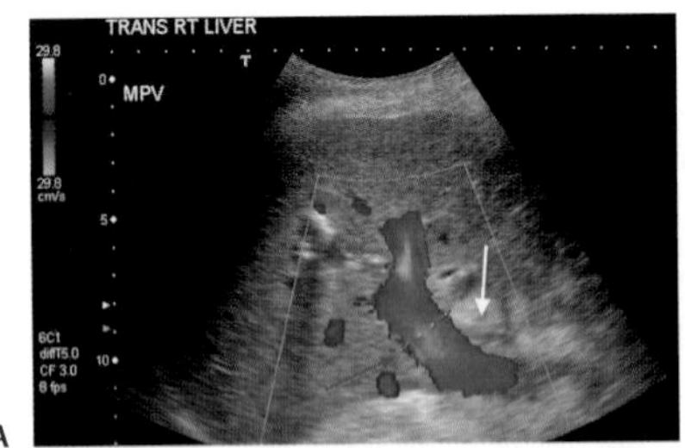

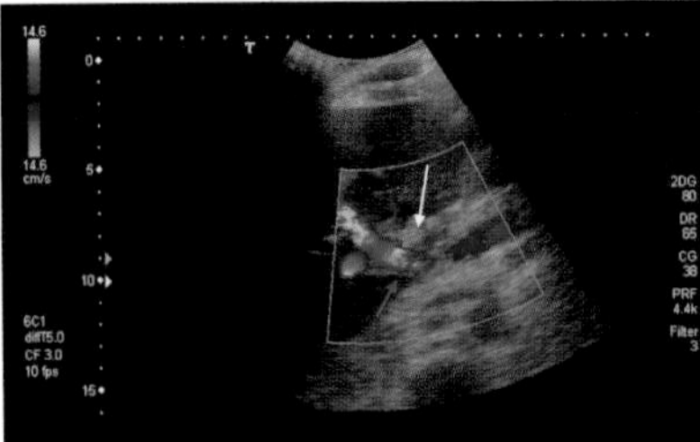
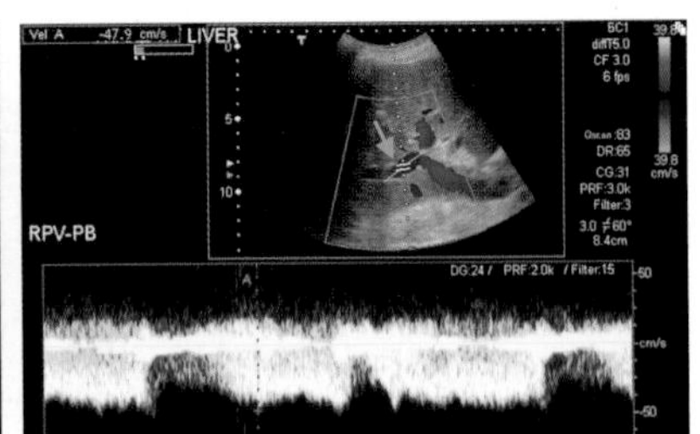

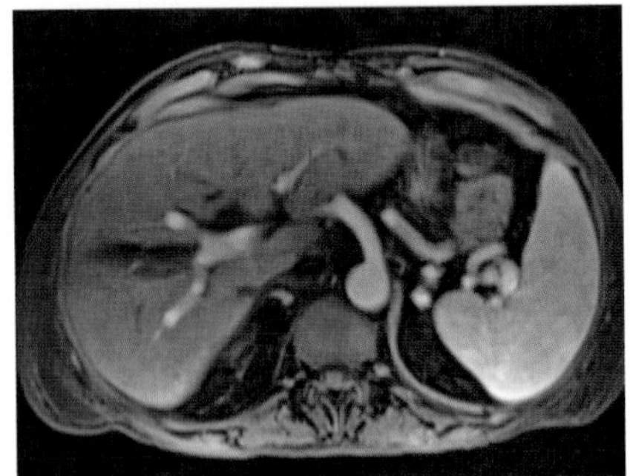
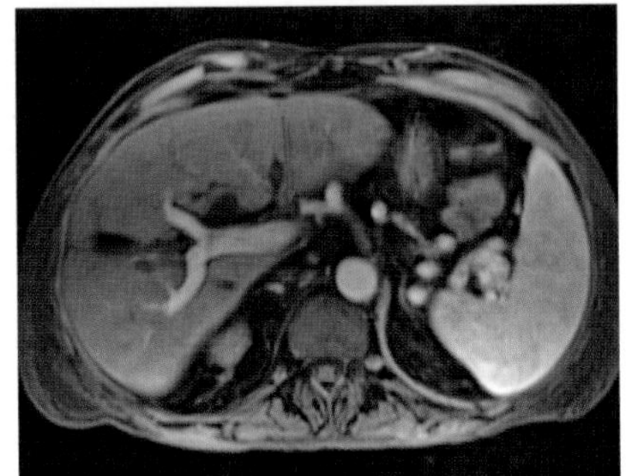

(A–C) Ultrasound of the liver with Doppler shows very good flow in the portal vein (*red arrow*). No definite evidence of arterial flow is noted in the excepted location of the hepatic artery (*white arrow*). The findings also confirmed with pulse Doppler tracing. **(D, E)** Magnetic resonance imaging of the liver with contrast shows sudden interruption of flow in the hepatic artery (*red arrow*). The celiac artery and portal veins are patent.

Differential Diagnosis

- ***Hepatic artery thrombosis:*** The single most common vascular complications in patients postliver transplant. The typical sonographic appearance is lack of visualization of the hepatic artery on Doppler ultrasound. An early and accurate diagnosis is critical in allograft survival.
- *Hepatic artery stenosis:* A common vascular complication posttransplant. Doppler ultrasound finding includes low resistance index (< 0.5), increased systolic velocity (> 200 cm/sec), and prolonged acceleration index (> 0.2 second).
- *Postsurgical hepatic artery spasm:* Usually occurs within the first 24 hours postliver transplant. Doppler ultrasound images demonstrate very high resistance flow within the hepatic artery, with occasional reversal of flow in diastole. The flow within the hepatic artery converts to a low-resistance flow after administration of vasodilators.

Essential Facts

- Hepatic artery thrombosis is the most common complication of liver transplant.
- The incidence is ~ 2 to 12% of cases.
- Risk factors include allograft rejection, type of anastomosis, and prolonged warm ischemic time.
- Doppler ultrasound is limited technically in the postoperative state, secondary to surgical dressing and or presence of free air.
- Lack of flow on Doppler ultrasound in the hepatic artery requires further assessment with computed tomography and or magnetic resonance angiography.
- Knowledge of the type of anastomosis is important, as complications usually originate at the anastomotic site.
- The biliary tree is only supplied by the hepatic artery; lack of flow could result in allograft loss.
- Early detection with revascularization helps in salvaging the transplant.

✓ Pearls & × Pitfalls

✓ The presence of intrahepatic arterial flow without documentation of main hepatic artery flow is not sufficient for the diagnosis of hepatic artery patency.

× Reduced flow within the hepatic artery secondary to spasm and/or secondary to low cardiac output could be misinterpreted as hepatic artery thrombosis.

Case 56

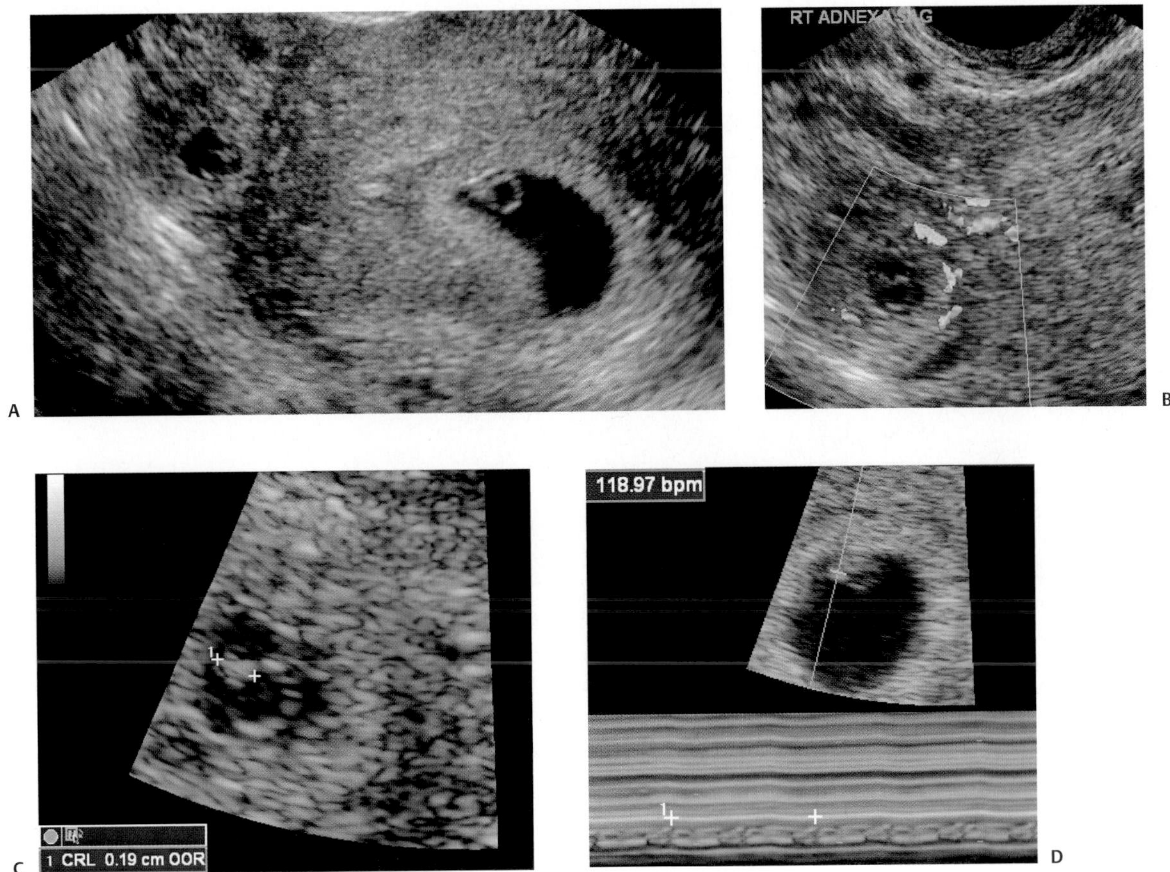

Clinical Presentation

A 39-year-old woman with right lower quadrant pain who is 6 weeks pregnant after fertility treatment.

Imaging Findings

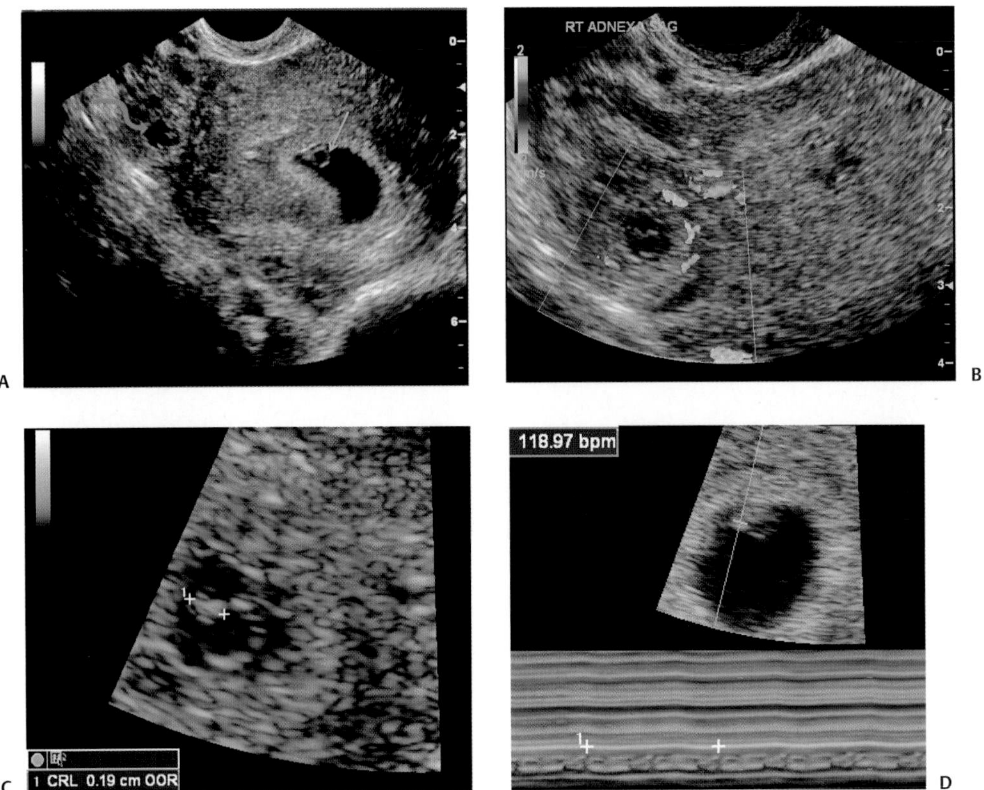

(A) Transvaginal scanning reveals an intrauterine gestation with a yolk sac and tiny embryo (*straight arrow*). A cystic structure is present in the right adnexa (*curved arrow*). **(B)** Higher resolution image of the right adnexa with color Doppler imaging demonstrates peripheral flow surrounding a cystic structure. **(C)** Even higher resolution image of the cystic region seen centrally in the right adnexa. **(D)** M mode tracing obtained within the right adnexa.

Differential Diagnosis

- ***Heterotopic twin pregnancy:*** An intrauterine pregnancy (IUP) and coexistent right adnexal ectopic pregnancy (EP) is consistent with a heterotopic twin pregnancy. Gestational sacs containing a yolk sac and embryo are present in the right adnexa and in the uterus.
- *Right adnexal EP with a pseudosac:* A pseudosac would not contain a yolk sac as is seen in the intrauterine sac above. The presence of a yolk sac distinguishes a gestational sac from a pseudosac.
- *IUP and a right corpus luteum:* Intense peripheral vascularity (ring of fire) is seen in both a corpus luteum and EP. A yolk sac would not be present in a corpus luteum. EPs are extraovarian; corpus lutea are intraovarian.

Essential Facts

- Heterotopic pregnancy is the simultaneous occurrence of two implantation sites. It is most often manifested as an IUP and EP.
- Heterotopic pregnancy (HP) is a rare entity that is usually seen in fertility patients.
- Incidence of HP is 1 in 7,000 fertility patients; it occurs spontaneously in 1 in 30,000 pregnancies.
- The incidence of HP has increased due to assisted reproduction and increased incidence of pelvic inflammatory disease.
- Risk factors for HP are the same as EP.
- Treatment of HP is usually surgical (laparoscopy). Nonsurgical management with ultrasound-guided injection of potassium chloride may be used in a nonviable and nonruptured EP.

✓ Pearls & × Pitfalls

× A small amount of free fluid in the pelvis can be a normal finding in pregnancy but can also indicate an EP.

✓ Hemoperitoneum is a very specific finding for ruptured EP.

× The gestational sac of an EP is often not identifiable by ultrasound. The more common ultrasound findings of an EP include an adnexal mass and complex free fluid (hemoperitoneum).

✓ The beta HCG is often misleading and falsely reassuring in the setting of HP. The beta HCG is often in the normal range due to the coexisting IUP.

Case 57

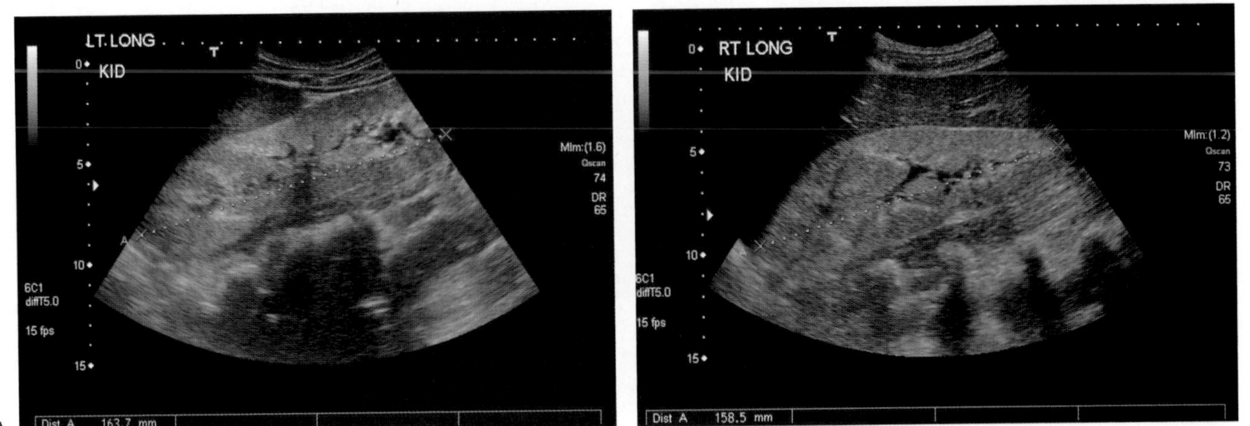

A B

Clinical Presentation

A 25-year-old man, human immunodeficiency virus (HIV) positive, presents with renal failure.

Further Work-up

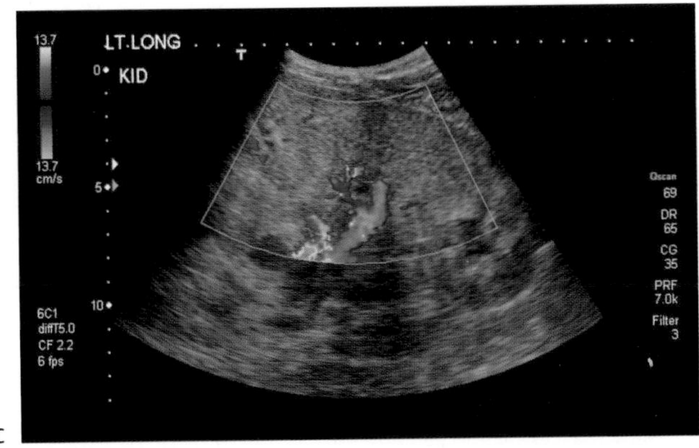

C

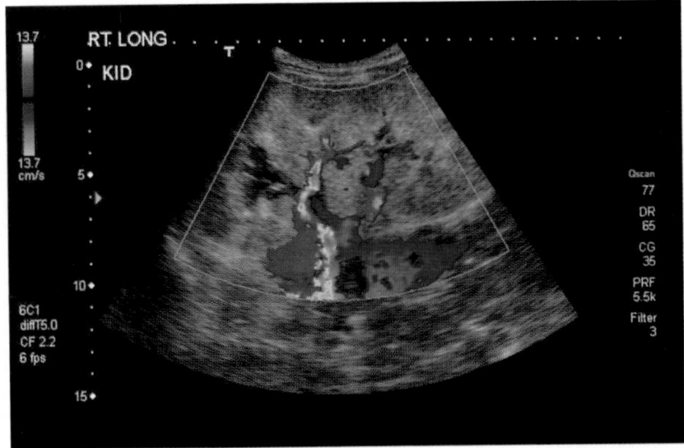

D

Imaging Finding

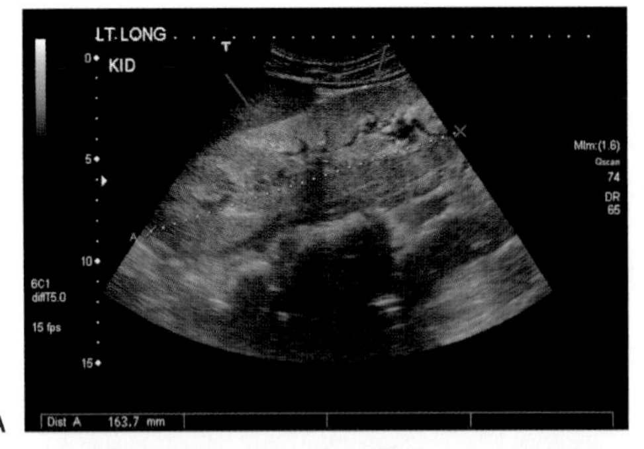

A

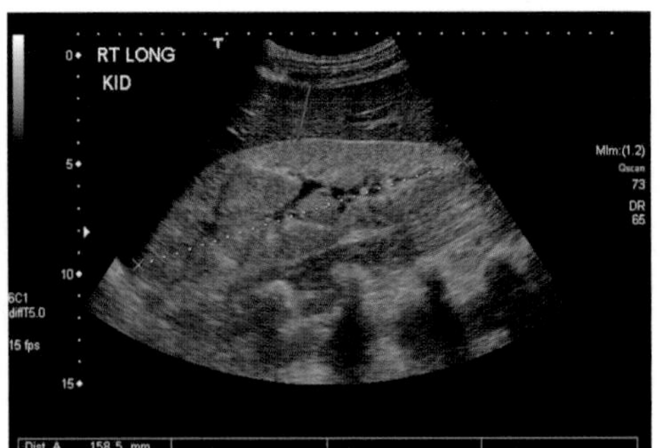

B

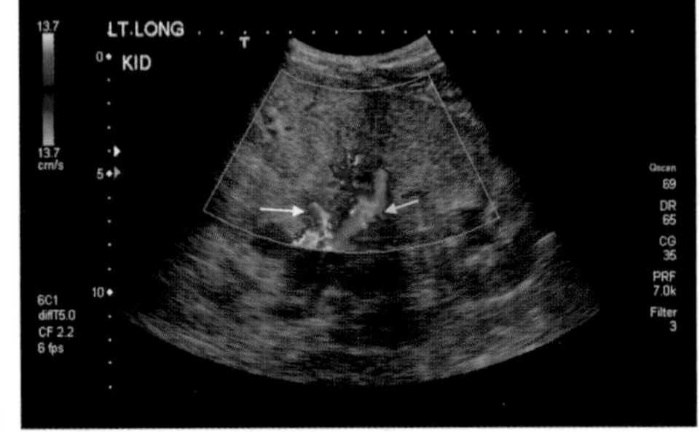

C

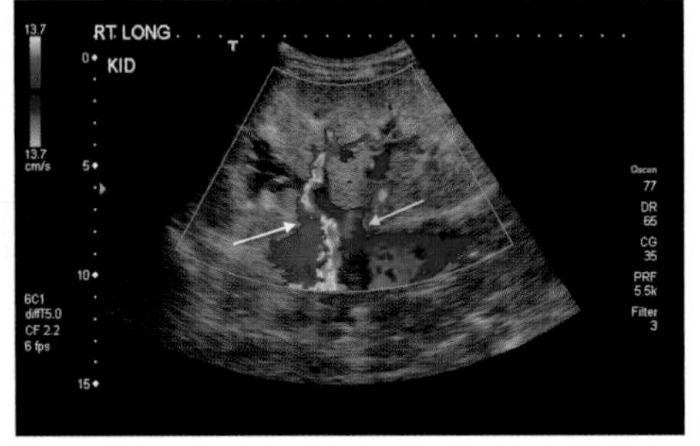

D

(A, B) Ultrasound (US) images of the kidneys demonstrate bilateral enlargement of the kidneys with increase in cortical echogenicity (*red arrows*). No definite evidence of hydronephrosis and or perinephric fluid is seen. Paucity of fat in the renal hilum is also noted. **(C, D)** Further Doppler images demonstrate normal flow in the renal artery (*white arrow*) and renal vein (*yellow arrow*) bilaterally. No definite evidence of aliasing is seen to suggest the presence of stenosis.

Differential Diagnosis

- ***HIV nephropathy:*** Involvement of the kidneys occurs in ~ 10% of HIV-positive patients. The kidneys appear enlarged and echogenic in early stages of HIV nephropathy and progress to small echogenic kidneys in end-stage disease. Paucity of sinus fat is also seen.
- *Diabetic nephropathy:* On US, within the early stages, the kidneys appear enlarged and hypoechoic in appearance. In end-stage disease, the kidneys become echogenic and small.
- *Interstitial nephritis:* Interstitial nephritis accounts for 25% of patients presenting with acute renal failure. The most common etiology is drug induced. The sonographic appearance includes enlarged kidneys with increased echogenicity of the cortex. Cortical medullary differentiation could be maintained.

Essential Facts

- HIV nephropathy occurs in ~ 10% of HIV-positive patients.
- More commonly affects African American males.
- Renal involvement could be related to direct involvement with HIV and/or secondary to antiviral drug nephrotoxicity.
- The patients develop hypertension and proteinuria, with progression into nephrotic syndrome and/or renal failure later on.
- US demonstrates bilaterally enlarged kidneys with increased cortical echogenicity. Loss of corticomedullary differentiation is also present.
- Other imaging findings include renal pelvicalyceal thickening and loss of renal sinus fat appearance.
- On computed tomography, the kidneys appear enlarged with striated enhancement seen after administration of intravenous contrast secondary to dilated tubules with protein.
- Visualization of abnormal kidney US in HIV-positive patients raises the concern for interstitial renal disease.

✓ Pearls & × Pitfalls

✓ There is increased incidence of atypical infection and malignancy (HIV-related lymphoma) in HIV-positive patients. A more detailed evaluation of the kidneys should be undertaken in these patients.

× The presence of enlarged echogenic kidneys in an HIV patient does not always imply HIV nephropathy. Renal biopsy is required for appropriate diagnosis.

Case 58

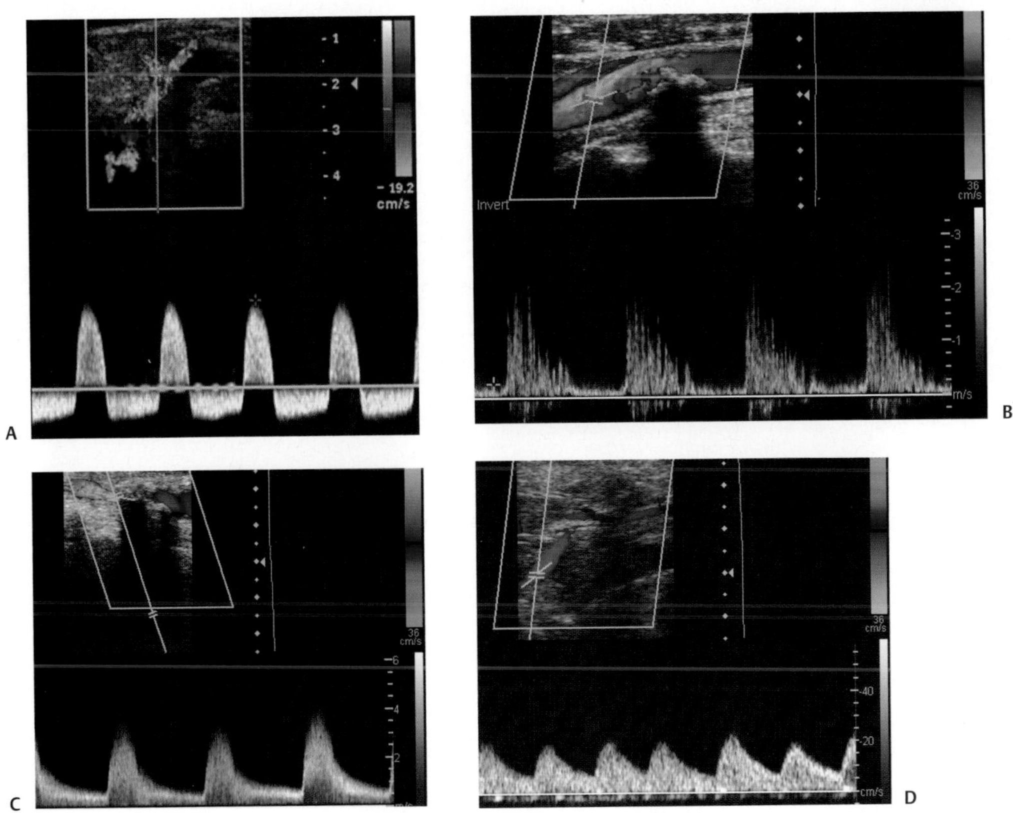

Clinical Presentation

Above are abnormal arterial waveforms from four different patients. Below are the etiologies resulting in such waveforms. Can you match each waveform with each condition?

Waveform waveform

DIAGNOSES

Parvus tardus waveform
Pseudoaneurysm
High grade stenosis
Post stenotic turbulence

Imaging Findings

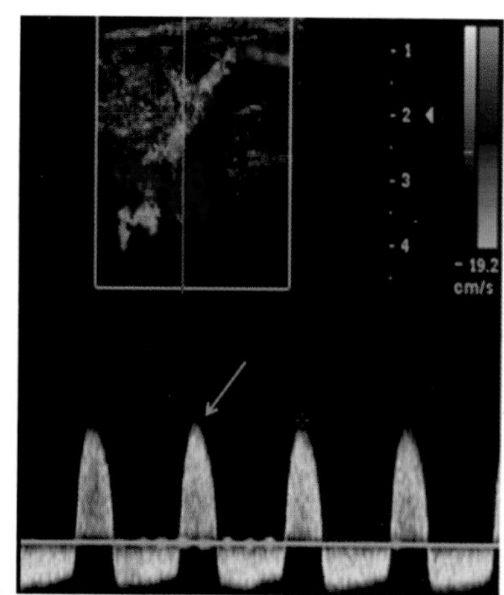

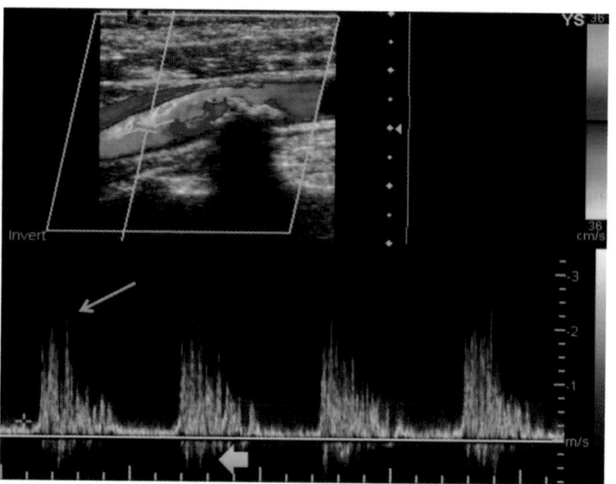

(A) To-and-fro flow seen in the neck of a pseudoaneurysm. Blood flows into the PSA during systole (*arrow*) and returns back into the artery during diastole when the pressure in the PSA becomes greater than the artery. Note the very high velocities in systole and spectral broadening. Note diastole is much longer than systole.

(B) Post stenotic turbulence. The featured appearance of the systolic peak (*thin arrow*) is typical of the post stenotic waveform with high velocities. Note a small amount of flow below the baseline (*thick arrow*) often seen with turbulence.

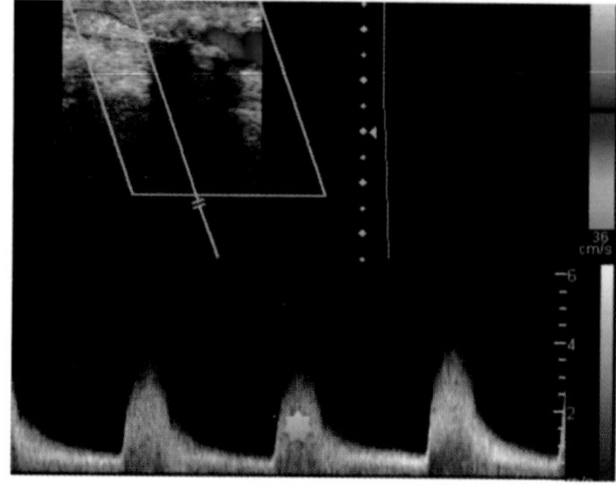

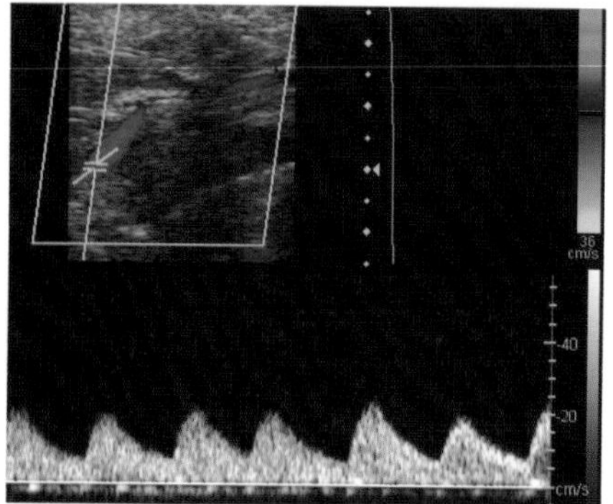

(C) Stenotic jet with spectral broadening: Elevated systolic velocity of 408 cm/sec is consistent with a high-grade stenosis (> 70%). Note the spectral broadening or filling in under the curve (*asterisk*) indicating a large spectrum of velocities typical of flow through a stenosis.

(D) Parvus tardus waveform distal to high-grade stenosis. Note the delayed upstroke, diminished amplitude, and delayed downstroke typical of a parvus tardus waveform. Note the velocity of only 23 cm/sec in the ICA. This waveform will be found distal to a high-grade stenosis.

Case 59

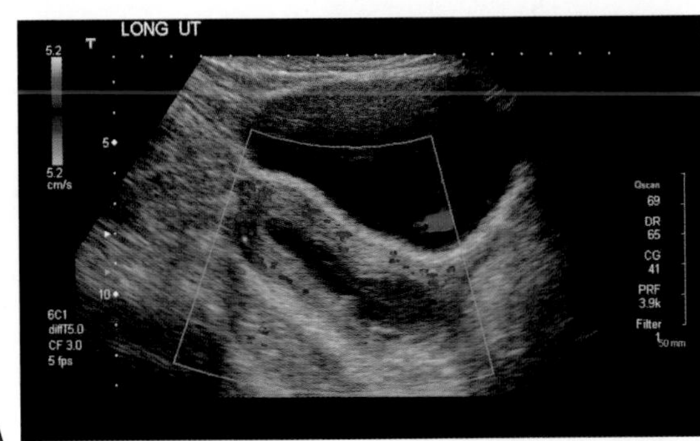

A

Clinical Presentation

A 25-year-old female, status post dilation and curettage (D&C), presents with abdominal pain and fever.

Further Work-up

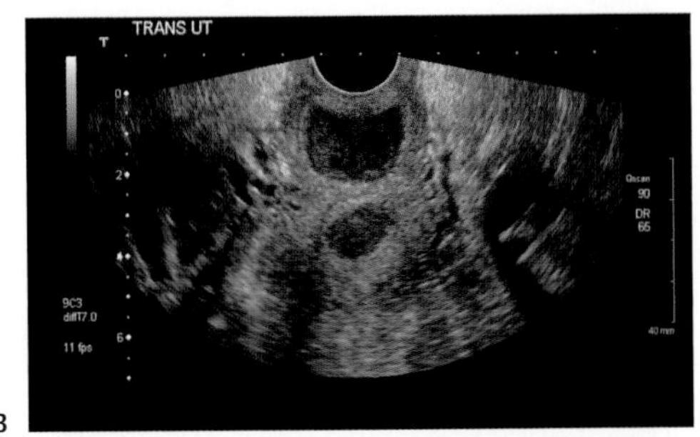

B

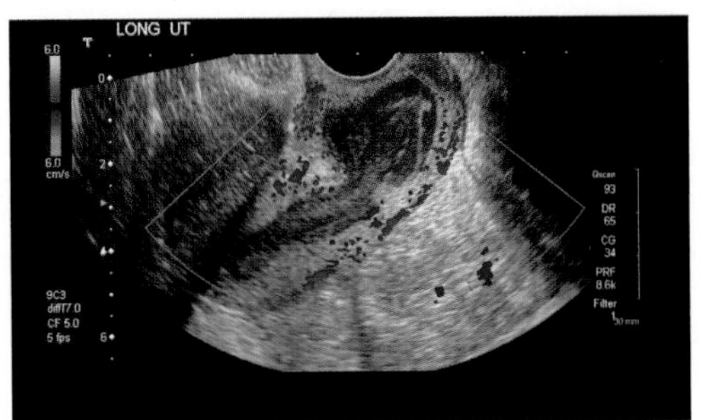

C

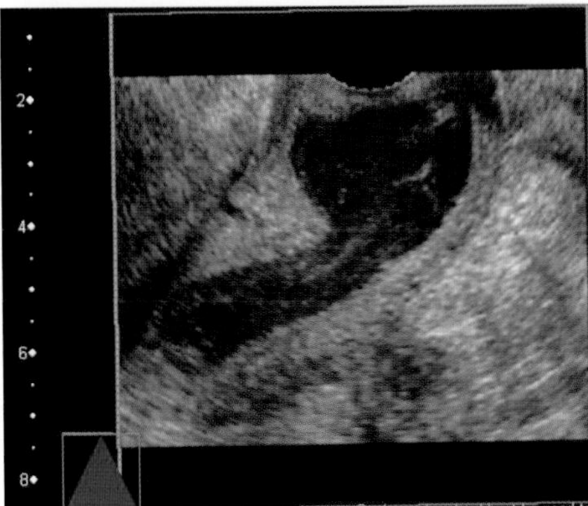

D

Imaging Finding

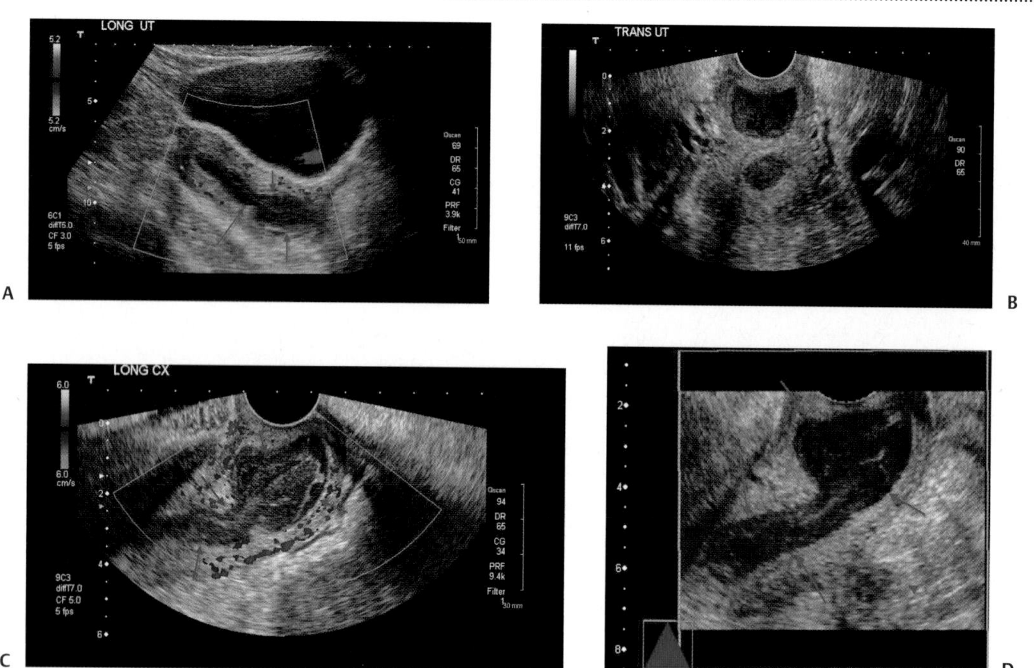

(A) Ultrasound (US) images of the uterus using transabdominal US demonstrate complex fluid within the endometrium as well as the cervical canal (*red arrows*). The endometrium appears distended. **(B, C)** Transvaginal US confirms the finding of complex endometrial fluid. No gross evidence of vascular flow is seen on Doppler imaging. The cervical canal is also distended with complex fluid; however, the cervical os remains closed. **(D)** Similar findings are noted on three-dimensional (3-D) US of the uterus.

Differential Diagnosis

- ***Endometritis/pyometrium:*** The patient presents with a history of intervention, instrumentation, and/or pelvic inflammatory diseases. Patients present with thickened endometrium, fever, cervical motion tenderness, and elevated white count. The sonographic appearance is variable and includes normal endometrium; thickened, poorly defined endometrium; and endometrial complex fluid and/or gas. Motion tenderness is usually present.
- *Retained products of conception:* The patient presents with persistent vaginal bleeding after delivery and or after D&C. The endometrium appears to be thickened and heterogeneous with possible visualization of endometrial vascular flow. A retained product is a clinical diagnosis and US helps in determining the need for surgical therapy.
- *Endometrial hematoma:* The patient usually has a history of recent intervention performed. Cervical stenosis and/or imperforated hymen (hematometrocolpos) could also be a causal factor. Pelvic US demonstrates heterogeneous, complex fluid within the endometrial cavity without definite evidence of flow centrally. The endometrium is normal sonographically.

Essential Facts

- Endometritis could be seen after delivery, D&C, instrumentation, intrauterine device placement, and pelvic inflammatory diseases.
- Pelvic US is the study of choice for evaluation of pelvic inflammatory disease and/or pelvic infection.
- Abnormal US of the pelvis is present in ~ 25% of cases of endometritis.
- The presence of motion tenderness despite normal US improves the positive predictive value of US.
- The uterus could be enlarged, with indistinct outline.
- The endometrium may be thickened with increased and/or decreased echogenicity. Endometrial hyperemia occasionally is present.
- The endometrium demonstrates irregular outlines, with the presence of internal echoes and/or debris.
- Gas could be seen in case of gas-producing organism.
- An extrauterine manifestation includes pelvic fluid, adnexal masses, and/or tubo-ovarian abscess.
- The presence of air improves the accuracy of US in diagnosing infection.

✓ Pearls & × Pitfalls

✓ The presence of a negative US does not exclude endometritis/pyometrium. The presence of uterine tenderness is suggestive of the diagnosis.

× Gas can be seen in up to 21% of clinically normal woman following vaginal delivery; clinical correlation with the patient's symptoms and laboratory results is needed to differentiate the two entities.

Case 60

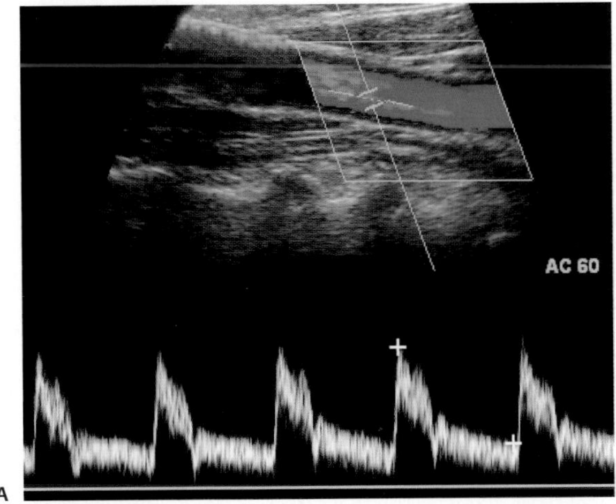

A

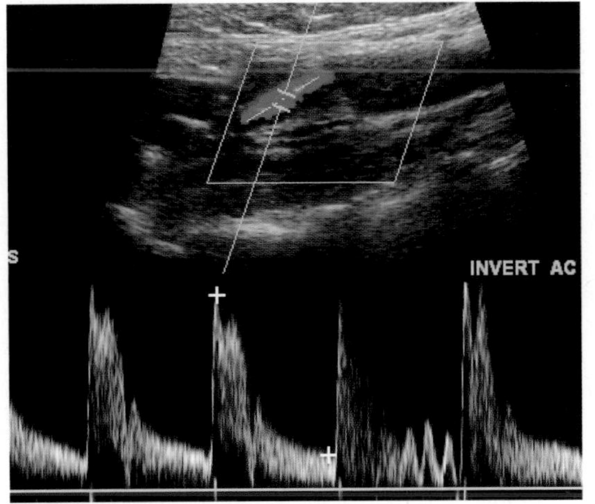

B

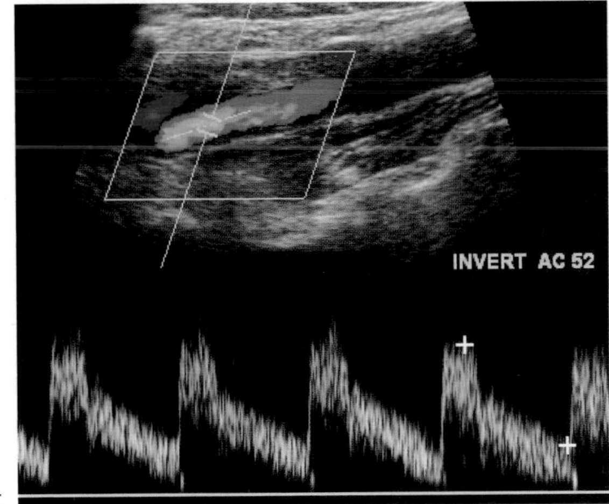

C

Clinical Presentation

Above are normal carotid artery waveforms obtained from the same patient. Can you identify which is the common, internal and external carotid artery?

Imaging Findings

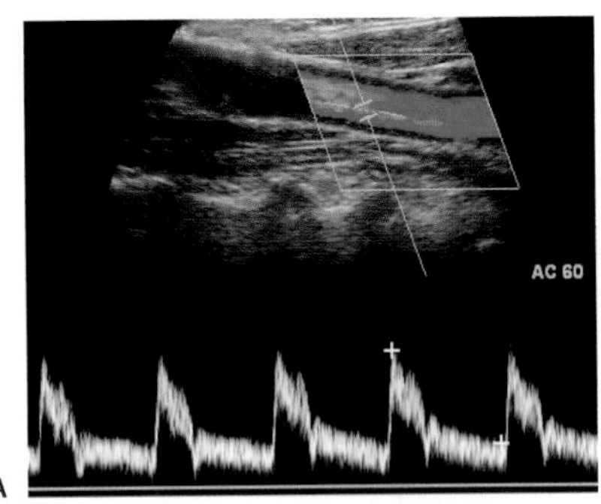

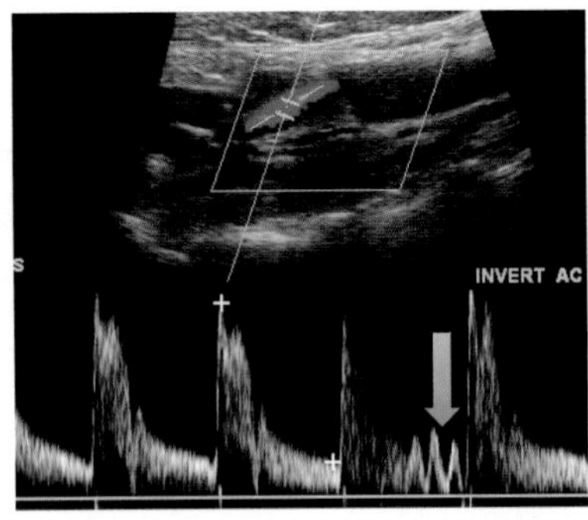

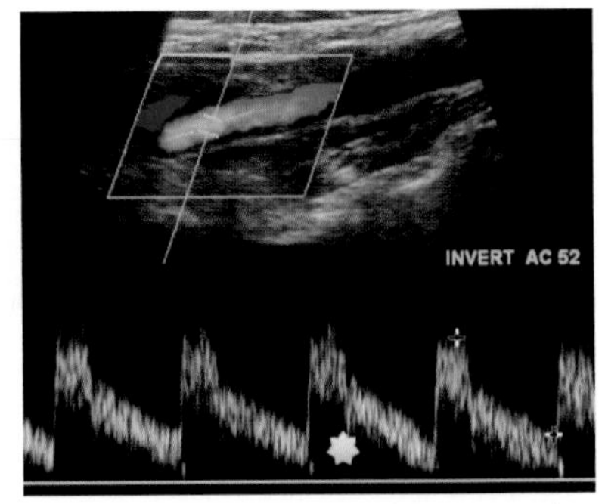

(A) The CCA waveform is intermediate resistance. **(B)** The external carotid artery waveform is high resistance. Note the temporal tap, oscillating waveforms during diastole that result from tapping on the superficial temporal artery at the lateral forehead. **(C)** The internal carotid artery waveform is low resistance with abundant forward flow in diastole. Note the presence of laminar flow with no filling in under the curve (*asterisk*).

Essential Facts

- The carotid arteries have signature waveforms. The ICA supplies the metabolically active brain and therefore is a low-resistance waveform.
- The ECA feeds the muscular bed of the face and has a high-resistance waveform. The CCA waveform is therefore intermediate resistance.
- Externalization of the CCA occurs with occlusion or a high-grade stenosis of the ICA. Flow in the CCA should be fairly symmetric bilaterally including velocities and waveforms.
- The circle of Willis allows for collateral flow to supply the contralateral hemisphere.
- Atherosclerotic vascular changes result in areas of turbulent flow related to bifurcations or branching of vessels. Carotid disease is most concentrated at the bifurcation (visible by ultrasound US) and the siphon (not visible by US).
- The temporal tap differentiates the ECA from the ICA. Tapping on the superficial temporal artery produces waves that are transmitted down to the ECA. (*arrow* in image **B**)
- For velocity criteria to determine stenosis, see **Case 200.**

✓ Pearls & × Pitfalls

× Tandem lesions can underestimate stenosis of the proximal lesion because of a dampening effect.

× In the setting of a high-grade stenosis, elevated velocities (as a result of collateral flow) may be present in the contralateral ICA mimicking stenosis.

× Elevated baseline velocities can be seen in tortuous vessels, hypertensive, and athletes without carotid stenosis.

× Doppler US is not very accurate for detecting vertebral artery stenosis. Vertebral artery velocities and waveforms vary.

Case 61

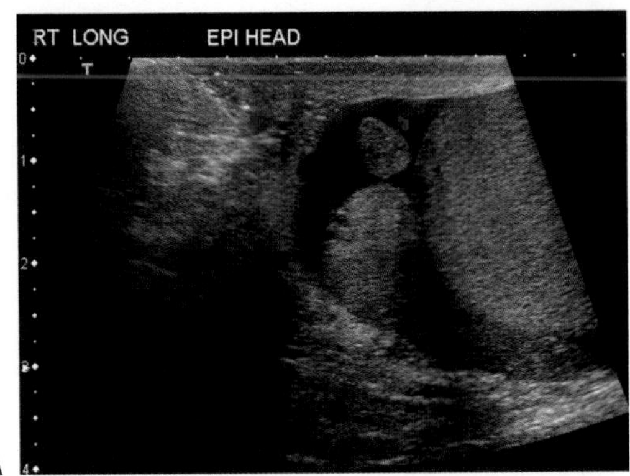

A

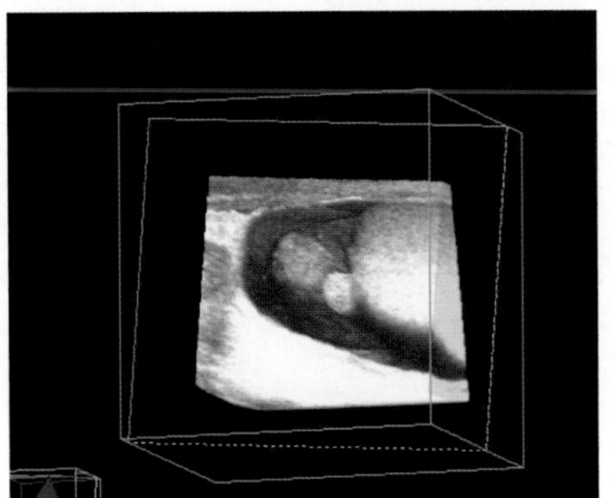
B

Clinical Presentation

A 20-year-old man presents with right testicular pain.

Further Work-up

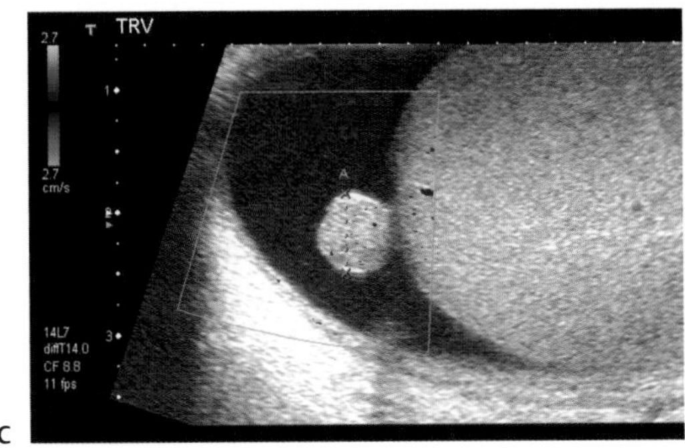

C

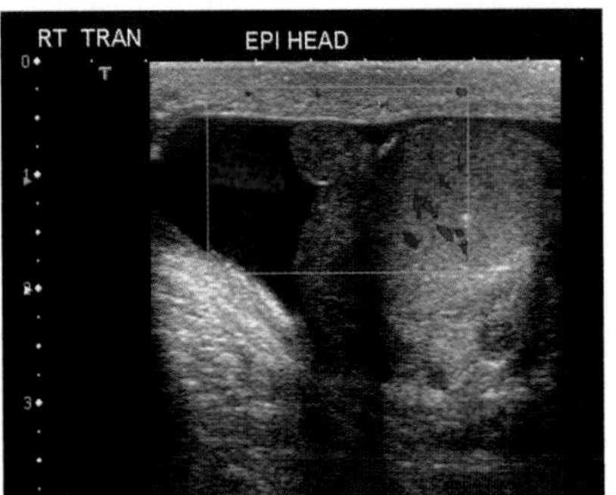

D

Imaging Findings

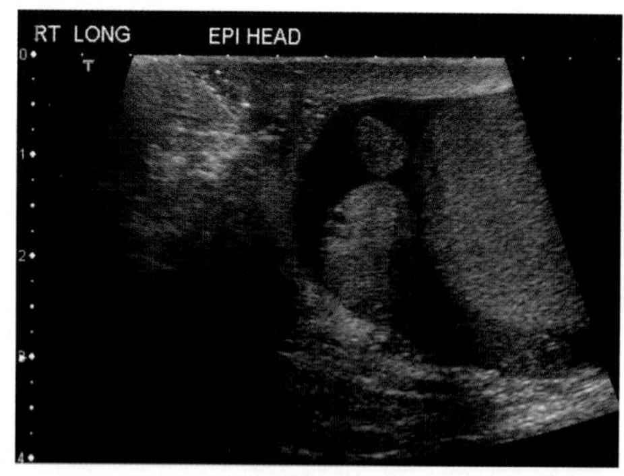

A

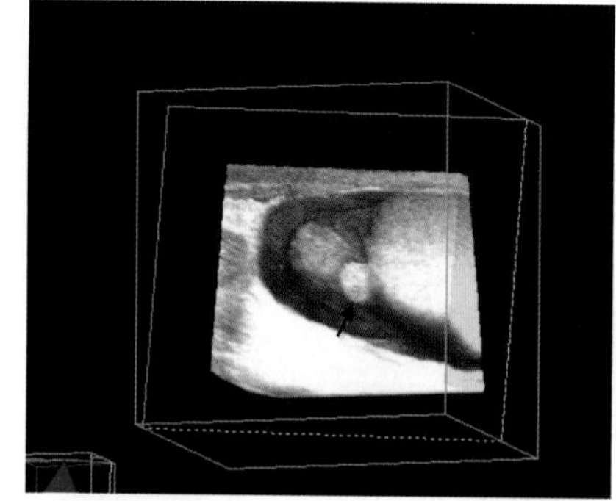

B

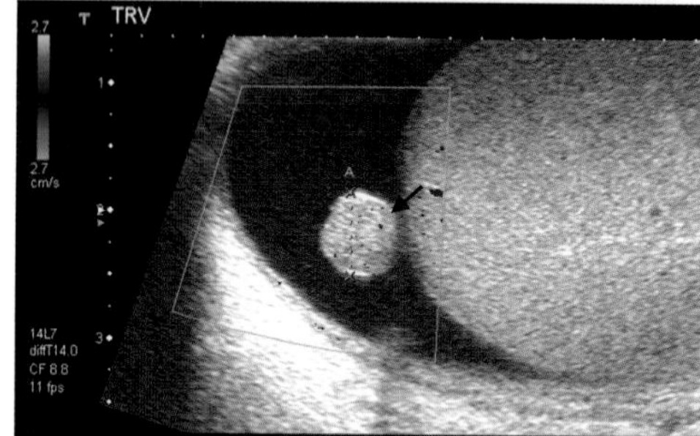

C

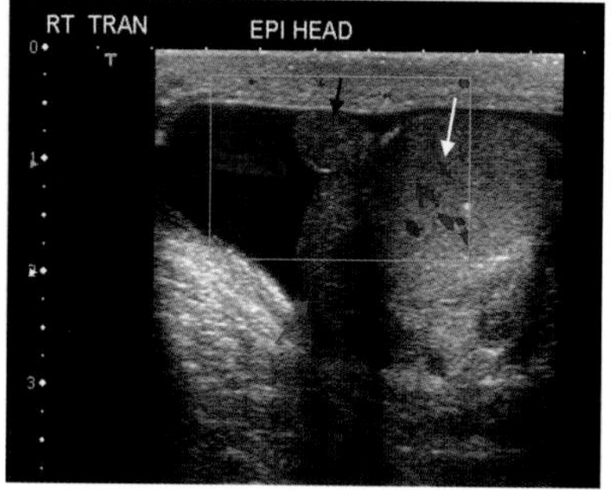

D

(A–D) Ultrasound evaluation of the right and left testicles demonstrates normal-appearing left testicle. On the right side, small to moderate hydrocele is noted with what appears to be paratesticular iso/mildly echogenic mass (*black arrow*). The mass appears to be separate from the epididymis (*red arrow*) and from the testicle. The separate structures are well seen on the three-dimensional image. No significant flow is noted within the paratesticular mass. Mild hyperemia is noted in the testicle adjacent to the mass (*white arrow*).

Differential Diagnosis

- ***Torsed testicular appendage:*** More commonly seen in pediatric patients who present with acute testicular pain. The typical sonographic appearance is paratesticular echogenic/isoechoic mass located in the groove between the epididymal head and testicle. Reactive hydrocele is a common associated finding. Doppler ultrasound shows no evidence of flow; focal hyperemia in the ipsilateral testicle could be seen.
- *Epididymitis:* Is the most common etiology of testicular pain in adults. Associated fever and pyuria could be seen. The typical sonographic appearance is enlarged heterogeneous epididymis with hyperemia. Associated orchitis could also be seen. Reactive hydrocele is a common associated finding. Close attention to exclude the possibility of abscess formation should be made.
- *Extratesticular mass:* The majority of extratesticular masses are benign, with estimated malignancy in 3% of cases. Ultrasound has 100% accuracy in distinguishing intratesticular from extratesticular masses. The most common extratesticular masses are spermatic cord lipoma and adenomatoid tumor. Lipoma appears as echogenic extratesticular mass with no associated pain, the lesion might be palpable on physical examination. Adenomatoid tumor appears as variable echogenicity tumor; however, smaller lesions are usually echogenic.

Essential Facts

- It is a common cause of testicular pain, especially in pediatric patients.
- It is a remnant of the paramesonephric duct, oval in shape, measures < 6 mm.
- It appears as medially located appendix in the groove between the testis and the head of the epididymis.
- The most sensitive sonographic appearance is enlarged (> 6 mm) and spherical testicular appendage.
- Torsed testicular appendage is usually hyperechoic on ultrasound; it also could appear as isoechoic or hypoechoic mass.
- Reactive hydrocele and/or scrotal wall thickening are common associated findings.
- Doppler ultrasound usually shows no evidence of flow within the normal and torsed testicular appendage; surrounding testicular hyperemia commonly seen.

✓ Pearls & × Pitfalls

✓ Doppler ultrasound is very helpful in differentiating testicular appendage from the epididymis head; this is especially valuable in isoechoic testicular appendage.

× Detection of flow within the testicular appendage is difficult on Doppler imaging, even in normal testicular appendage. Lack of Doppler flow within the testicular appendage is not diagnostic of torsed testicular appendage.

Case 62

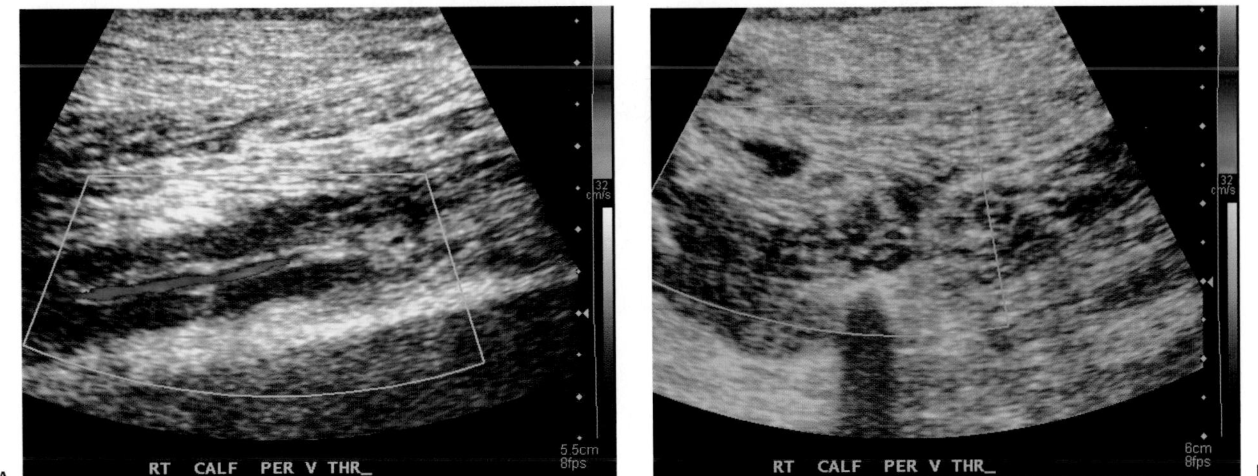

■ Clinical Presentation

A 40-year-old man with recent knee surgery presents with right calf pain and swelling.

Imaging Findings

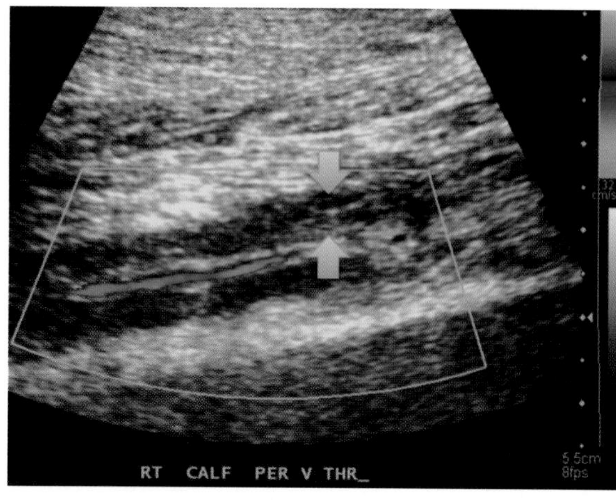

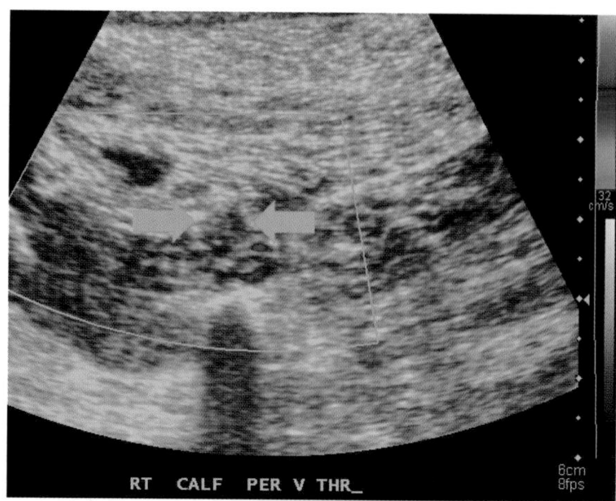

(A, B) Longitudinal and transverse color Doppler image of the right calf reveals a patent peroneal artery (*red*) surrounded by paired veins. *Arrows* denote the more anterior of the peroneal veins. The veins contain internal echoes and do not demonstrate any flow with color. Note the discrepancy in diameters between the artery and veins.

Differential Diagnosis

- ***Acute calf deep venous thrombosis:*** The distended, completely occluded paired calf veins are consistent with acute calf deep venous thrombosis.
- *Acute superficial thrombosis of the calf:* Superficial veins do not have an accompanying artery. Superficial veins are located in the subcutaneous tissues immediately deep to the skin.
- *Chronic calf deep venous thrombosis:* Chronic thrombus would not distend the vein. It would not be completely occluding as in this case.

Essential Facts

- Calf vein imaging is controversial. Below are the organizational recommendations for calf imaging:
- American College of Radiology (ACR): Currently, calf vein imaging is optional but may soon be required in symptomatic patients.
- Intersocietal Commission for the Accreditation of Vascular Laboratories (ICAVL): Calf vein imaging should be performed when appropriate or required by laboratory protocol.
- Gastrocnemius and soleal veins are considered deep veins.
- A small calf clot can be a normal occurrence. Most are asymptomatic.
- Calf veins are often treated to prevent the post phlebitic syndrome.

✓ Pearls & × Pitfalls

✓ Calf veins, unlike thigh veins, are usually paired.

✓ Serial examination of calf thrombosis is performed to evaluate for propagation. Twenty percent of calf veins propagate.

Case 63

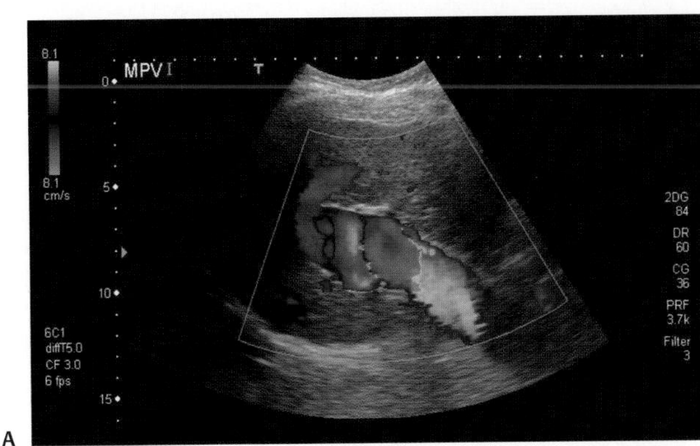

A

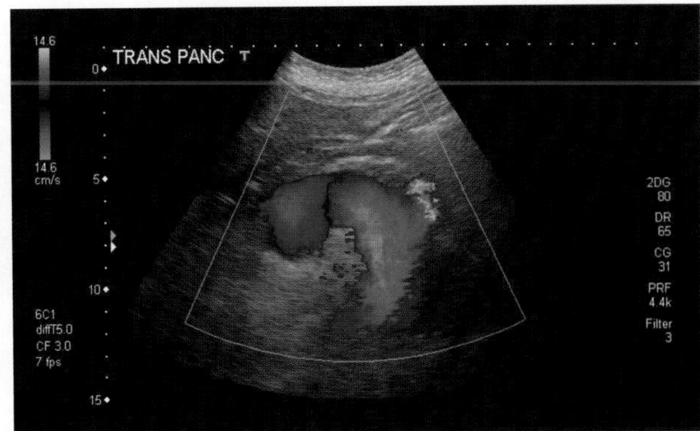

B

Clinical Presentation

A 55-year-old woman with history of hepatitis C presents for Doppler evaluation.

Further Work-up

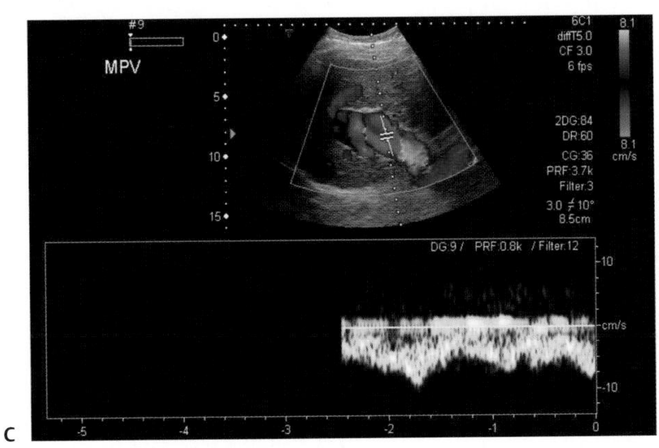

C

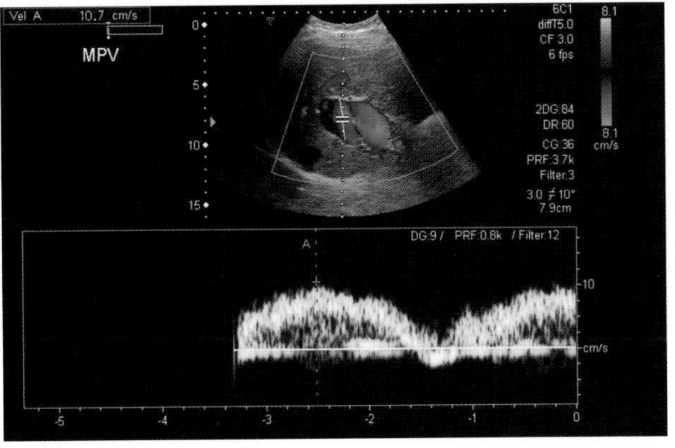

D

Imaging Findings

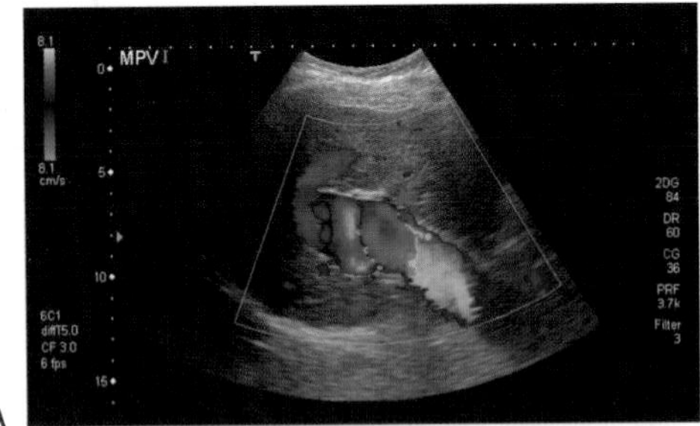

A

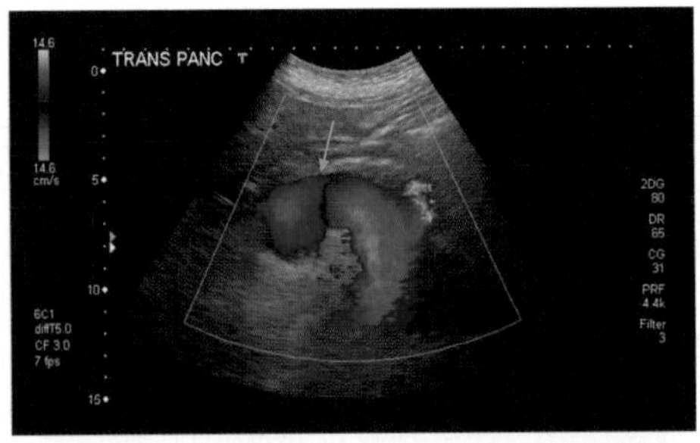

B

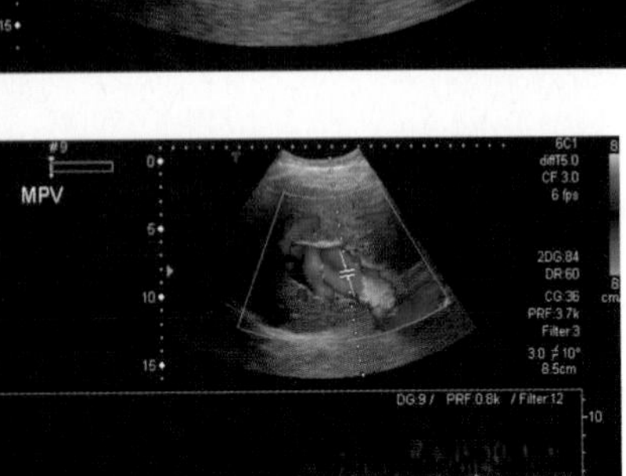

C

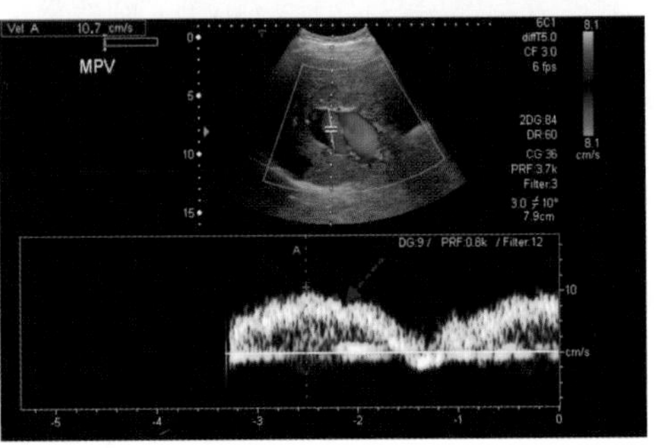

D

(A, B) Doppler ultrasound evaluation of the portal vein demonstrates what appears to be bidirectional flow within the main portal vein in the porta hepatis (*green arrow*). Doppler evaluation of the splenic vein as well as portal confluence demonstrates normal direction of flow. The portal vein appears to be enlarged. **(C, D)** Doppler tracing demonstrates retrograde as well as antegrade flow within the main portal vein in the porta hepatis (*blue arrow*).

Differential Diagnosis

- ***Helical flow in the portal vein:*** Helical flow within the portal system represents changes from the normal laminar flow in the portal vein, and the changing color representing bidirectional flow is noted in the portal vein depending on the location of the cursor within the helix. The presence of helical flow should prompt further assessment of possible underlying liver disease.
- *Bidirectional flow in the portal vein:* Bidirectional flow in the portal vein usually presents as a sequela of portal hypertension. Doppler tracing above and below baseline is present in the same location of the portal vein, clearly visualized during real-time ultrasound Doppler tracing. Other signs of portal hypertension might be seen and help to narrow the differential diagnosis.
- *Portal vein stenosis with poststenotic turbulence:* Narrowing in the portal vein could be related to extrinsic mass impression, partial clot, and/or anastomotic narrowing in patients with a history of liver transplant. The sonographic appearance demonstrates an area of narrowing in the portal vein on gray scale imaging, with focal area of increased velocity noted on color Doppler at and after the area of stenosis. Turbulence of flow is noted on pulse Doppler tracing.

Essential Facts

- Normal flow in in the portal system is hepatopedal with minimal pulsatility.
- Helical flow is an unusual finding in normal patients.
- In helical flow, Doppler ultrasound shows alternating bands of red and blue within the portal vein.
- The direction of flow on duplex ultrasound tracing depends on the location of the cursor within the helix.
- Helical flow is usually associated with abnormal findings in the liver (seen only in 2% of normal patients). The associated abnormalities range from liver cirrhosis, portosystemic shunt, patients with liver transplant, and in patients status post transjugular intrahepatic portosystemic shunt (TIPS).
- Helical flow is occasionally associated with intrahepatic portosystemic shunt.
- Helical flow seen in patient status post liver transplant is more apparent in the early postoperative stages.

✓ Pearls & × Pitfalls

✓ The presence of alternating bands of red and blue in the portal vein is highly suggestive of helical flow; the changes associated with bidirectional flow are more apparent during breathing.

× The presence of mixed bands of color on Doppler ultrasound noted in helical flow could be misinterpreted as bidirectional flow and reversal of flow in the portal vein.

Case 64

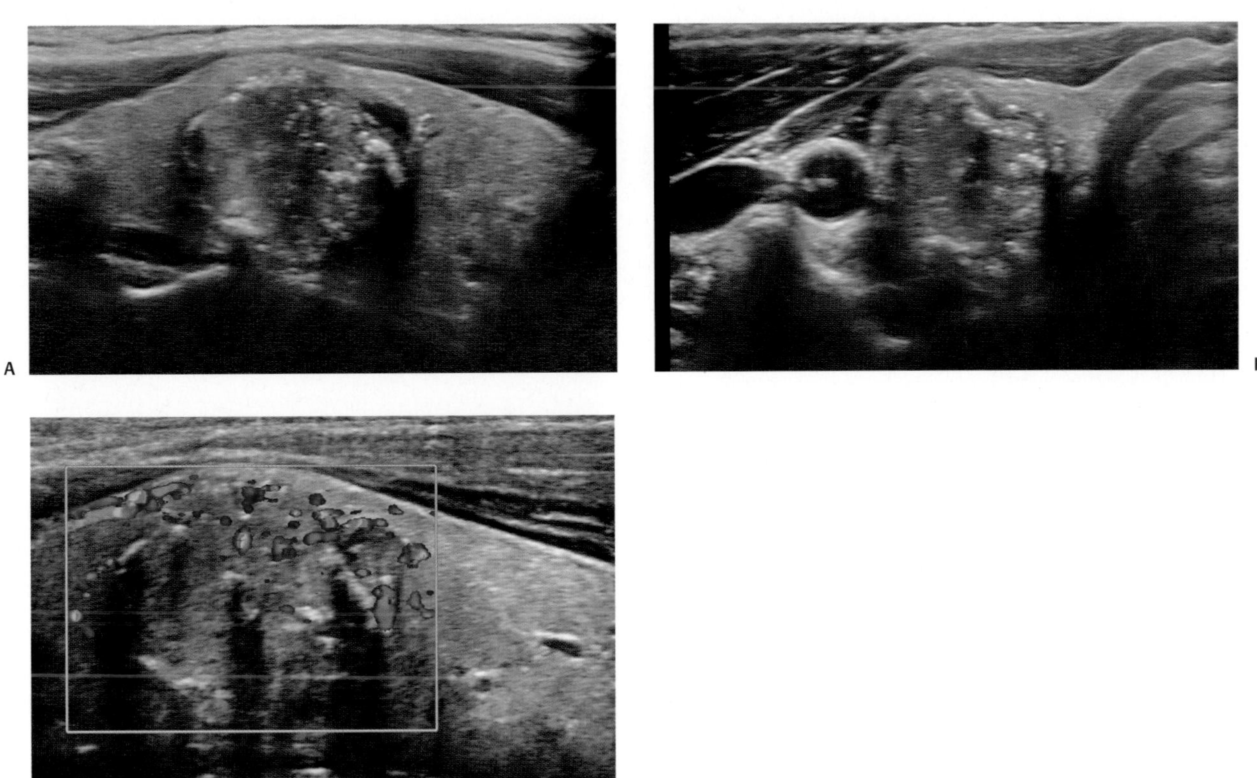

Clinical Presentation

A 40-year-old man with a palpable right thyroid nodule noted on physical exam.

Imaging Findings

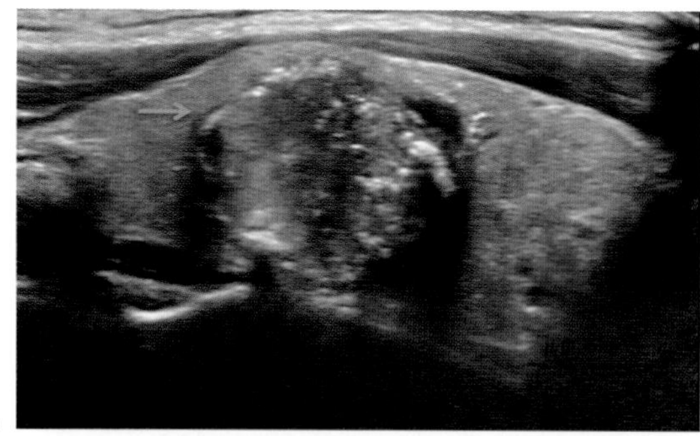

A

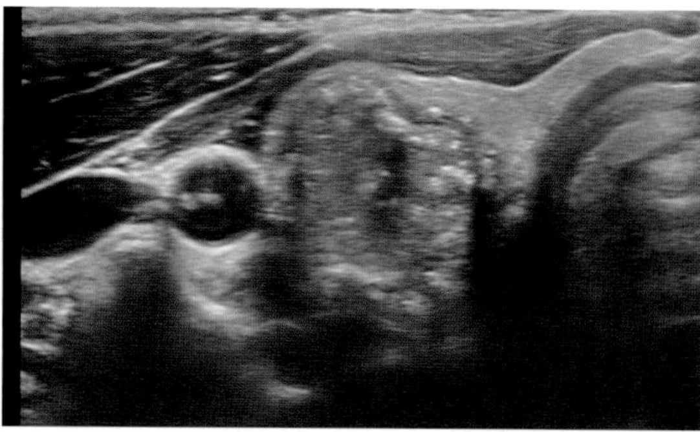

B

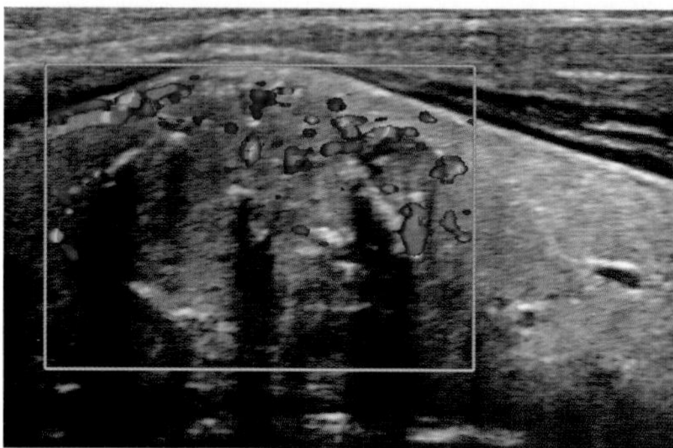

C

(A) Longitudinal view of the right thyroid reveals a lesion with coarse and psammomatous calcifications. Rim calcifications are seen superiorly (*arrow*). **(B)** Transverse image demonstrates a lobular contour of the lesion anteriorly. **(C)** With color Doppler imaging, the lesion is hypervascular. Note the dense shadowing from the coarse calcifications. Left lobe was normal.

Differential Diagnosis

- ***Papillary thyroid cancer:*** Psammomatous calcifications (PCs) in a solid lesion are suspicious for papillary carcinoma and should be biopsied regardless of size.
- *Multinodular goiter (MNG):* Multiple similar-appearing nodules are present in an MNG. These nodules are not usually calcified. MNG is usually bilateral.
- *Indeterminate lesion:* A lesion with psammomatous or coarse calcifications is suspicious, not indeterminate.

Essential Facts

- Psammomatous calcifications, also referred to as microcalcifications are the most specific finding of malignancy, with specificities reported up to 95%.
- Solid lesions with coarse central calcifications are suspicious for malignancy.
- Coarse calcifications and microcalcifications can be seen together as in this case.
- Coarse calcifications will shadow but psammomatous calcifications will not.
- Peripheral (eggshell) calcifications are less suspicious for malignancy.
- Psammomatous calcifications are typical of papillary carcinoma. Coarse central calcifications can be seen with medullary carcinoma.
- Thyroid nodules are extremely common. They are present in 50% of autopsies.
- Thyroid cancer is rare. It represents 1% of cancers. Cell types include:
  - Seventy-five to 80% papillary carcinoma
  - Ten to 20% follicular carcinoma
  - Three to 5% medullary carcinoma
  - One to 2% anaplastic carcinoma
- Risk factors for thyroid cancer include radiation, family history, and hereditary syndromes (MEN 2, Cowden syndrome, familial polyposis)

✓ Pearls & × Pitfalls

✓ A solid nodule with calcification is suspicious for malignancy regardless of size.

✓ Suspicion for malignancy: psammomatous calcifications> coarse calcifications> rim calcifications.

× There is controversy regarding biopsy of subcentimeter suspicious lesions. Subcentimeter solid lesions with definite microcalcifications are often biopsied.

× Psammomatous calcifications can be confused with the comet tail artifact seen in colloid lesions.

× Both benign and malignant lesions can demonstrate increased vascularity.

× Thyroid cancer can be stable for years. Benign lesions can grow.

Case 65

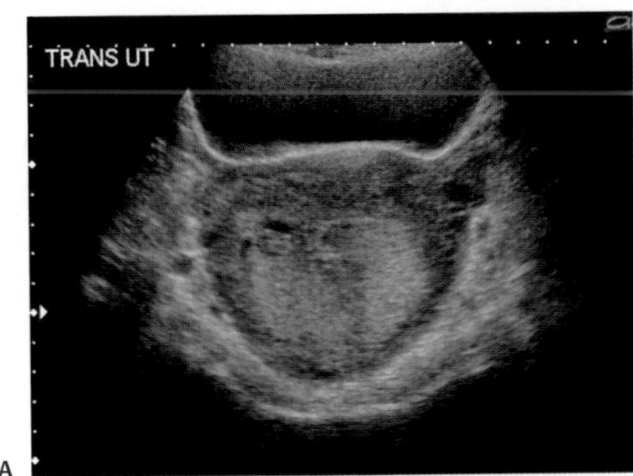

A

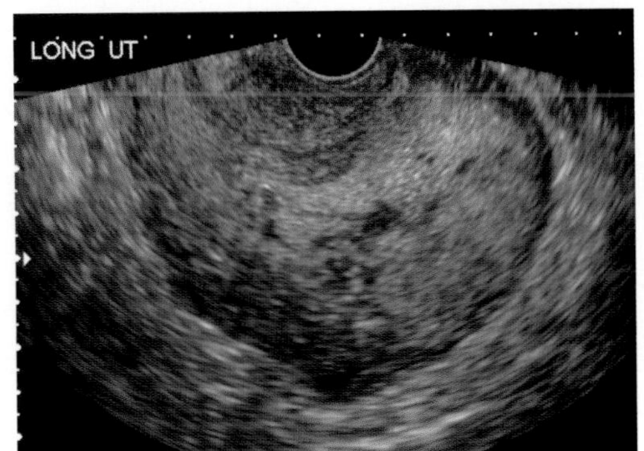

B

■ Clinical Presentation

A 25-year-old woman, 10 days postpartum, presents with persistent vaginal bleeding.

■ Further Work-up

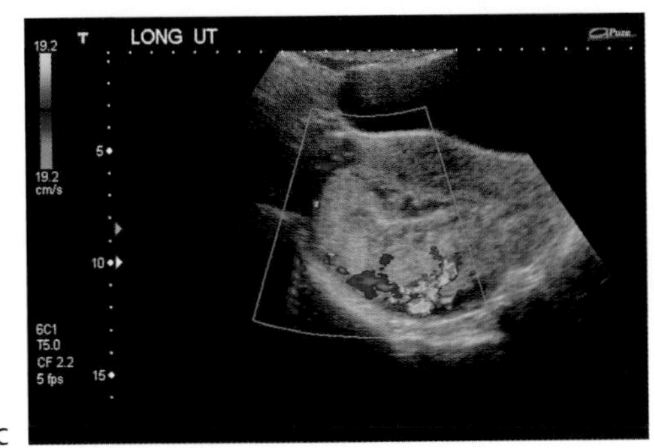

C

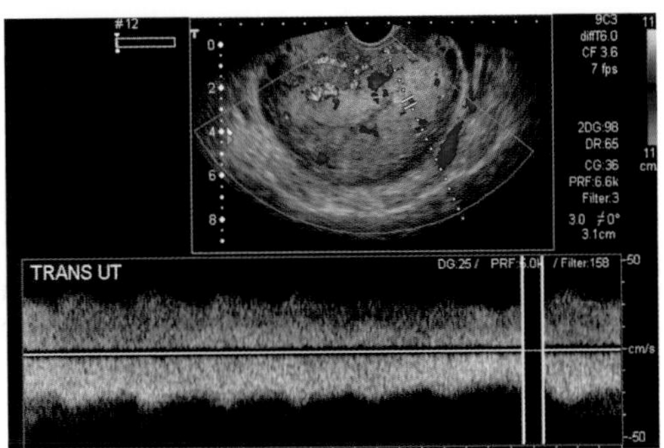

D

Imaging Findings

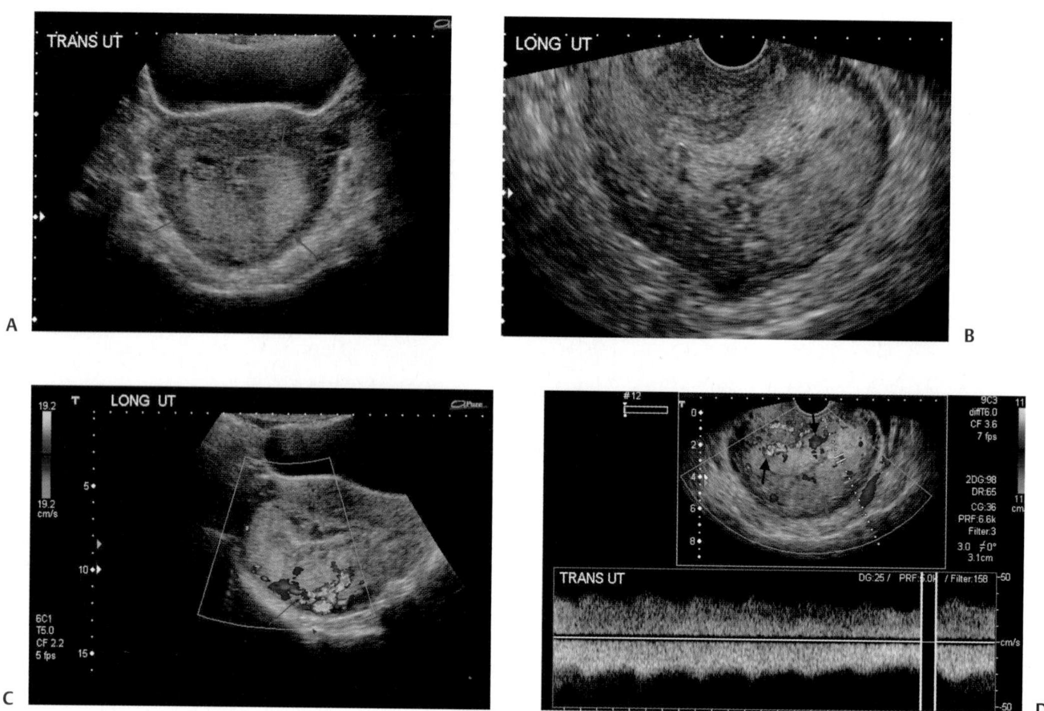

(A–D) Images of the pelvis using transabdominal and transvaginal ultrasound demonstrate markedly thickened endometrium (*red arrows*) with cystic changes. The junctional zone is poorly defined on the current study. Doppler images demonstrate extensive vascular flow with predominately low-resistance waveform within the endometrium (*black arrows*).

Differential Diagnosis

- ***Retained products of conception:*** The patient usually presents with postpartum bleeding; the typical sonographic appearance is a thickened echogenic endometrium with vascular flow. The diagnosis is usually clinical and the value of ultrasound is to assess the need for surgical therapy.
- *Arteriovenous fistula/malformation:* The condition could be congenital and/or acquired. The most common presentation is bleeding in a patient status post dilation and curettage. Heterogeneous appearance of the myometrium with dominant vessel is noted on gray scale images. Doppler assessment of the vessel demonstrates very low resistance waveform with dominant draining vein.
- *Endometritis:* The patient usually presents with foul vaginal discharge, fever, and leukocytosis. The presence of air/twinkle artifact within the endometrium in a patient with no history of recent delivery and/or intervention is suggestive of the diagnosis. Air could be present after recent delivery; the presence of air is not diagnostic in postpartum state.

Essential Facts

- Uncommon complication of conception, patient presents with prolonged bleeding and endometritis.
- Could be seen after miscarriage and/or full-term gestation.
- In postpartum uterus with bleeding, lack of echogenic endometrial lesion or only endometrial fluid has high negative predictive value.
- The sonographic appearance is endometrial cystic mass, complex fluid in the endometrium, thick endometrium with cystic changes.
- The presence of vascular flow on Doppler imaging improves the diagnostic accuracy; lack of flow does not exclude retained products.
- The value of ultrasound is to assess the need for additional surgical intervention. No surgical intervention is required when ultrasound is normal.

✓ Pearls & × Pitfalls

✓ The presence of normal endometrium does not exclude retained products; however, it helps to exclude the need for surgical intervention.

× The implantation site will remain vascular in postpartum, the presence of blood clot adjacent to implantation site could be misinterpreted as retained products with endometrial flow.

Case 66

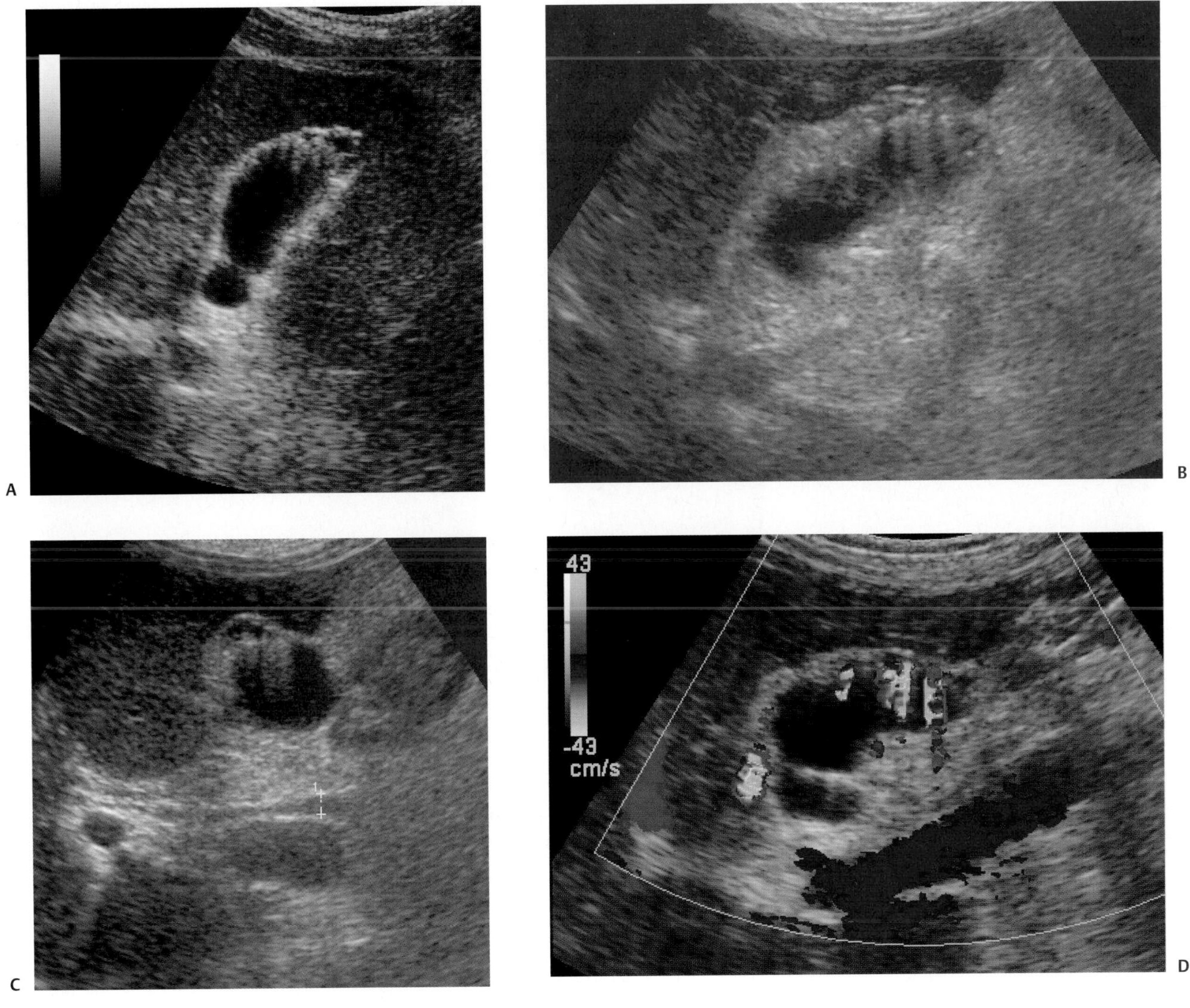

A B C D

Clinical Presentation

An 80-year-old man with abdominal pain.

Imaging Findings

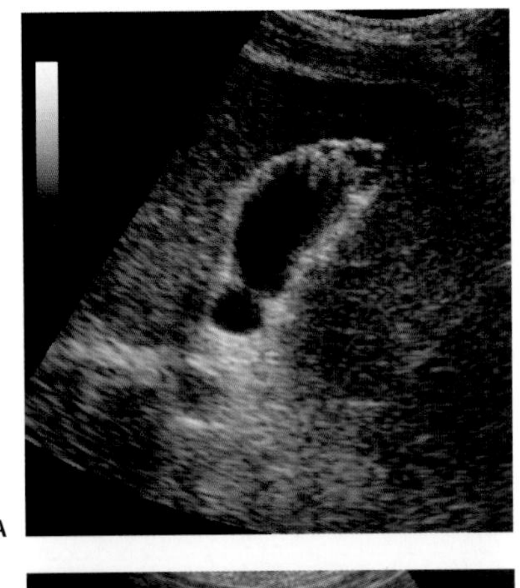
A

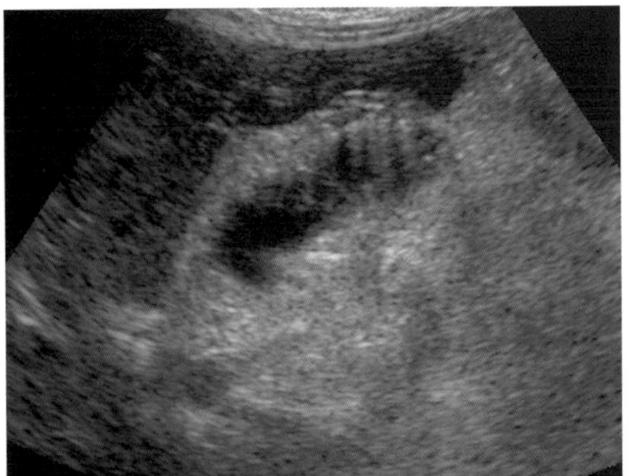
B

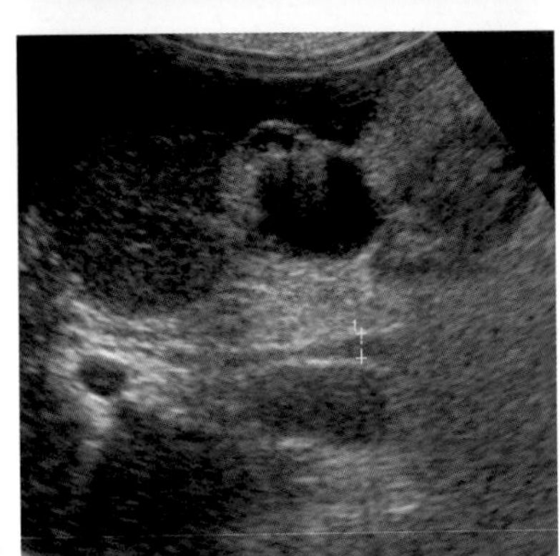
C

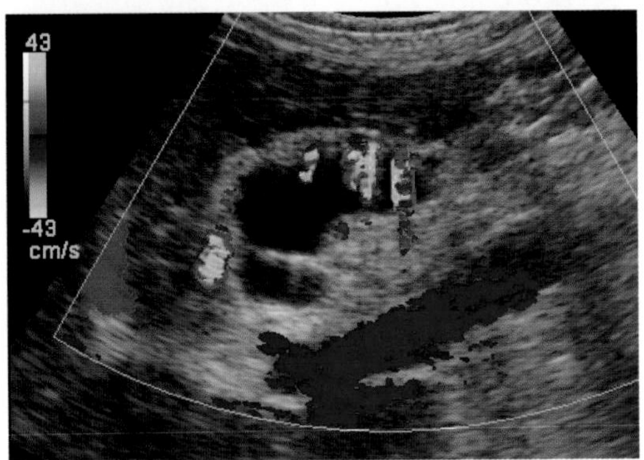

D

(A–D) Longitudinal view of the right upper quadrant reveals linear echoes extending into the gallbladder lumen. Cystic changes are present in the gallbladder wall near the fundus. Twinkle artifact from the anterior wall of the gallbladder is noted with color Doppler.

Differential Diagnosis

- ***Adenomyomatosis of the gallbladder (GA):*** Focal thickening of the gallbladder fundus with cystic changes and comet tail artifacts is consistent with adenomyomatosis of the gallbladder.
- *Malignant mass of the gallbladder fundus:* Focal thickening of the gallbladder with flow would be suspicious for a mass. However, color Doppler in this case is so intense despite the high-flow scale, it can only be twinkling artifact and not internal vascularity.
- *Shadowing gallstones:* Gallstones would be located in the dependent portion of the gallbladder and would demonstrate shadowing, not the echogenic comet tail artifact seen within the lumen of the gallbladder above.

Essential Facts

- Adenomyomatosis of the gallbladder is an incidental finding reported in up to 9% of cholecystectomy specimens. It is usually asymptomatic but
  - Ninety percent of patients have coexistent gallstones.
  - GA is more commonly focal than diffuse. Focal GA usually involves the fundus.
- Sonographic features of adenomyomatosis of the gallbladder include:
  - Focal or diffuse thickening of the gallbladder wall
  - Cystic changes within the gallbladder wall (Rokitansky-Aschoff sinuses)
- Echogenic foci in the gallbladder wall with or without comet tail artifact or shadowing
  - Twinkling artifact with color Doppler ultrasound
- GA is more common in women and not considered premalignant.
- The echogenic foci in the wall seen with GA represent concretions or tiny stones and cause twinkling artifact. Computed tomography will not usually reveal calcification in these lesions.
- Hyperplastic cholecystosis includes two different entities:
  - Adenomyomatosis of the gallbladder
  - Cholesterolosis: Multiple cholesterol polyps. This usually occurs without wall thickening.

✓ Pearls & × Pitfalls

× Gallbladder wall thickening is nonspecific, but cystic changes within a thickened wall are specific for adenomyomatosis.

✓ The intramural cystic changes of GA can be tiny and a high-frequency transducer is essential for identification of the cysts.

× Focal GA is most commonly present in the fundus. Because the fundus is anterior (near field) it can be difficult to visualize with ultrasound.

× Focal GA can mimic malignancy and surgery may be needed to exclude malignancy.

Case 67

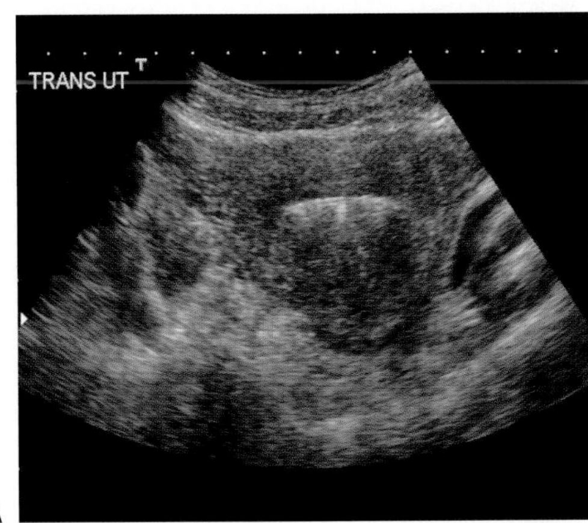

A

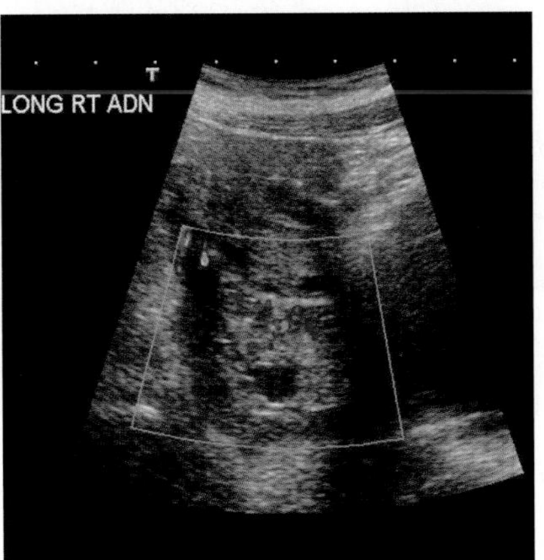

B

Clinical Presentation

A 35-year-old woman, gravida 3, para 3, presents with right-sided pelvic pain.

Further Work-up

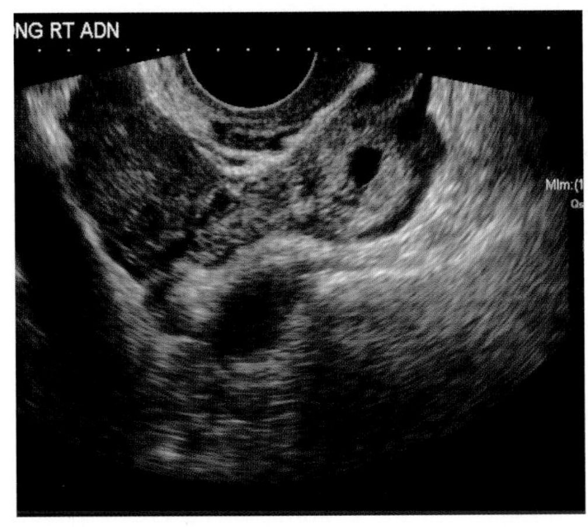

C

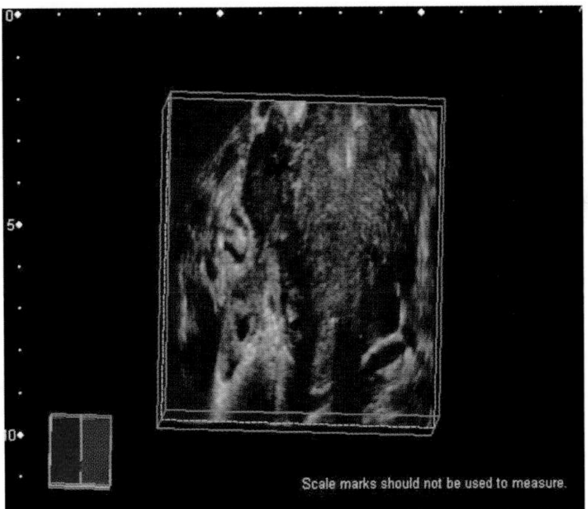

D

Imaging Findings

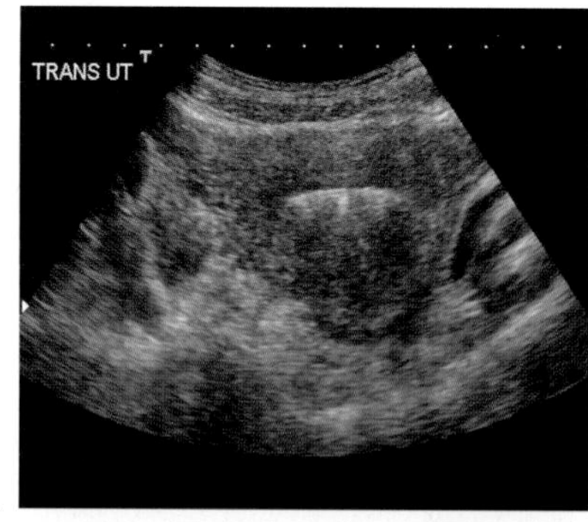

A

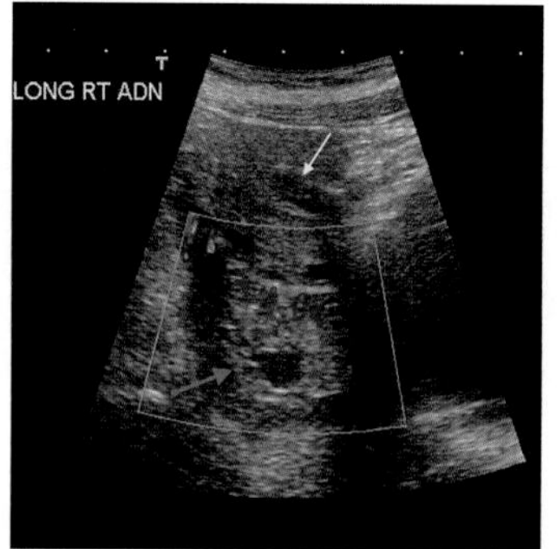

B

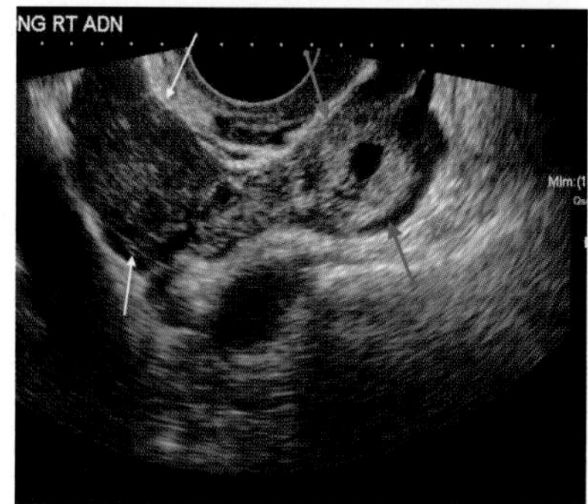

C

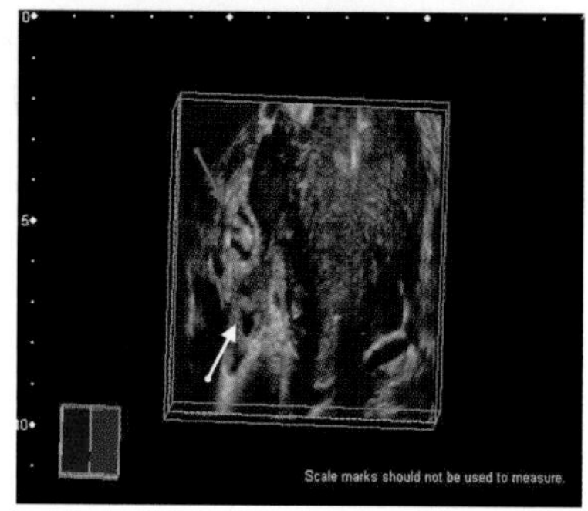

D

(A–D) Ultrasound images of the pelvis using a transabdominal approach demonstrate an intrauterine device (IUD) located in the endometrium (*red arrow*). Right-sided adnexal mass is also present (*green arrow*). Follow-up transvaginal ultrasound images of the pelvis demonstrate a right-sided adnexal mass, which appears to be paraovarian in location (*white arrow*). The right ovary appears grossly unremarkable. The IUD (*red arrow*), right ovary (*white arrow*), and right adnexal mass (*green arrow*) are clearly visualized on a single three-dimensional ultrasound image.

Differential Diagnosis

- ***IUD with right-sided ectopic pregnancy:*** The typical clinical presentation includes vaginal bleeding, pain, and positive pregnancy test. Ultrasound shows an IUD in the endometrium, without visualization of endometrial gestational sac. An adnexal mass is visualized; the presence of yolk sac and/or fetal heart rate within the adnexal mass is diagnostic.
- *IUD with right-sided tubo-ovarian abscess:* IUDs are associated with increased incidence of pelvic inflammatory disease . The patient presents with pelvic pain, elevated white blood cells, fever, and vaginal discharge. Ultrasound shows an IUD in the endometrium, as well as possible visualization of complex adnexal lesion. The presence of a negative pregnancy test favors the diagnosis.
- *IUD with right-sided paraovarian mass:* The incidence of tubal malignancy is very low. The patient usually presents with pelvic pain and palpable adnexal lesion on physical examination. Ultrasound evaluation demonstrates an adnexal lesion, likely separate from the ovary. The presence of intraluminal, low-resistance flow on Doppler ultrasound favors the diagnosis of possible adnexal mass.

Essential Facts

- The clinical presentation of ectopic pregnancy includes vaginal bleeding, abdominal pain, positive pregnancy test, and palpable adnexal lesion.
- IUDs are associated with increased incidence of ectopic pregnancies.
- Among patients with IUDs, 16% of pregnancies are ectopic.
- The incidence of ectopic pregnancy in patients with IUDs is ~ 5%.
- The sonographic appearance includes IUD without evidence of intrauterine gestation. An adnexal mass is visualized.
- The presence of yolk sac and/or heart rate in the adnexa is diagnostic of ectopic pregnancy.
- The presence of echogenic fluid within the cul-de-sac may represent ectopic rupture.
- Other secondary signs includes enlargement of the uterus and thickening of the endometrium with possible visualization of pseudosac.

✓ Pearls & × Pitfalls

✓ An ectopic pregnancy should be considered in patients with IUDs that present with irregular vaginal bleeding. Pregnancy test and pelvic ultrasound should be performed to rule out ectopic pregnancy.

× Lack of visualization of intrauterine pregnancy in a patient with intrauterine device and positive pregnancy test could be attributed to shadowing from the device, obscuring the endometrium. Both adnexa should be closely evaluated to exclude the possibility of ectopic pregnancy.

Case 68

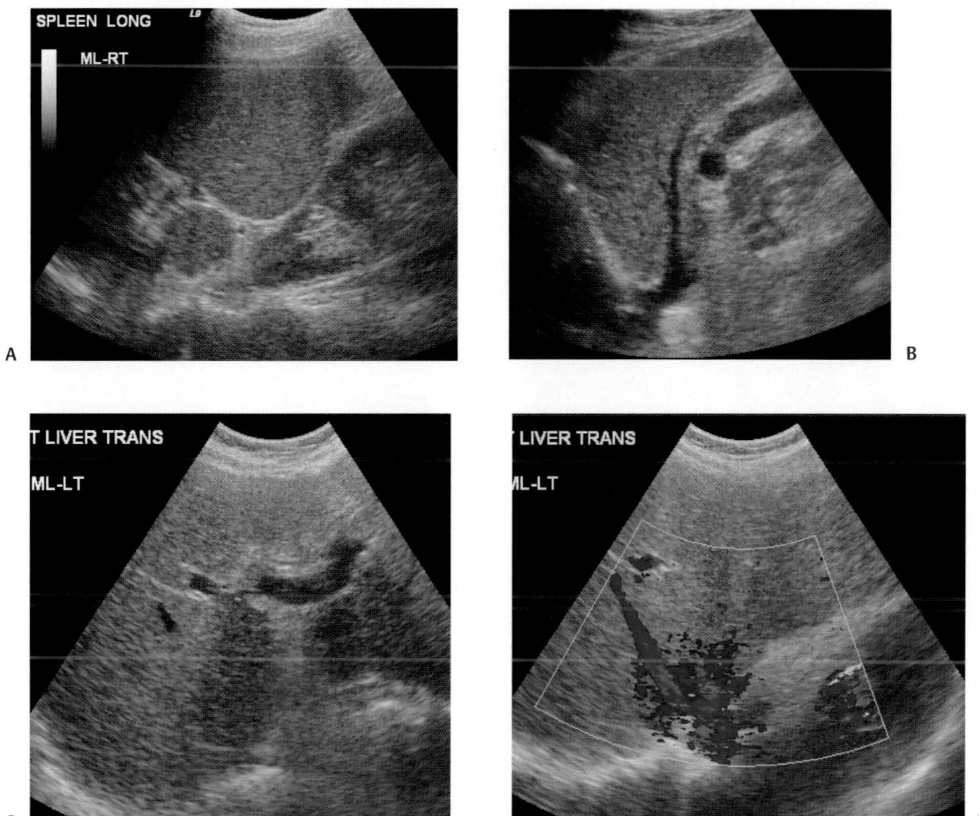

A B C D

Clinical Presentation

A 60-year-old woman with abdominal pain.

Further Work-up

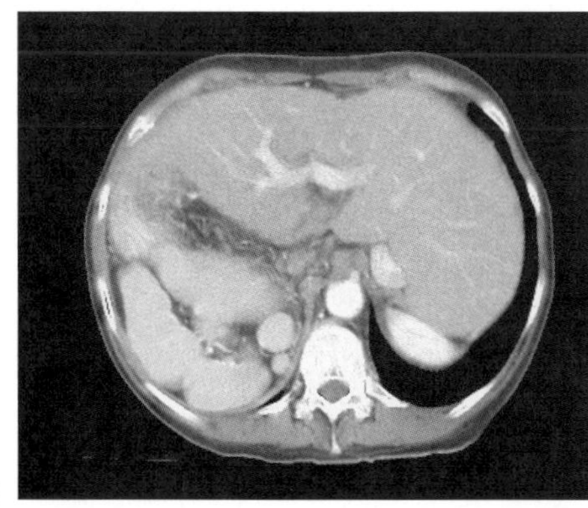

E

Imaging Findings

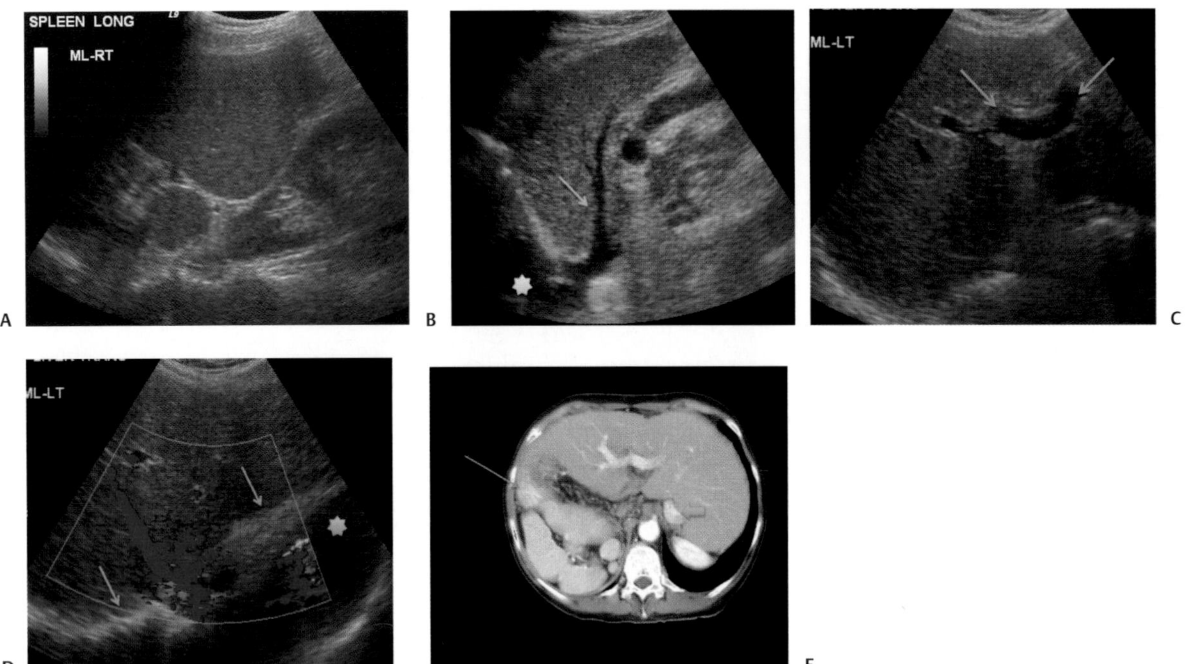

(A) Longitudinal view of the right upper quadrant reveals multiple solid masses in the expected location of the liver. **(B)** Longitudinal image of the left upper quadrant demonstrates a draining vein (*arrow*) into the heart (*asterisk*). **(C)** Transverse image in the midepigastrium demonstrating the right and left portal veins (*arrows*). **(D)** Transverse color Doppler image in the left upper quadrant reveals the confluence of the hepatic veins adjacent to the heart. *Asterisk* denotes the cardiac apex. *Arrows* denote the diaphragm. **(E)** Multiple solid masses are present in the right upper quadrant on CT. The liver is predominantly left sided. There is a right-sided stomach (*thin arrow*). The intrahepatic cava (*thick arrow*) is to the left of the aorta. Multiple spleens are present in the right upper quadrant.

Differential Diagnosis

- ***Polysplenia with abdominal heterotaxy:*** Multiple small spleens in the right upper quadrant, midline or left-sided liver, right-sided stomach, and left-sided IVC are consistent with polysplenia and abdominal heterotaxy.
- *Polysplenia without heterotaxy:* Polysplenia can occur without abdominal heterotaxy, but the spleens would be present in the left upper quadrant.
- *Wandering spleen:* A wandering spleen is usually a solitary spleen often located in the lower, abdomen or pelvis. In the setting of a wandering spleen the liver would be present in the right upper quadrant.

Essential Facts

- Heterotaxy syndrome includes polysplenia and asplenia. There are overlapping findings in asplenia and polysplenia.
- Polysplenia is a complex congenital syndrome characterized by variable visceral heterotaxia (situs ambiguous). Associated cardiovascular anomalies are variable.
- Situs inversus is complete mirror image of situs solitus. Situs ambiguous (heterotaxy) can be bilateral right or left sided. Polysplenia is bilateral left sidedness, asplenia is bilateral right sidedness.
- The multiple spleens in polysplenia can vary in size and number. There can be multiple similar-sized spleens or a dominant spleen with multiple much smaller spleens.
- As seen in this case, polysplenia typically has multiple spleens in the right upper quadrant, a right-sided stomach, left-sided or midline liver, and a short pancreas.

✓ Pearls & × Pitfalls

× Polysplenia can occur with left-sided spleens.
× Multiple accessory spleens can mimic polysplenia with normal situs.
× There is no single pathognomonic anomaly seen with polysplenia, though an interrupted IVC is the most common finding.
✓ The spleens are always on the same side as the stomach with heterotaxy.
✓ Cardiac anomalies are less common in polysplenia and not as complex as asplenia.

Case 69

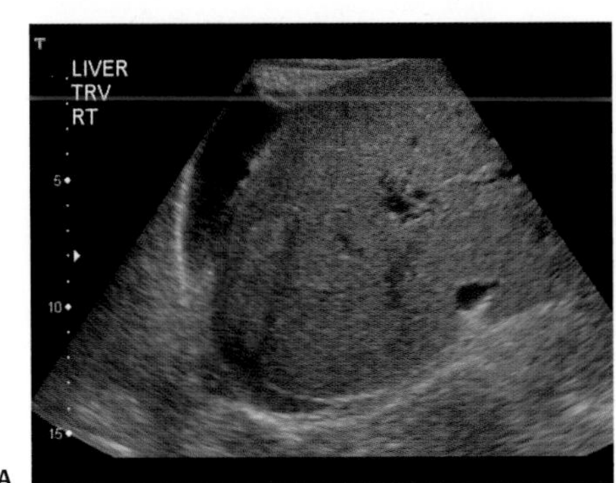

A

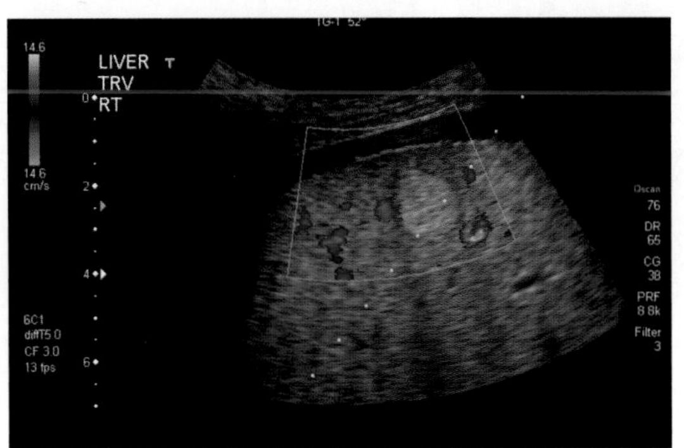

B

Clinical Presentation

A 47-year-old man with history of hepatitis C presents for evaluation of focal hepatic lesion.

Further Work-up

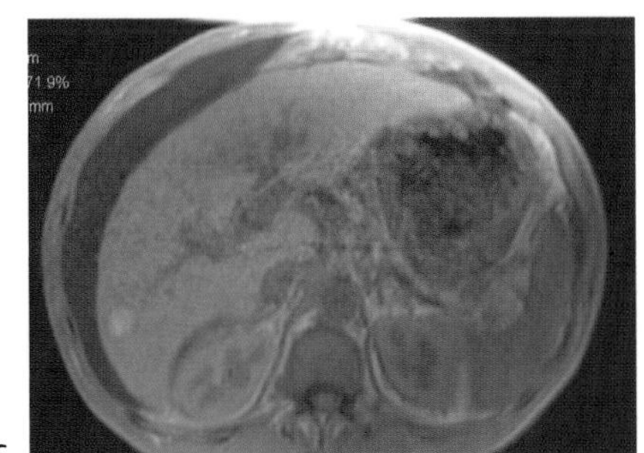
C

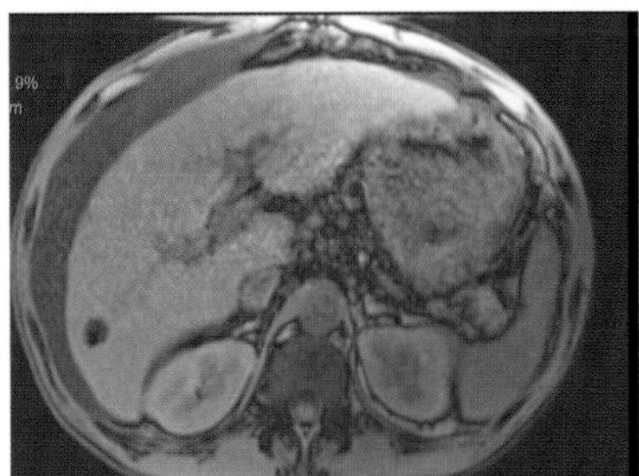
D

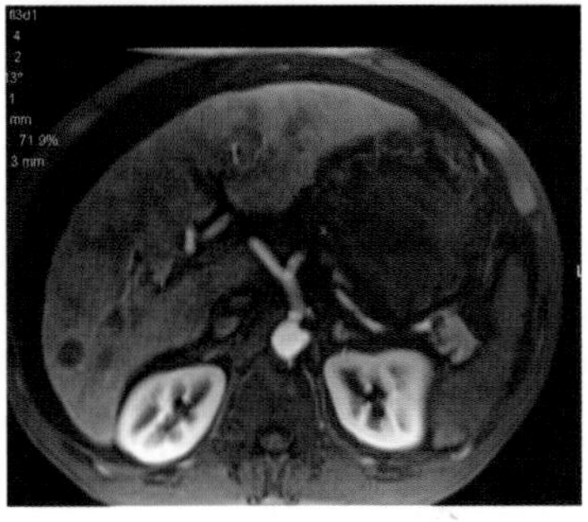
E

Imaging Findings

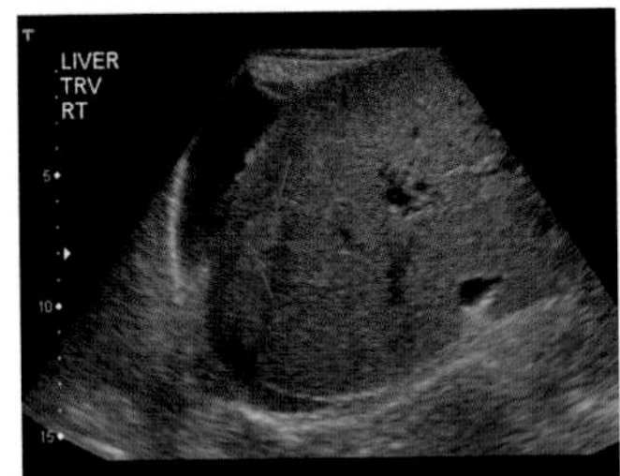

A

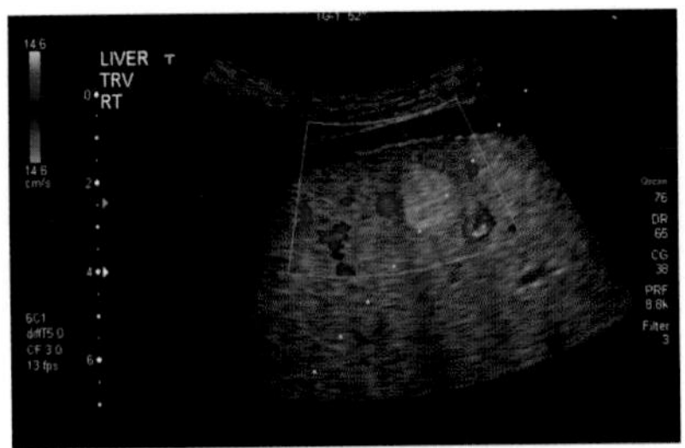

B

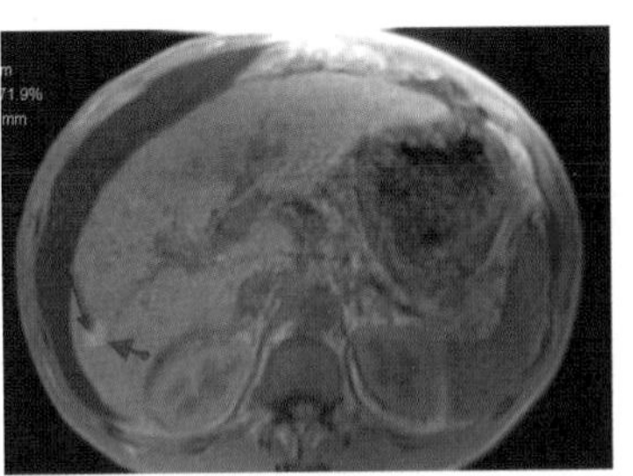

C

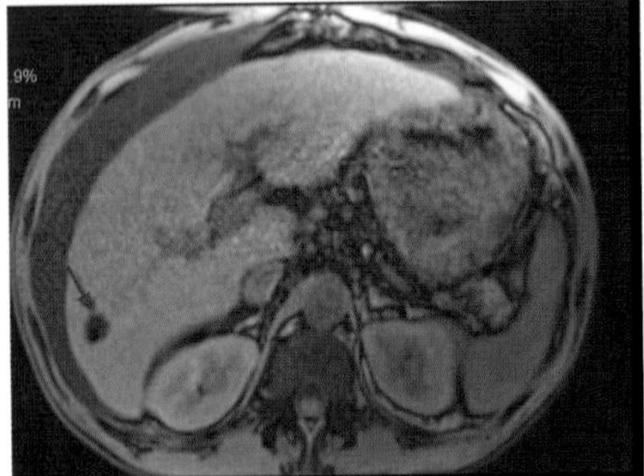

D

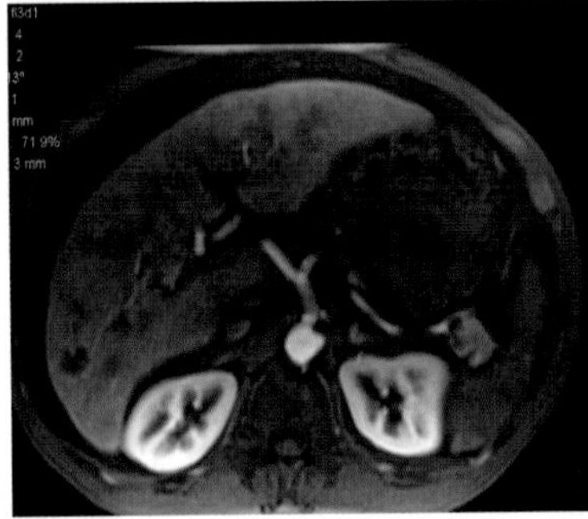

E

(A, B) Ultrasound images of the liver demonstrate echogenic mass in segment 6 of the liver (*red arrows*) with possible hypoechoic rim (*green arrow*). Doppler ultrasound images demonstrate no significant flow within the mass. **(C–E)** Magnetic resonance imaging (MRI) of the liver demonstrates hyperintense lesion on T1-weighted images, with heterogeneous loss of signal on the out-of-phase images suggestive of patchy deposit of fat within the lesion (*red arrow*). The postcontrasted images demonstrate what appears to be peripheral enhancement. A hypointense rim is also visualized on the T1-weighted images (*green arrow*).

Differential Diagnosis

- ***Fat-containing hepatocellular carcinoma:*** Fat could be visualized mainly in small hepatocellular carcinoma. The deposit of fat is usually patchy and irregular within the lesion. The lesion appears echogenic on ultrasound, with occasional visualization of enhanced through transmission. Signal loss on the out-of-phase images, with hyperintense appearance on the in-phase images is noted on MRI, confirming the presence of fat. The enhancement pattern could be atypical.
- *Hepatic hemangioma:* The most common benign hepatic tumor. The most common sonographic appearance is an echogenic, well-defined mass with enhanced through transmission. An isoechoic and/or hypoechoic appearance is less likely. On MRI images, hemangiomas are bright on T2 images with peripheral nodular interrupted enhancement on the postcontrasted images. The lesion retains contrast on the delayed postcontrast images.
- *Hepatic adenoma:* More common in young women with a history of oral contraceptive usage. The sonographic appearance of hepatic adenomas is nonspecific; it could be hypoechoic, hyperechoic, and/or isoechoic to the liver. The lesion appears more complex in cases of superimposed complications such as hemorrhage. A homogeneous distribution of fat within the lesion is noted on MRI imaging, which in the appropriate clinical setting is suggestive of the diagnosis.

Essential Facts

- Hepatocellular carcinoma is the most common primary hepatic malignancy.
- Smaller lesion (< 1.5 cm) could be associated with fatty deposits.
- Fatty deposits in the tumor could be seen in up to 35% of small hepatocellular carcinomas.
- The presence of fat in hepatocellular carcinoma is usually patchy, in contrast to adenoma where fatty deposition is more uniform.
- Fat-containing hepatocellular carcinoma appears echogenic on ultrasound, with increased signal intensity on T1-weighted images. Asymmetric loss of signal on the out-of-phase image is noted.
- The hyperintense appearance on T1-weighted images could also be related to presence of glycogen and/or hemorrhage within the lesion.
- The presence of hypoechoic rim along the margins of the lesions could be related to surrounding edema and usually implies aggressive lesion.

✓ Pearls & × Pitfalls

✓ The presence of a hypoechoic rim along hepatic lesion implies surrounding edema; an aggressive lesion-like infection and/or malignancy should be considered.

× The presence of an echogenic mass lesion in the liver should not be always interpreted as a benign lesion. An echogenic malignancy such as fat-containing hepatocellular carcinoma and/or echogenic metastasis (likely renal cell carcinoma) should be in the differential diagnosis.

Case 70

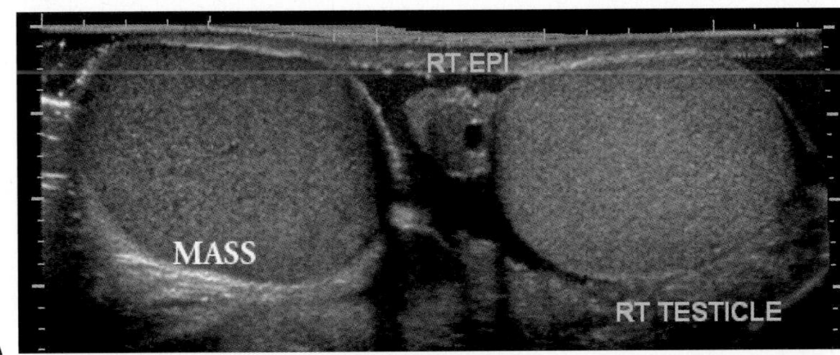

A

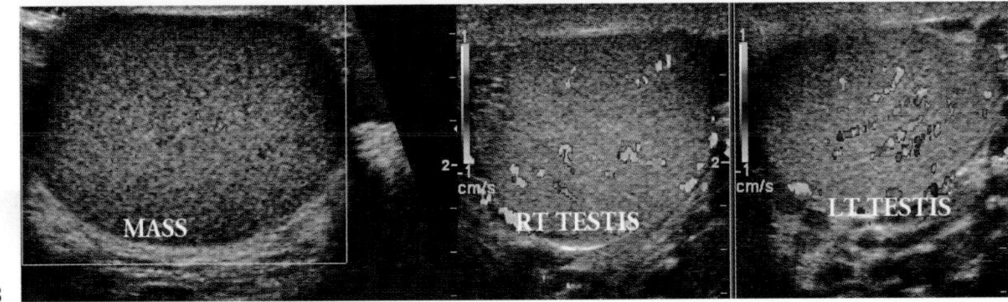

B

■ Clinical Presentation

A 58-year-old man with a slowly enlarging right scrotal mass located superior and lateral to the right testicle.

Imaging Findings

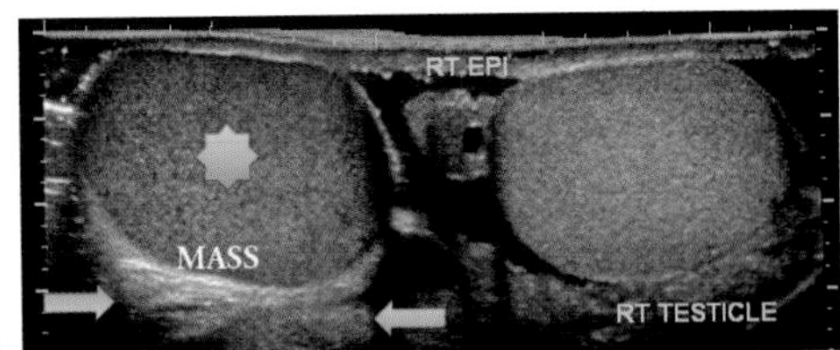

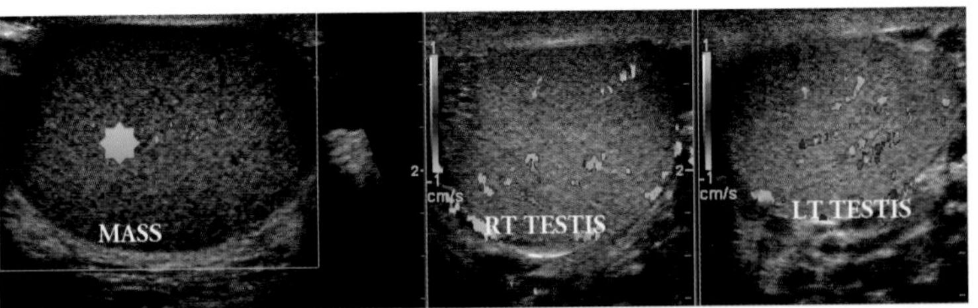

(A) Transverse image through the palpable lesion (*asterisk*) immediately deep to the skin. It is clearly separate from the epididymis (marked) and right testicle. Note the acoustic enhancement deep to the lesion (*arrows*). **(B)** Color Doppler images through the lesion (*asterisk*) and both testicles demonstrates normal and symmetric flow in the testicles but no flow in the lesion. The palpable lesion is otherwise very similar in appearance to the testicles.

Differential Diagnosis

- ***Pseduotestis appearance of an epidermoid:*** A nonvascular lesion that mimics a testicle in a hair-bearing area is consistent with epidermal inclusion cyst. It has been described as a pseudotestis in appearance.
- *Spermatocele*: Spermatoceles are less echogenic and are located within the epididymis.
- *Polyorchidism:* Although the gray scale appearance of the lesion mimics a testicle, no internal vascularity is identified as would be present in a testicle.

Essential Facts

- An epidermal cyst is formed by the inclusion of squamous epithelium into the subcutaneous tissues. It slowly enlarges with proliferation of keratinous debris, cholesterol, or sebaceous materials.
- They arise in hair-bearing areas including the scalp, face, neck, trunk, extremities, and scrotum. They can be congenital or acquired.
- The lesions are slow growing and usually asymptomatic. They can rupture and become painful.
- The sonographic appearance of epidermal cysts is varied. A classic appearance is the "pseudotestis pattern," as in this case. The shape and echogenicity of epidermal cyst mimic a testis.
- Subcutaneous epidermal cysts are common and benign.

Other Imaging Findings

- On computed tomography (CT) and magnetic resonance imaging, epidermal cysts are well circumscribed, low density on CT, and demonstrate signal intensities characteristic of simple cysts. They may be hyperintense on T1. They are contiguous with or extend to the skin.

✓ Pearls & × Pitfalls

✓ Epidermal cysts contain internal echoes mimicking a solid lesion.

✓ No internal vascularity should be detectable in an epidermal inclusion cyst.

× Swirling debris within an epidermal inclusion cyst can mimic flow.

× *Epidermal cyst*, *epidermal inclusion cyst*, and *epidermoid* refer to the same entity. They are often erroneously referred to as sebaceous cysts.

✓ Multiple epidermal cysts can be seen in Gardner syndrome, particularly in the face and scalp.

✓ Malignant transformation (squamous cell) is extremely rare.

Case 71

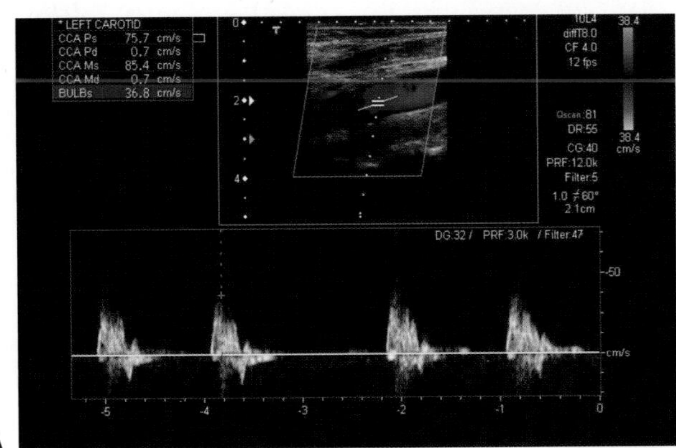

A

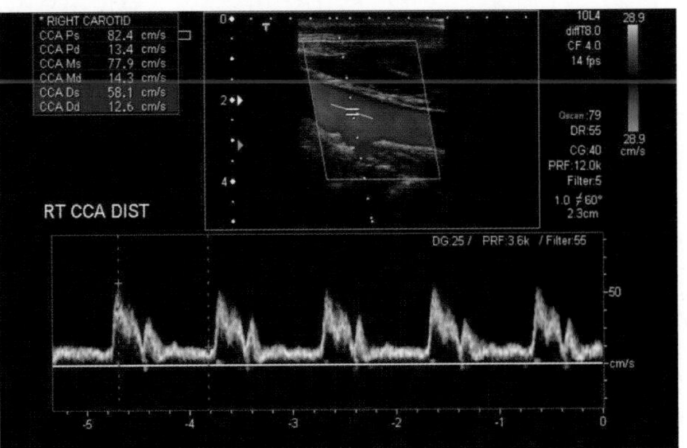

B

Clinical Presentation

An 85-year-old woman presents with a history of left retinal artery occlusion.

Further Work-up

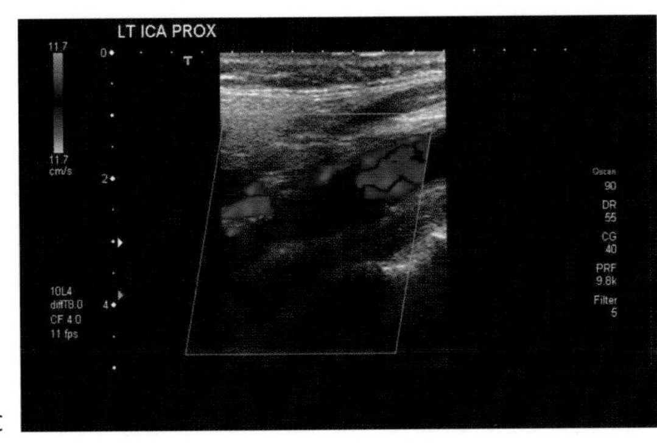

C

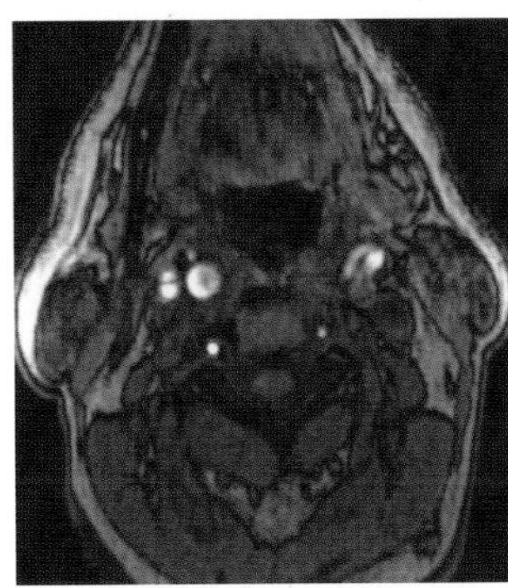
D

Imaging Findings

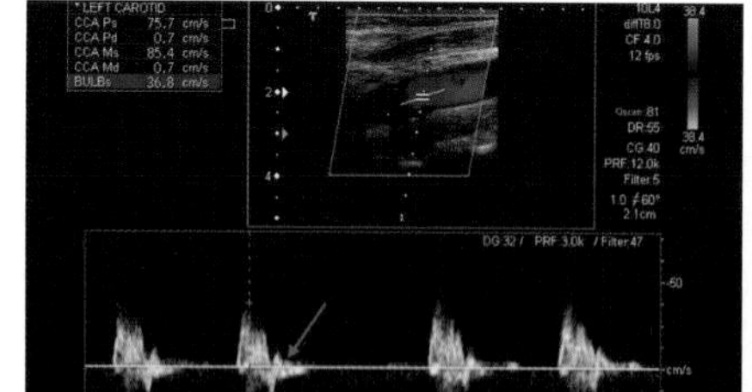

A

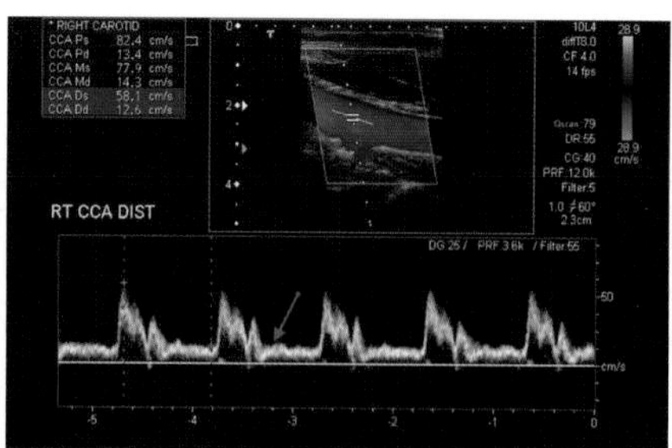

B

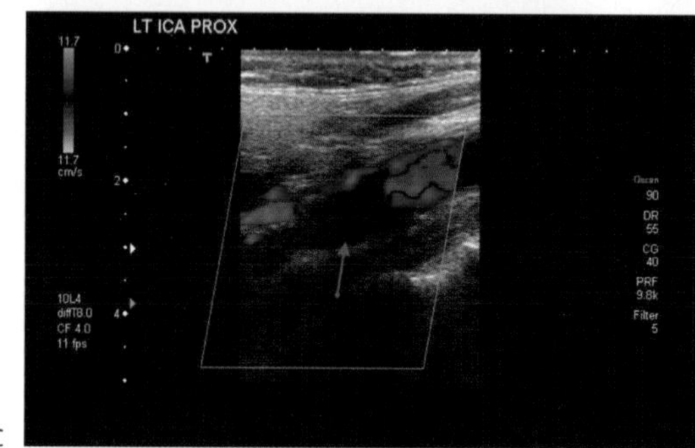

C

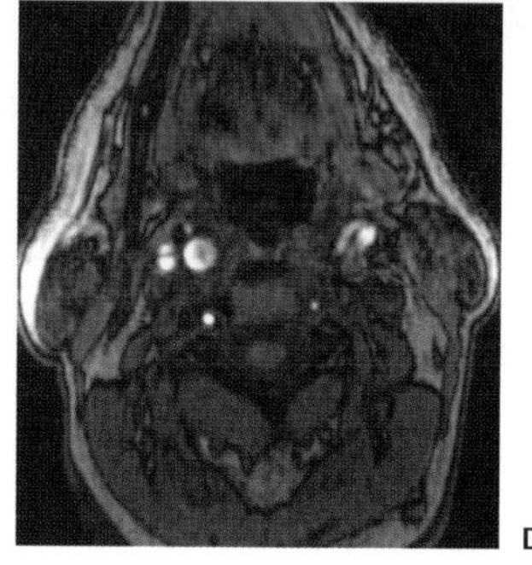

D

(A, B) Doppler ultrasound tracing of the left common carotid artery demonstrates abnormal, high-resistance waveform within the vessels with no flow/minimal reversal in diastole (*red arrow*). The flow within the right common carotid artery is a normal, low-resistance waveform with antegrade flow in diastole. **(C, D)** Further Doppler assessment of the left internal carotid artery demonstrates no evidence of flow with findings suggestive of complete occlusion (*green arrow*). No definite evidence of intimal flap was noted on ultrasound. Further evaluation with magnetic resonance angiography (MRA) of the neck confirms the sonographic findings of complete occlusion of the left internal carotid artery. No definite evidence of false lumen and/or intimal flap is visualized on MRA (*green arrow*).

Differential Diagnosis

- ***Reversal of diastolic flow secondary internal carotid occlusion:*** Doppler ultrasound demonstrates a high-resistance waveform within the carotid artery proximal to the stenosis/occlusion. This is more apparent closer to the stenosis, distal to the heart. No Doppler flow is noted within the occluded segment of the vessel. Other signs of occlusion/near occlusion include internalization of the external carotid artery and tardus parvus waveform distal to the near occlusion. Bilateral involvement of both carotids could be seen.
- *Reversal of diastolic flow secondary to internal carotid artery dissection:* The patient usually presents with episodes of headache preceding the ischemic events. Other presentations include transient ischemic attack, ptosis, neck swelling, and pulsatile tinnitus. The most common sonographic appearance is the presence of high-resistance flow or no flow on Doppler ultrasound within the occluded artery. The intimal flap is occasionally visualized on Doppler ultrasound. The false lumen is noted in 40% of cases on Doppler ultrasound.
- *Reversal of diastolic flow secondary to aortic regurgitation:* Is noted in patient with severe aortic valvular regurgitation. Abnormal reversal of flow within the common carotid artery is visualized during diastole. Depending on the severity of the aortic regurgitation, reversal of flow may be limited to early diastole or noted throughout diastole. Reversal of flow is noted bilaterally, more apparent when tracing obtained closer to the heart.

Essential Facts

- Stroke is one of the leading causes of death in developed countries, the majority related to atherosclerotic disease.
- The Doppler tracing demonstrates low-amplitude waveform with reversal and/or absent antegrade diastolic flow.
- Usually visualized proximal to complete and/or near complete occlusion of the carotid artery.
- Could also be visualized as a sign of aortic dissection; an attempt to visualize the intimal flap should be made.
- Bilateral high-resistance waveform can be seen secondary to increased intracranial pressure and/or diffuse vasospasm.
- Bilateral high-resistance waveform could also be seen secondary to bilateral carotid atherosclerotic disease.
- In case of diastolic flow reversal associated with aortic regurgitation, the reversal of diastolic flow is more pronounced closer to the heart.
- Parvus tardus waveform is visualized distal to critical stenosis, high-resistance proximal to the stenosis.
- Internalization of the external carotid artery also could be a sign of complete occlusion of the internal carotid artery

✓ Pearls & ✗ Pitfalls

✓ Reversal of flow in diastole secondary to aortic regurgitation is more apparent closer to the heart; however, reversal of flow in diastole secondary to stenosis is more apparent distal to the heart, closer to the stenosis.

✗ To-and-fro flow secondary to pseudoaneurysm in the neck could be reflected into the carotid tracing and misinterpreted as reversal of flow in diastole. Close attention should be made to exclude a pseudoaneurysm.

Case 72

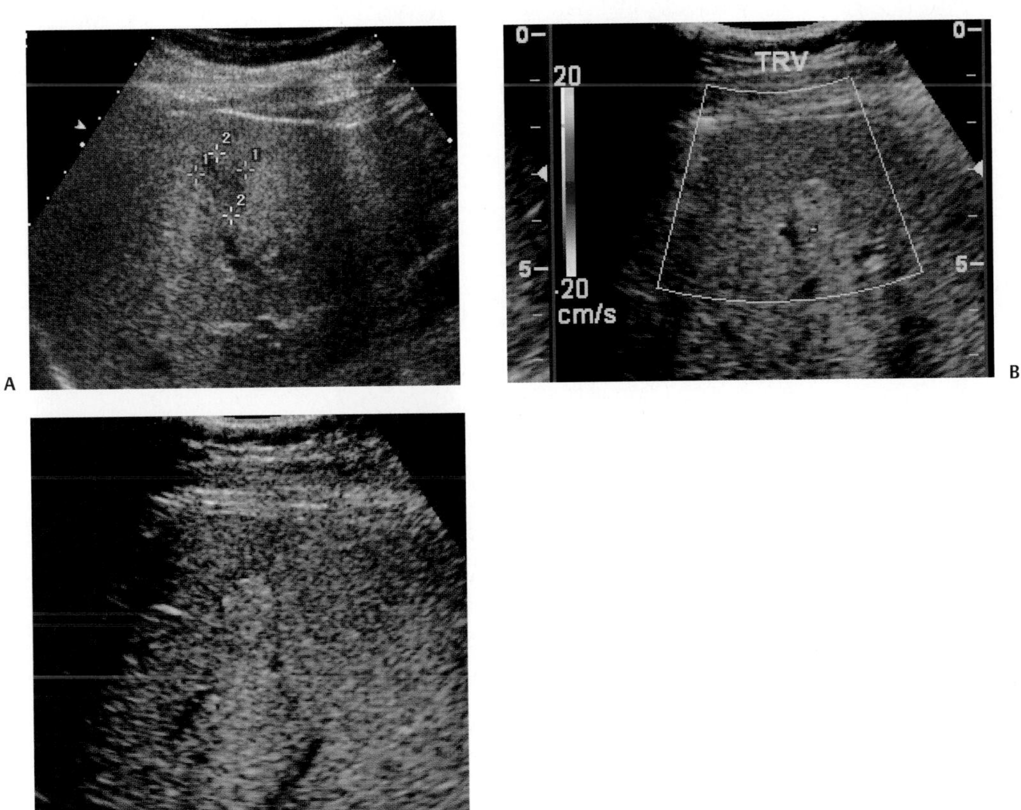

Clinical Presentation

A 55-year-old woman with newly diagnosed diabetes mellitus. In review of prior studies, images **B** and **C** were performed one year earlier.

Further Work-up

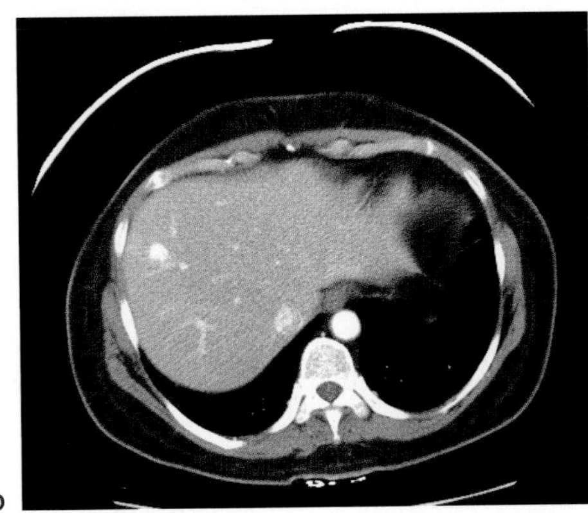

Imaging Findings

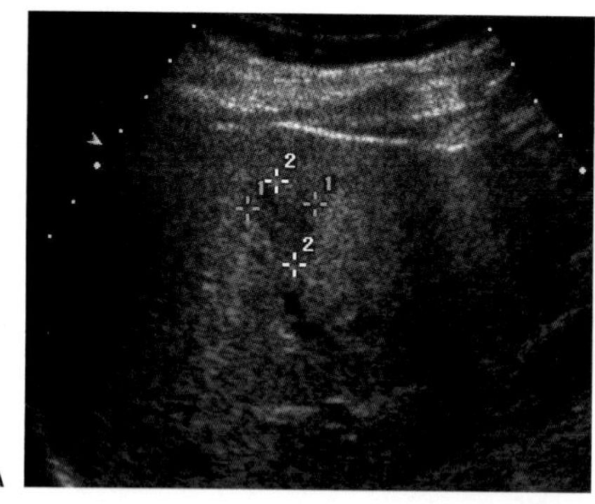
A

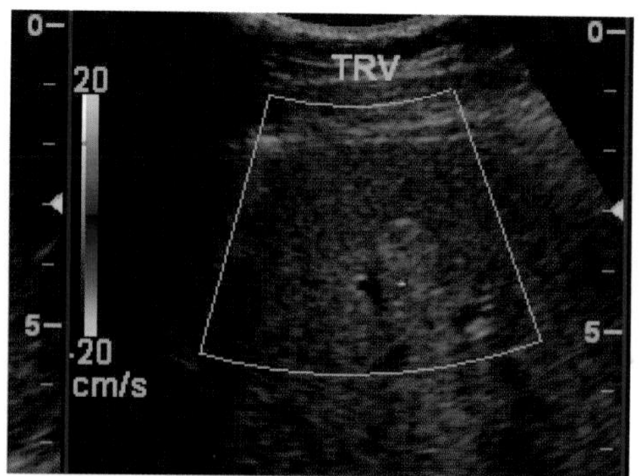

B

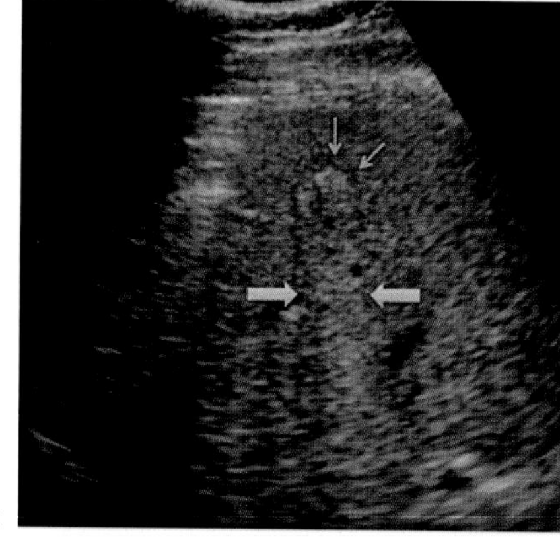
C

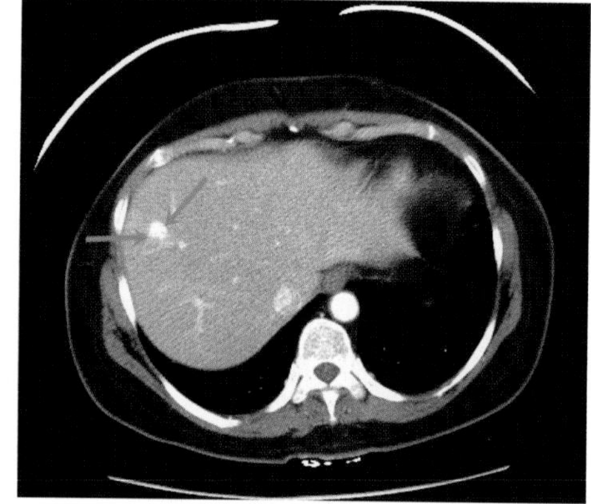
D

(A) There is a 2 cm hypoechoic lesion in a background of a fatty liver. In review of prior studies **(B, C)** the lesion was previously echogenic, well-circumscribed and faceted in configuration. *Thin arrows* denote the angulated margins. Note acoustic enhancement (*thick arrows*) **(D)** Post contrast CT reveals an enhancing lesion (*arrows*) which is isodense with the venous pool.

Differential Diagnosis

- ***Hemangioma in a fatty liver:*** A stable lesion that is well circumscribed, faceted in configuration, and demonstrates acoustic enhancement is consistent with a hemangioma. A hemangioma may appear hypoechoic in a fatty liver.
- *Hepatic metastasis:* The most common echogenic metastases are from a colon primary. They will not be geographic in configuration or stable over time. Metastases are usually multiple.
- *FNH:* Usually isoechoic to liver and therefore difficult to detect. They may contain a central scar.

Essential Facts

- Hepatic hemangiomas are the most common benign hepatic neoplasm and occur in 1 to 4% of the population. They are more common in females.
- They are usually asymptomatic, but large hemangiomas can cause symptoms related to mass effect.
- Sonographic features of hemangiomas include the following:
  - Usually echogenic
  - Well circumscribed with geographic or angulated margins
  - Exhibit distal sonic enhancement
  - Internal vascularity can be detected in about half of all lesions.
- With newer ultrasound machines and enhanced imaging, hemangiomas contain tiny anechoic regions representing the vascular channels. Additionally, a very thin hypoechoic halo may be detectable.

✓ Pearls & × Pitfalls

✓ Hemangiomas can be hypoechoic in the setting of fatty infiltration of the liver but echogenic in a normal liver without fatty infiltration as in this case.

✓ Classic hemagiomas in a patient with no risk factors do not require further evaluation.

× Hemangiomas can be atypical, and further imaging may be required to exclude malignancy.

✓ Subcentimeter hemagiomas detected by ultrasound may not be detectable by computed tomography or magnetic resonance imaging.

× Flow can be detected with color Doppler in 50% of hemangiomas but not hypervascular to the liver.

Case 73

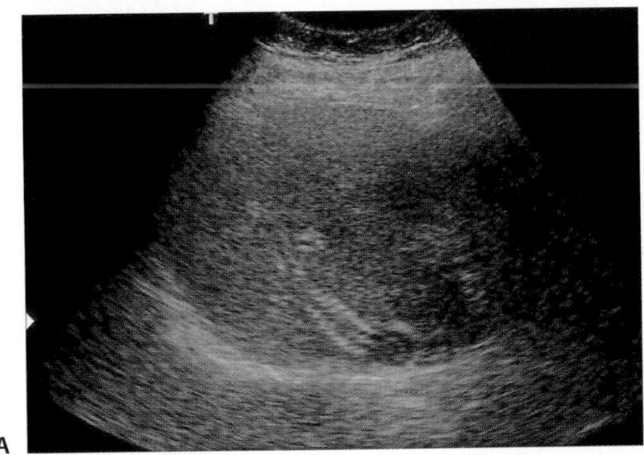
A

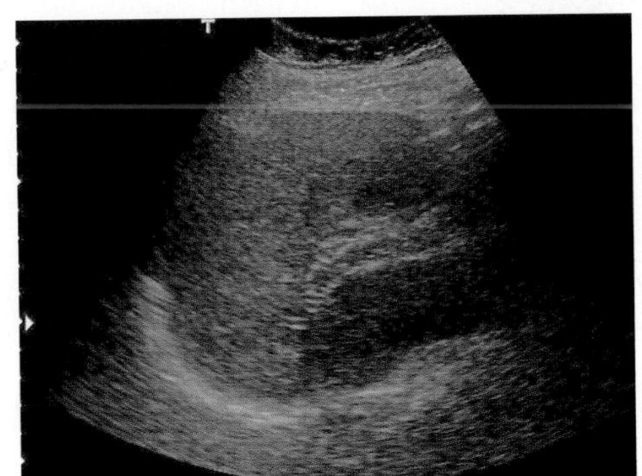
B

Clinical Presentation

A 70-year-old man with a history of portal hypertension, status post transjugular intrahepatic portosystemic shunt (TIPS) placement, presents for evaluation of TIPS patency.

Further Work-up

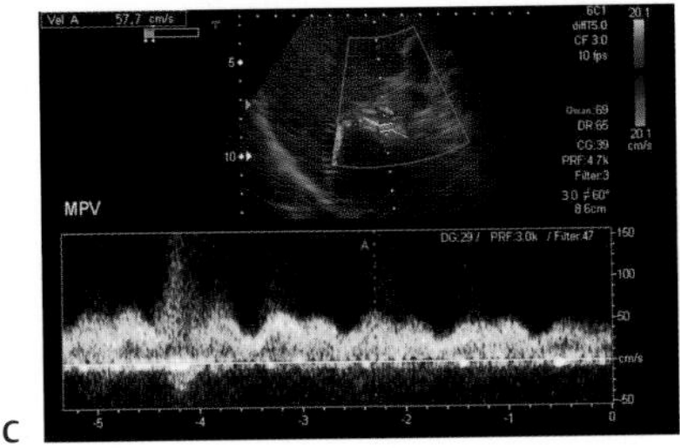

C

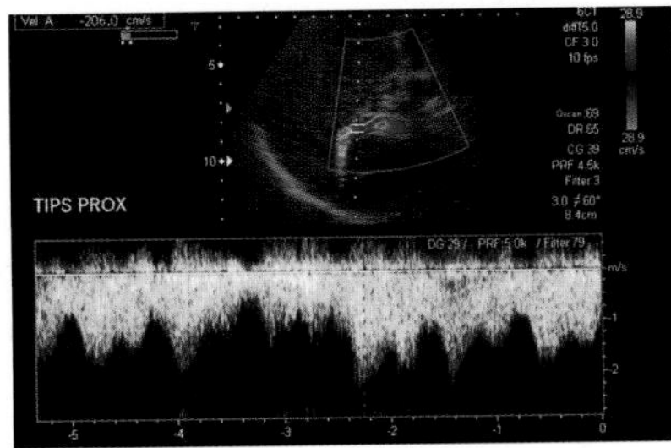

D

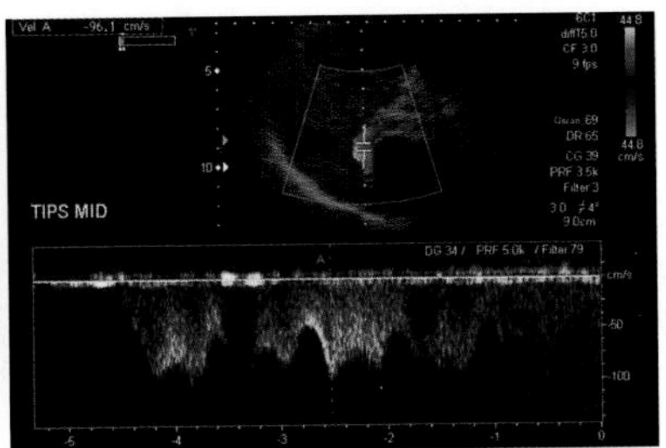

E

Imaging Findings

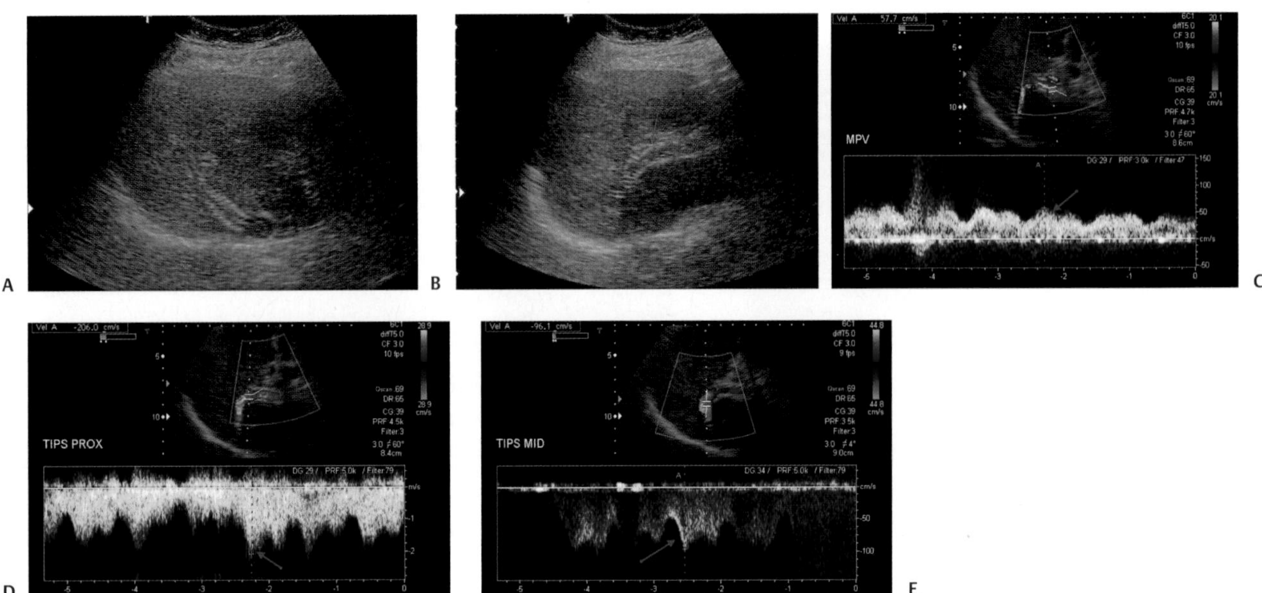

(A, B) Gray scale images of the liver demonstrating TIPS extending from the right portal vein into the right hepatic vein (*red arrows*). No significant narrowing is noted on the gray scale images. **(C–E)** Further evaluation using Doppler imaging demonstrates normal direction, antegrade flow within the main portal vein (*green arrow*, image **C**). Increased velocity is noted in the proximal segment of the TIPS (*green arrows*, images **D**, **E**), with a normal velocity present in the mid and distal segment. Pulsatile waveform within the TIPS is noted.

Differential Diagnosis

- ***Early TIPS malfunction:*** Doppler ultrasound is a reliable, noninvasive, and sensitive method for evaluation of early TIPS malfunction. The sonographic signs of early TIPS malfunction includes a focal area of increased velocity within the TIPS and/or a velocity gradient > 50 cm/sec. Secondary signs of portal hypertension are not seen.
- *Normal Doppler evaluation of TIPS:* The sonographic signs suggestive of normal flow in the TIPS includes normal velocity (< 200 cm/sec and > 50 cm/sec), a velocity gradient < 50 cm/sec throughout the TIPS, pulsatile waveform within the main portal vein, and reversal of flow within the intrahepatic portal system distal to the TIPS. The velocity in the portal vein is > 30 cm/sec.
- *TIPS malfunction*: The clinical presentation includes ascites, splenomegaly, and/or gastrointestinal bleeding. The sonographic signs of TIPS malfunction are detected before the clinical manifestations. This includes the presence of focal areas of increased velocity within the TIPS (> 200 cm/sec), no flow within the TIPS on color and/or power Doppler, antegrade flow within the intrahepatic portal vein distal to the TIPS, and secondary signs of portal hypertension as a delayed manifestation of TIPS malfunction.

Essential Facts

- TIPS is a widely accepted treatment for portal hypertension complications.
- Early detection of TIPS malfunction enables revision with subsequent maintaining patency of the shunt.
- Doppler ultrasound is a noninvasive, sensitive way for early assessment of TIPS malfunction.
- Venogram with pressure gradient measurement is the gold standard for evaluation of TIPS malfunction.
- The most common site of TIPS malfunction is the distal side (venous side).
- Doppler velocity should be measured at the proximal, mid, and distal segment of the TIPS.
- Doppler criteria suggestive of TIPS malfunction includes:
  - Peak TIPS velocity > 200 cm/sec and/or < 50 cm/sec.
  - Velocity gradient > 50 cm/sec within the TIPS.
  - Main portal vein velocity < 30 cm/sec.
  - Antegrade flow within the intrahepatic portal system, distal to the TIPS.
  - Loss of pulsatility within the main portal vein.

✓ Pearls & × Pitfalls

✓ Doppler tracing should be performed in any area of aliasing seen on color Doppler throughout the TIPS.

× The presence of antegrade flow within the left portal vein secondary to recannulized paraumbilical vein could be misinterpreted as antegrade flow within the left portal vein secondary to TIPS malfunction.

Case 74

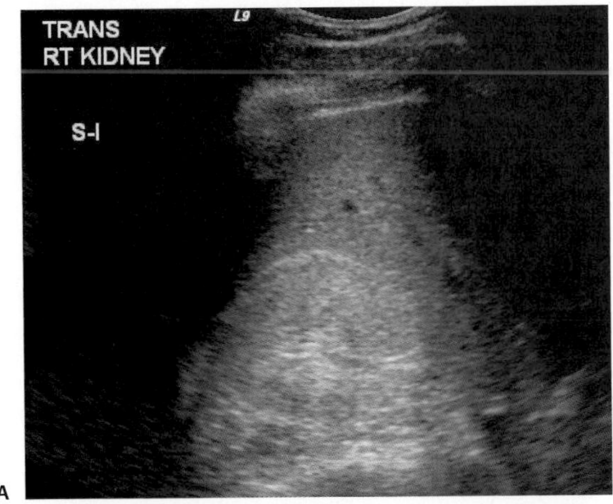

A

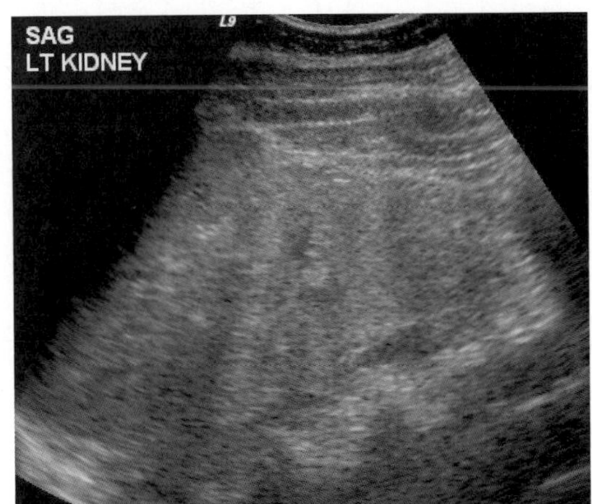

B

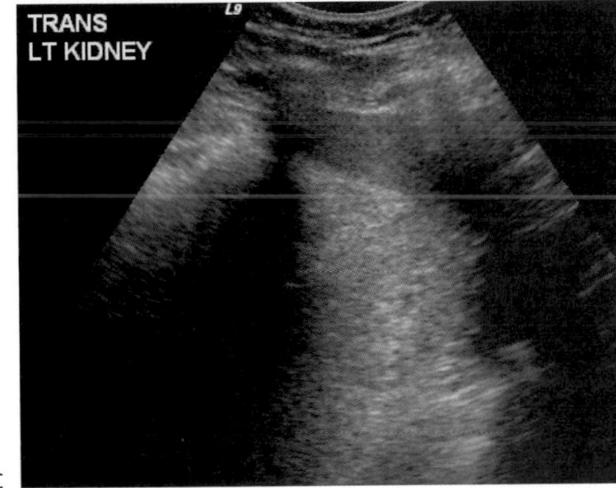

C

■ Clinical Presentation

A 51-year-old man with history of intravenous (IV) drug abuse presents to the emergency department with vomiting and is found to have markedly elevated BUN and creatinine.

Imaging Findings

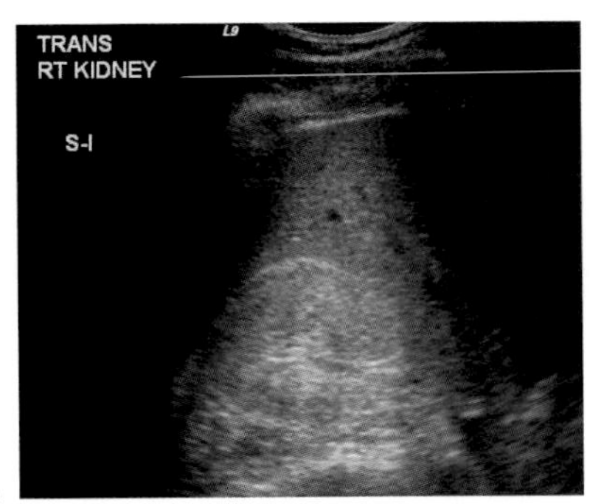

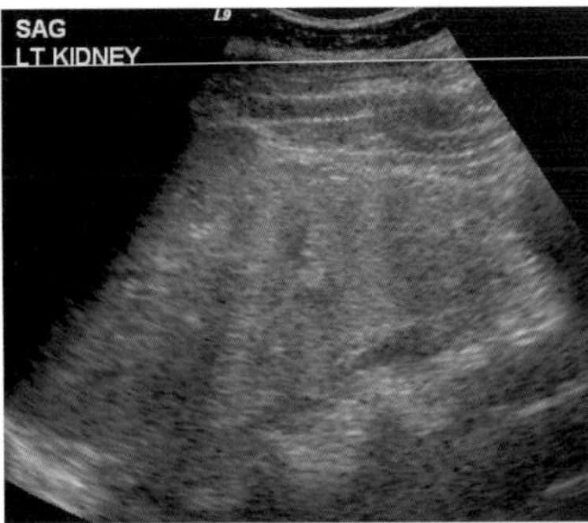

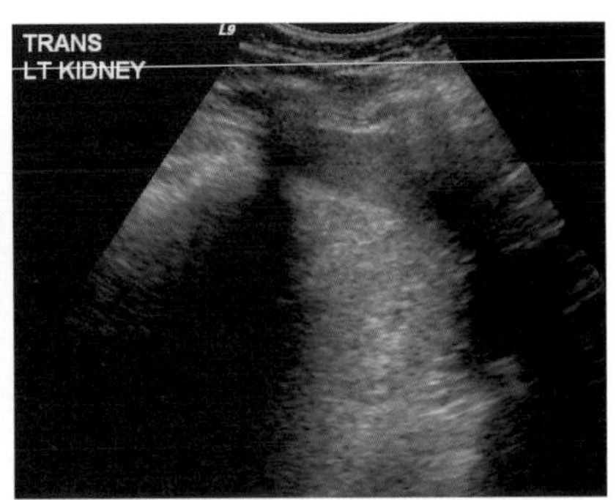

Transverse **(A, C)** and longitudinal **(B)** views of the kidneys demonstrate increased cortical echogenicity, significantly greater than the liver and spleen. It is difficult to distinguish the renal cortex from the sinus fat. The kidneys are normal in size and smooth in contour. A noncontrast computed tomography (not shown) demonstrated normal-appearing kidneys without cortical thinning. No calcifications were seen.

Differential Diagnosis

- ***Acquired immunodeficiency syndrome (AIDS) nephropathy:*** Echogenic kidneys in a patient with a history of IV drug abuse can be consistent with AIDS nephropathy.
- *Amyloidosis:* The kidneys would be enlarged and less echogenic.
- *Acute intersitial nephritis:* Usually drug induced; results in echogenic kidneys and, unlike the above kidneys, have well-defined hypoechoic pyramids.

Essential Facts

- Echogenic kidneys indicate the presence of parenchymal renal disease. Generally, ultrasound cannot distinguish one cause of parenchymal renal disease from another.
- Causes of echogenic kidneys include
  - Diabetes (most common): Normal or enlarged kidney.
  - Hypertensive nephrosclerosis: Small kidney. Often asymmetric
  - Glomerulonephritis (GN): Normal or enlarged kidney.
  - Interstitial nephritis (usually drug induced): Normal or enlarged kidney.
  - Systemic lupus erythematosus: Kidney size variable.
  - AIDS: Normal or enlarged kidney.
  - Amyloidosis: Normal or enlarged kidney.
- AIDS nephropathy is multifactorial relatated to human immunodeficiency virus (HIV)–induced glomerulosclerosis, nephrotoxic drugs, infection (MAI or *Pneumocystis carinii*).
- The echogenicity of the kidneys should be equal to or less than that of the liver and less than the spleen.
- The kidneys decrease in size with duration of disease. Cortical echogenicity increases with progression of renal failure.
- The normal size of the kidneys ranges from 9 to 13 cm.
- The normal left kidney may be up to 2 cm longer that the right, whereas the right kidney may be as much as 1.5 cm longer than the left.

✓ Pearls & × Pitfalls

- × The kidneys can appear normal even in the setting of significant renal disease.
- × The abnormal appearance of the kidneys does not correlate with the degree of renal dysfunction.
- × Biopsy is usually needed to determine the cause of parenchymal renal disease in the setting of echogenic kidneys.
- ✓ The resistive index is often elevated in the setting of parenchymal renal disease.
- × Echogenic kidneys may be missed in the setting of a fatty liver.
- × Hypoechoic medullary pyramids usually indicate parenchymal renal disease but can also be a normal finding in thin and young patients.

Case 75

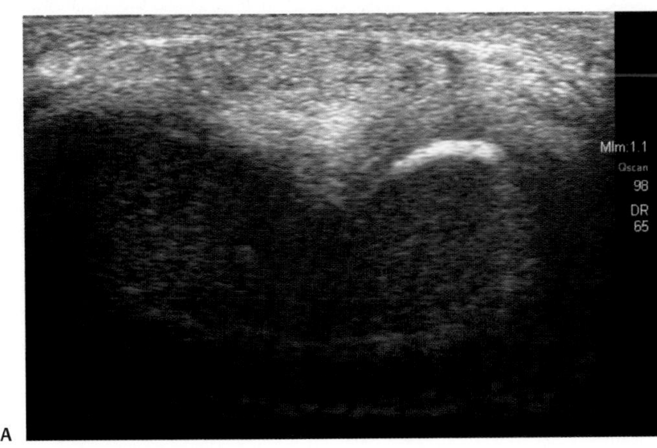

A

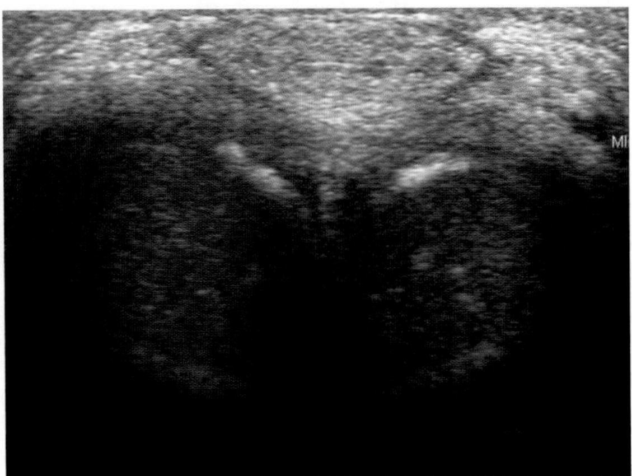

B

Clinical Presentation

A 39-year-old man presents with history of painful erection.

Further Work-up

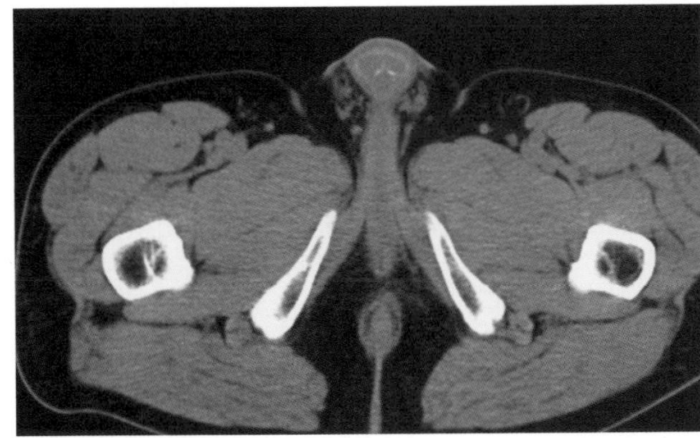

C

Imaging Findings

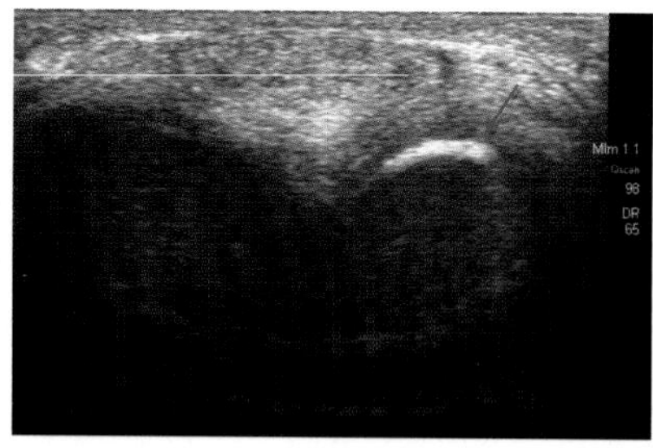
A

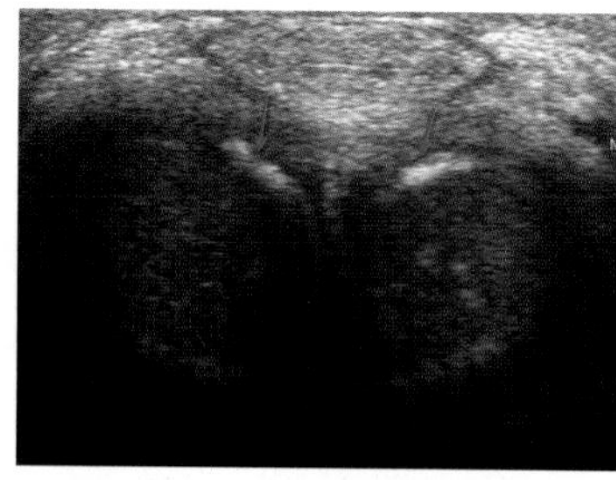
B

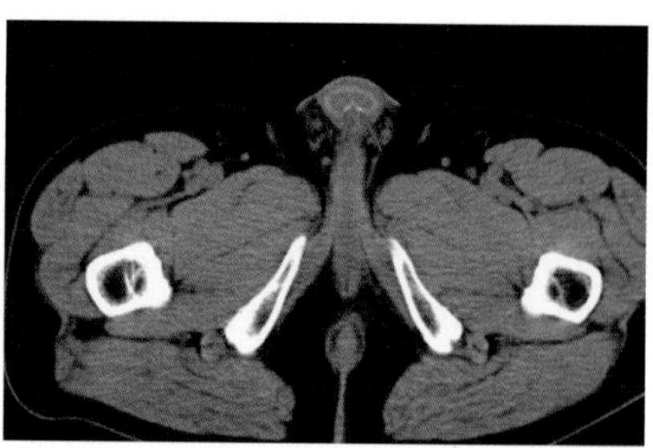
C

(A, B) Ultrasound images of the penis demonstrate multiple peripheral calcifications located predominantly medially and ventrally in the periphery of corpora cavernosa bilaterally (tunica albuginea) (*red arrows*). No definite evidence of additional masses is seen. **(C)** Computed tomography scan images of the pelvis confirm the sonographic finding of calcification within the ventral medial aspect of the corpora cavernosa (*red arrows*).

Differential Diagnosis

- ***Peyronie disease:*** The patient presents with painful erection, penile deformity, or shortening during erection. Plaque is usually felt on physical examination. Sonographically, calcified plaque within the tunica albuginea, predominantly dorsally in the corpora cavernosa, is noted. Deformities at the site of the plaque could also be present.
- *Cavernosal fibrosis secondary to local trauma:* Focal penile trauma could be related to prior invasive procedures, blunt injury, and/or injury during intercourse. The trauma could be single and/or repetitive resulting in flexion of the tunica albuginea with subsequent development of tears and bleeding. A clot formation with deposition of fibrin predispose for development of scar and plaque formation. Review of patient history reveals prior traumatic injury. Erectile deformity occasionally visualized. Sonographic evaluation of the penis demonstrates unilateral calcifications and/or focal thickening in the tunica albuginea at the site of injury. Doppler assessment usually reveals no abnormality.
- *Dorsal penile vein thrombosis:* The onset is insidious, occurring over 2 to 14 days. A palpable cord-like structure is noted on physical examination. The condition usually has no effect on erection and/or ejaculation. Doppler ultrasound evaluation demonstrates distended tubular structure at the location of the dorsal penile vein without evidence of flow. In rare cases, traumatic disruption of the dorsal penile vein could be seen with surrounding hematoma.

Essential Facts

- The incidence of Peyronie disease is 1 in 100; the average onset is 53 years.
- It is related to formation of fibrous plaque within the tunica albuginea with development of erectile pain, penile deformity, curvature, and occasionally, shortening.
- Pain is a common presentation during the early stage of Peyronie disease; painless erection is present when the scar matures.
- Ultrasound is valuable for confirmation and assessing disease extent and response to therapy.
- Tunica albuginea thickening could be visualized globally, when compared with normal patients.
- Calcified irregular plaque is visualized.
- Plaques are more often located on the dorsal aspect of the penis; however, they can occur ventrally and laterally.
- Circumscribed plaque with focal thinning of the corpora cavernosa corresponds to the site of penile bending.
- The girth of the tunica albuginea is reduced at the site of the plaque.
- Measurements of the thickness of the corpora cavernosa at multiple sides are critical in assessing the severity of the deformity.

✓ Pearls & × Pitfalls

✓ Sonographic evaluation during erection improves the diagnostic accuracy of ultrasound; multiple calcified plaques within the tunica albuginea predominantly dorsally and focal changes in thickness within the corpora cavernosa are suggestive of the diagnosis.

× The presence of a single calcified plaque within the tunica albuginea likely related to focal cavernosal fibrosis, however, could be misinterpreted as Peyronie disease; correlation with physical examination and the patient history improves the diagnostic accuracy.

Case 76

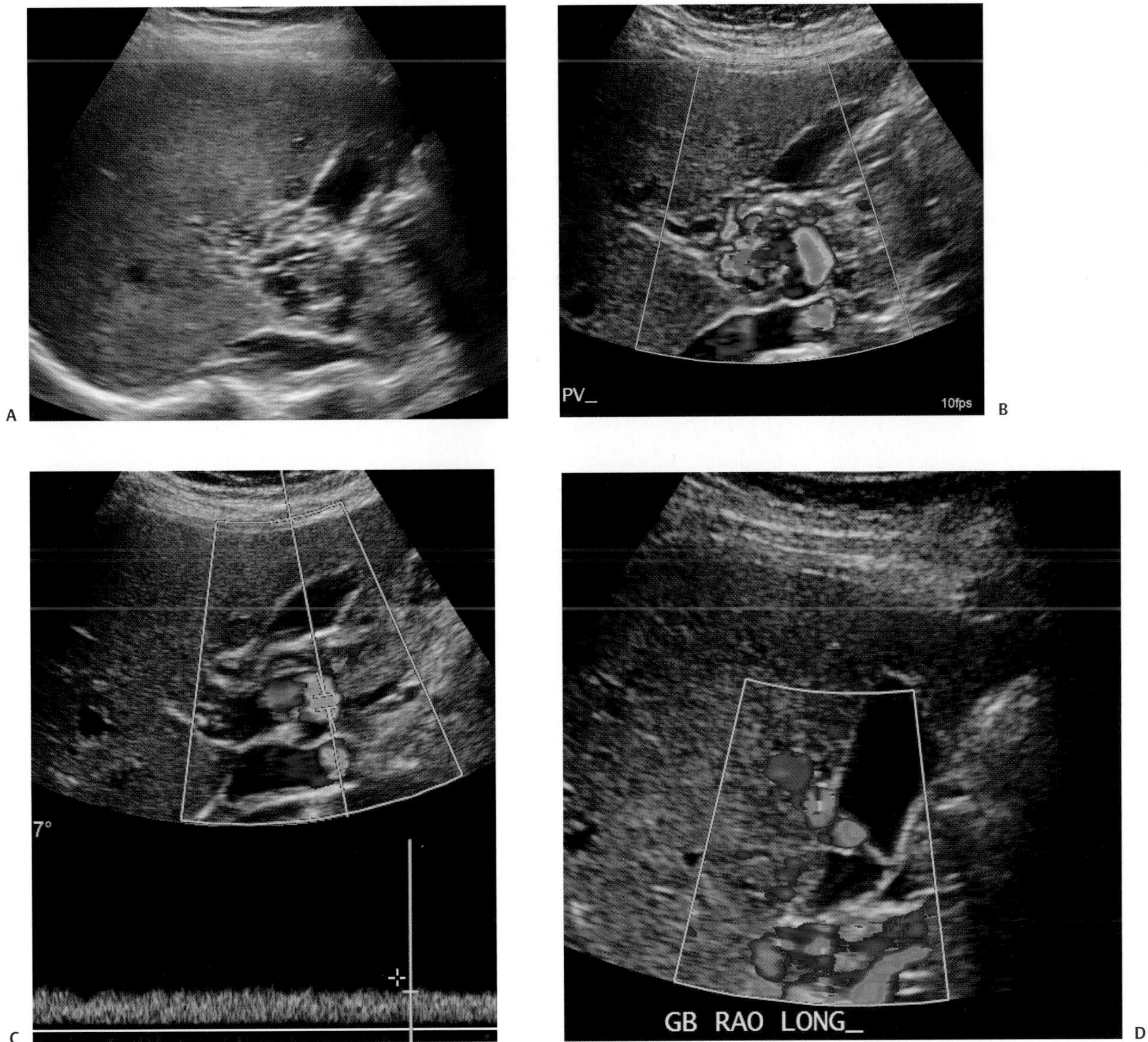

A B C D

Clinical Presentation

A 35-year-old woman recently postpartum with right upper quadrant (RUQ) pain.

Imaging Findings

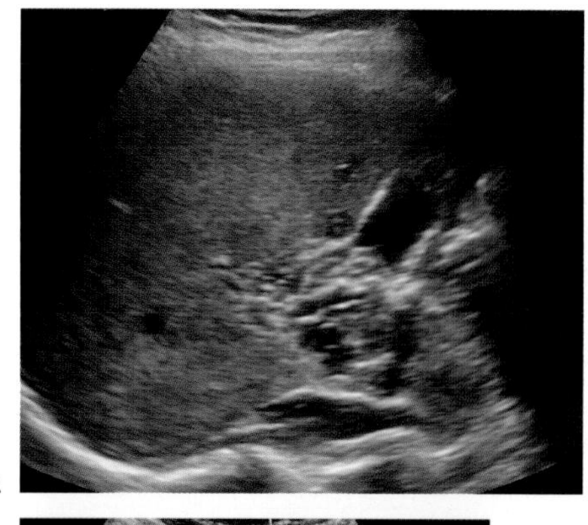
A

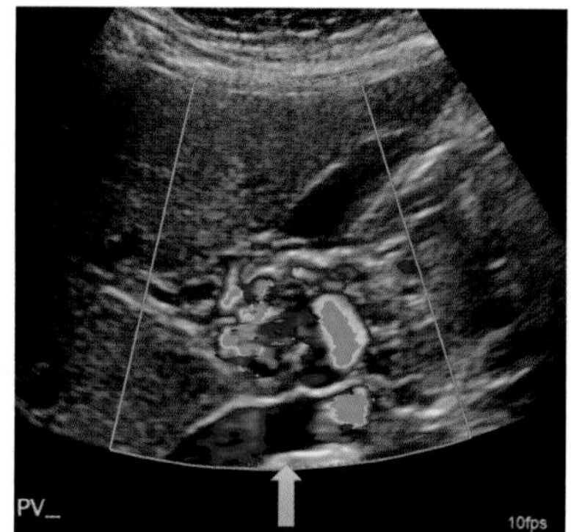

B

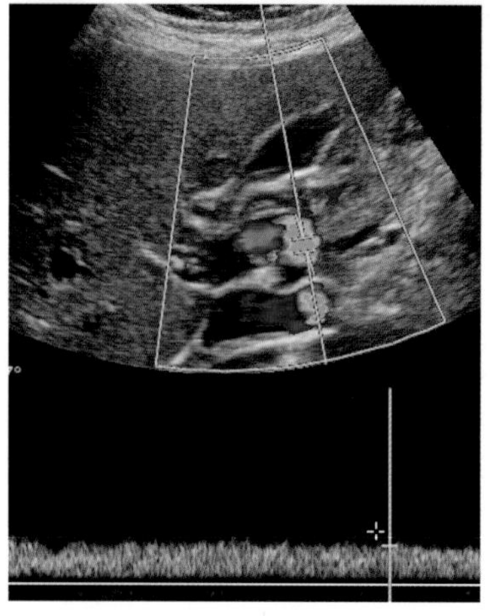
C

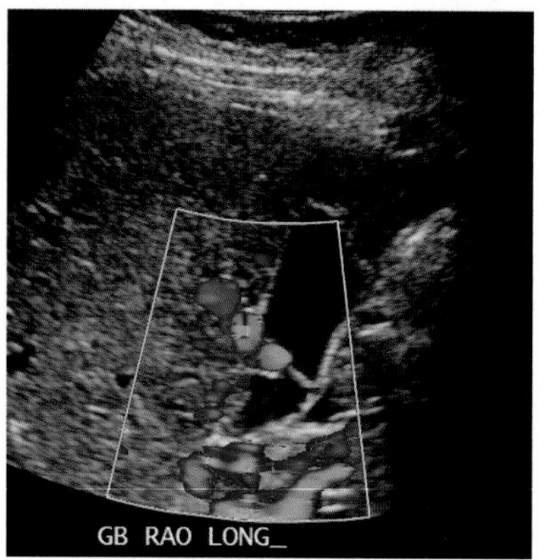

D

(A) Longitudinal view of the RUQ demonstrates a normal-appearing liver. Numerous small cystic areas are present expanding the porta hepatis. **(B)** Color Doppler confirms that these are vascular structures. A main PV is not identified. The IVC is present in the far field (*arrow*); it descends away from the porta. **(C)** Spectral Doppler demonstrates low-velocity hepatopetal flow. **(D)** Gallbladder varices are identified with color Doppler imaging.

Differential Diagnosis

- ***Cavernous transformation of the portal vein (CTPV):*** A cluster of tangled vessels in the porta that demonstrate hepatopetal venous flow and no identifiable portal vein is consistent with CTPV.
- *Vascular liver mass:* Discrete echogenic borders (see Image **D**) are seen separating this lesion from the surrounding liver indicating an extrahepatic origin.
- *Vascular tumor thrombus in the portal vein:* The portal vein enlarges when is contains tumor thrombus. Flow within malignant tumor thrombus (Striates sign) is very subtle, unlike the extensive flow seen in CTPV.

Essential Facts

- CTPV develops when venous collaterals replace an occluded portal vein. The occluded portal vein is not usually identifiable with ultrasound.
- Etiology of PV occlusion is usually unknown. In children, umbilical venous catheters in infancy are sometimes implicated, but most often the etiology is unknown. In this case the patient developed PV thrombosis with a recent pregnancy.
- CTPV appears as a mass of tubular anechoic vessels in the porta hepatis that demonstrate hepatopetal venous flow with spectral Doppler.
- CTPV is a portoportal collateral pathway and can include biliary and gastric branches of the portal vein. In this case gallbladder varices are present.
- These veins are usually insufficient to bypass the splenomesenteric inflow and therefore portal hypertension frequently coexists. Patients often present with gastroesophageal variceal bleeding. However, patients can be asymptomatic with normal liver function.
- The hepatic artery is recruited to supply the liver with oxygen. This can result in heterogeneous enhancement of the liver on computed tomography and magnetic resonance imaging.
- CTPV is a rare condition with various etiologies and diverse clinical presentations.
- Children or adults may present with complications of portal hypertension, but CTPV can also be asymptomatic.

✓ Pearls & ✗ Pitfalls

✓ Color Doppler ultrasound allows for rapid and accurate diagnosis of CTPV.

✗ Rarely CTPV can occur with a coexistent patent portal vein.

✓ Portal hypertension can be present with CTPV and therefore, when diagnosed, evaluation for ascites and splenomegaly should be conducted.

✓ Although liver disease and portal hypertension are risk factors, CTPV occurs commonly in normal livers.

Case 77

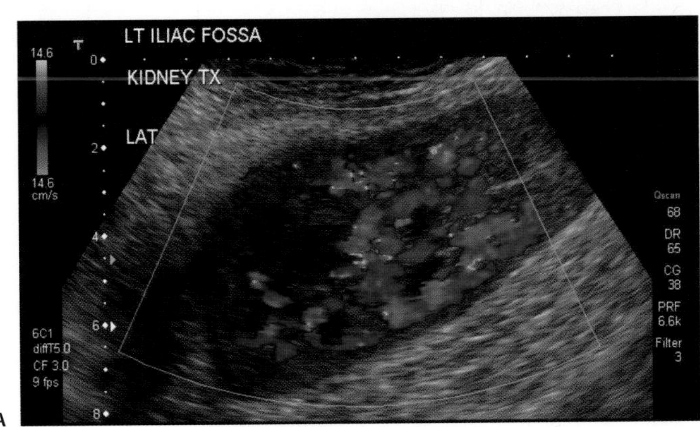

A

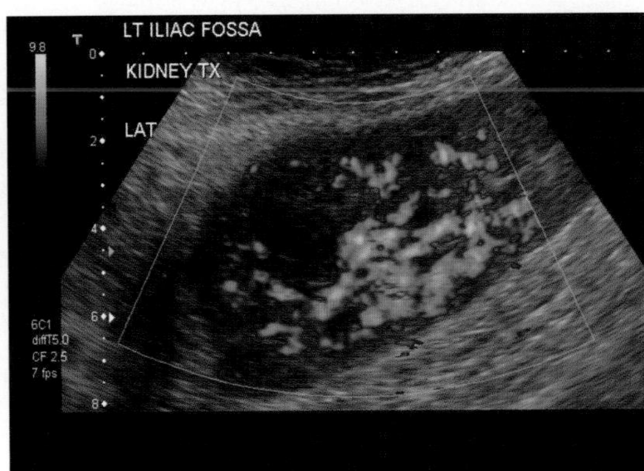

B

Clinical Presentation

A 22-year-old woman with history of renal transplant 3 years ago presents with fever and left-sided pelvic pain.

Further Work-up

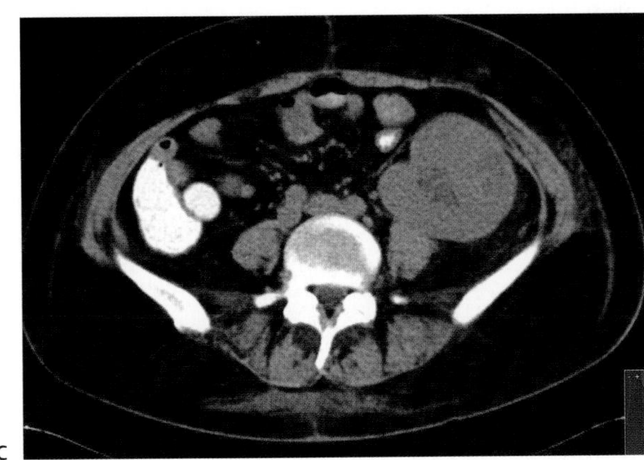

C

Imaging Finding

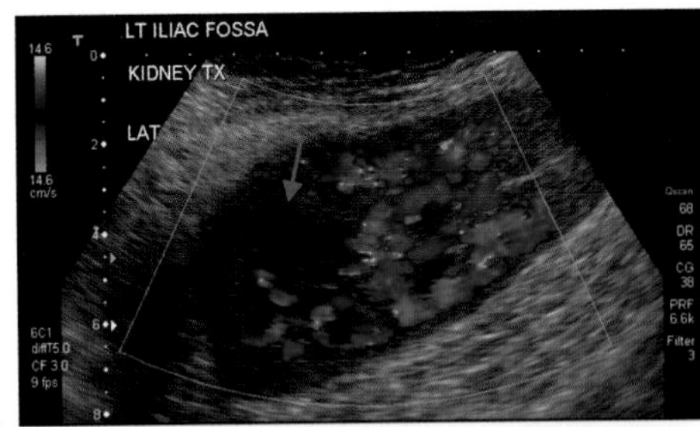

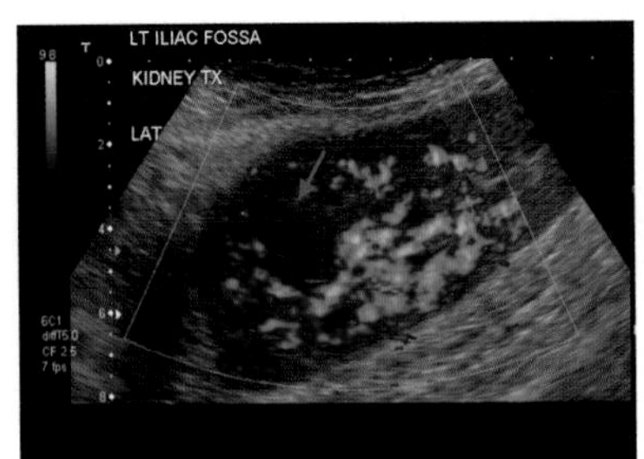

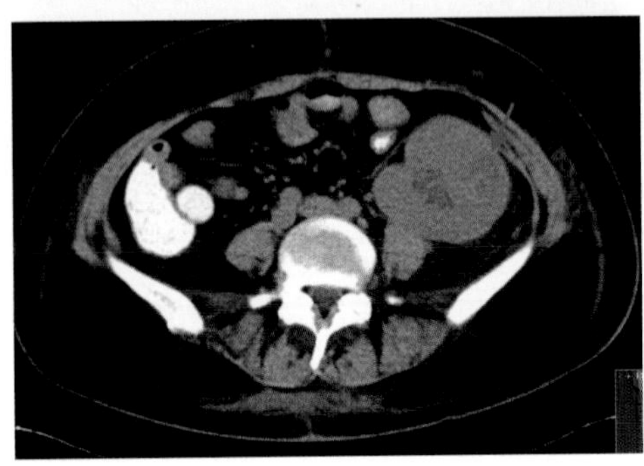

(A, B) Ultrasound images of the transplanted kidney with color demonstrate focal rounded hypoechoic area within the midpole of the transplanted kidney in the left iliac fossa (*green arrow*). No evidence of flow is noted within the questionable lesion on color Doppler. This finding was confirmed using power Doppler ultrasound. **(C)** Further evaluation using computed tomography scan without intravenous contrast of the transplanted kidney demonstrates hypodense lesion within the midpole of the transplanted kidney, corresponding to the abnormal findings seen on Doppler ultrasound (*green arrow*).

Differential Diagnosis

- ***Focal renal abscess/pyelonephritis:*** The patient presents with fever, pain, and occasionally pressure secondary to development of abscess. The sonographic appearance is nonspecific; however, the presence of complex cystic lesion with low-level echoes within the kidneys raises the suspicion of possible abscess. Early diagnosis and treatment is critical for graft survival.
- *Renal neoplasm:* Prolonged immunosuppression following renal transplant increases the risk of renal malignancy. The average reported malignancy is 6% in patients with renal transplant. The most common focal renal lesion is adenocarcinoma, with the majority of cases occurring in the native kidneys. This is presumably related to hemodialysis. The sonographic appearance is a hypoechoic renal lesion and or echogenic renal lesion. The lesion is usually hyperemic.
- *Renal infarct:* Could be segmental and/or diffuse. The etiologies include acute rejection, renal artery thrombosis, and/or vasculitis. Swelling and tenderness over the graft area is noted clinically. The typical sonographic appearance includes poorly marginated wedged-shaped hypoechoic area. Focal area of decreased flow is also present on Doppler and power ultrasound.

Essential Facts

- More than 80% of renal transplant recipients experience at least one episode of infection within the first year after transplantation.
- Early diagnosis and intervention minimize the risk of graft loss.
- Infections are divided into early posttransplant and late posttransplant infection.
- The patient presents with fever of unknown origin, pain, and/or symptoms related to pressure from abscess formation.
- In a transplanted patient with fever, any peritransplant fluid collection should be considered infected.
- The sonographic appearance is variable, including focal increased and/or decreased echogenicity.
- Abscesses usually have a complex cystic nonspecific appearance on ultrasound. The presence of gas improved the accuracy of ultrasound.
- The presence of an echogenic mass within a transplanted kidney raises the suspicion of fungal ball.

✓ Pearls & × Pitfalls

✓ Visualization of echogenic lesion within a transplanted kidney in a patient with sign of infection should raise the suspicion for possible fungal ball.

× The clinical presentation and imaging findings of renal infarct and focal pyelonephritis/abscess could overlap. The presence of complex rounded cystic lesion is suggestive of an abscess.

Case 78

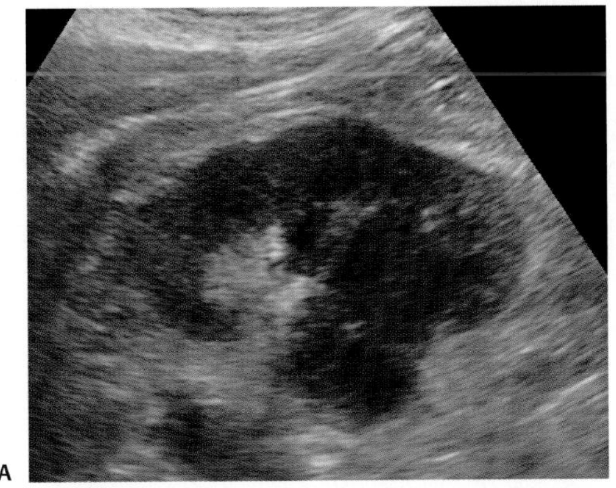
A

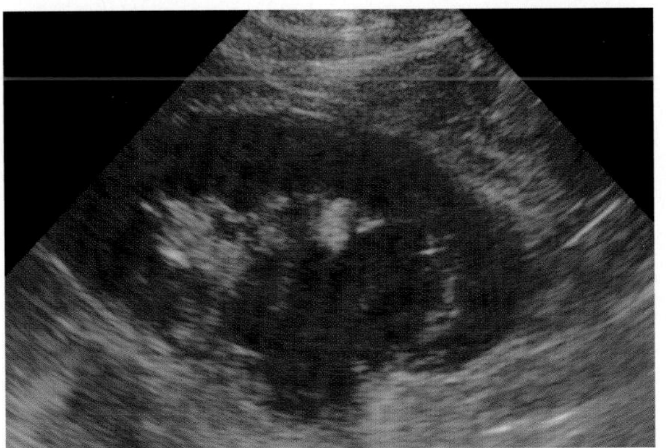
B

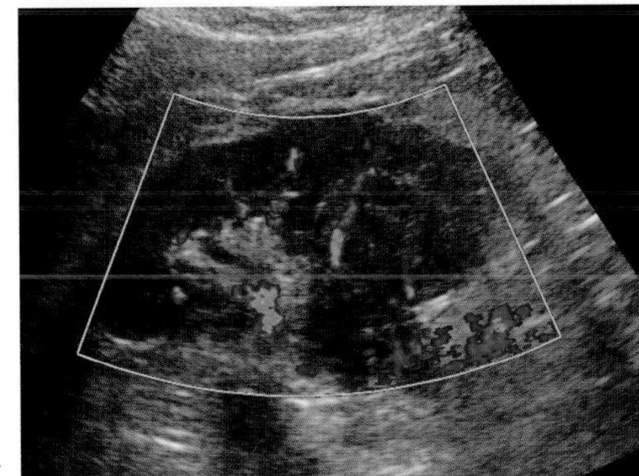
C

Clinical Presentation

A 55-year-old man with hematuria.

Further Work-up

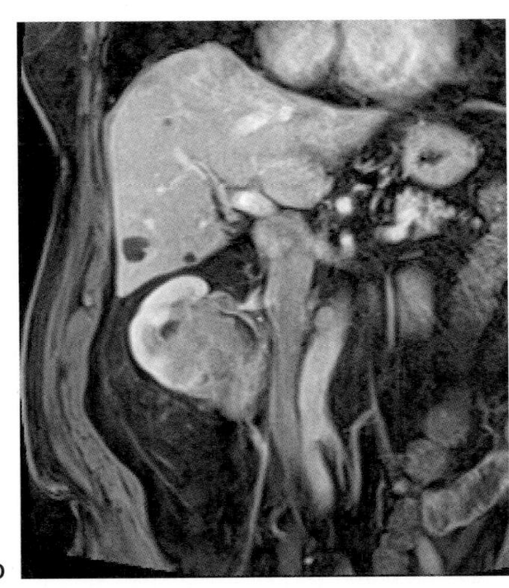
D

Imaging Findings

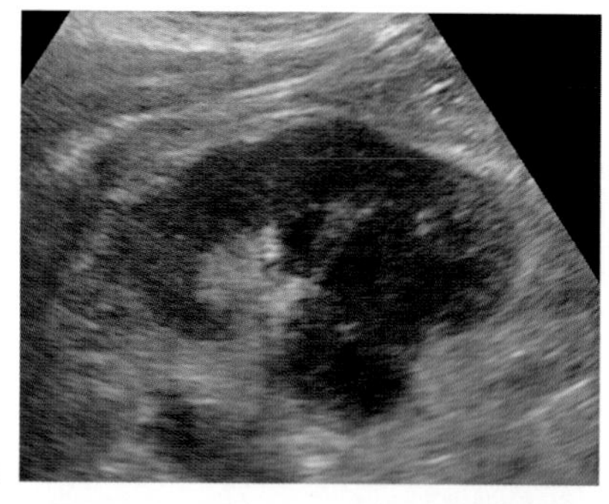

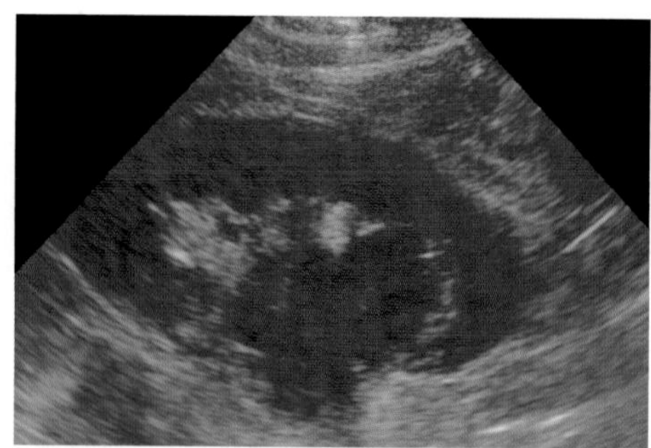

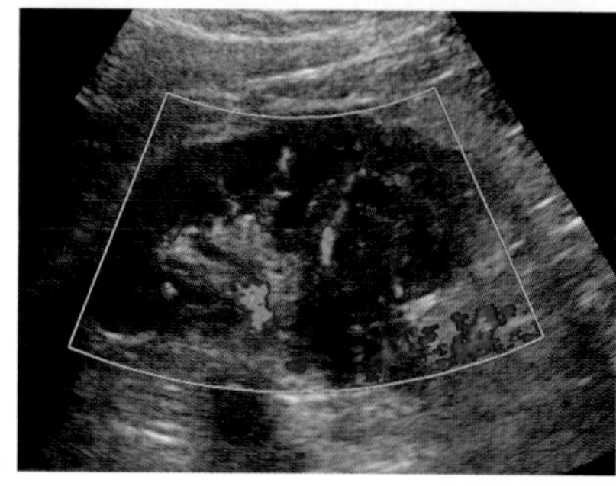

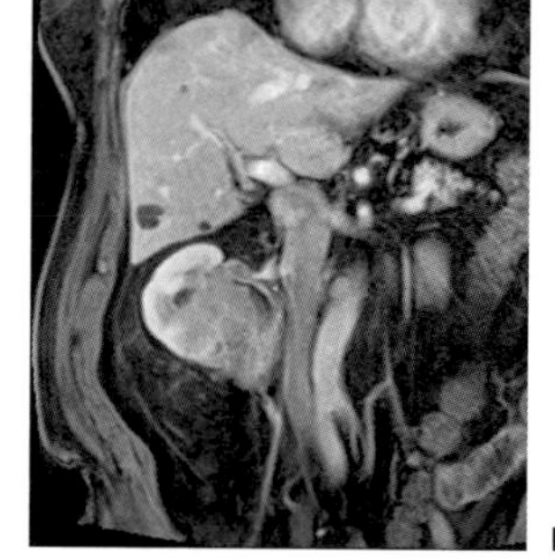

(A) The right kidney contains a hypoechoic mass within the lower pole extending into the renal pelvis. **(B)** Using a different color tint, the mass is clearly separate from the renal cortex. **(C)** With color Doppler imaging, flow is present within the lesion. **(D)** Coronal MR image of the right kidney demonstrate an irregular soft tissue enhancing mass. The mass extends medially within the expected location of the sinus fat and collecting system.

Differential Diagnosis

- ***Transitional cell carcinoma (TCC):*** A vascular mass occupying the collecting system and extending into the renal pelvis is consistent with a TCC.
- *Renal cell carcinoma (RCC):* Although an RCC may extend into the renal pelvis, it usually distorts the renal contour. Its epicenter would be the renal cortex. It may involve the renal vein.
- *Complex hydronephrosis:* Pus or blood can cause dilation of the collecting system and demonstrate internal echoes but would not demonstrate flow with color Doppler imaging.

Essential Facts

- TCC is commonly multifocal with a high incidence of recurrence. The bladder is the most common site for TCC followed by the renal pelvis.
- Only 2 to 4% of bladder TCCs develop upper tract TCC, but 40% of patients with upper tract TCC develop bladder cancer.
- TCCs represent 15% of renal tumors.
- Male female ratio is 2:1. Incidence peaks in the seventh decade.
- Smoking is the most significant risk factor for the development of TCCs.
- TCCs have the highest recurrence rate for any cancer.

✓ Pearls & × Pitfalls

✓ Color Doppler imaging is critical to distinguish soft tissue masses from complex fluid in the collecting system.

✓ When large, TCCs are infiltrative and may not distort the renal contour as in this case.

× Ultrasound has a very limited role in evaluating the ureter and periureteric tissues.

× Ultrasound is commonly requested for evaluation of patients with hematuria but has limited sensitivity for detection of small TCCs.

Case 79

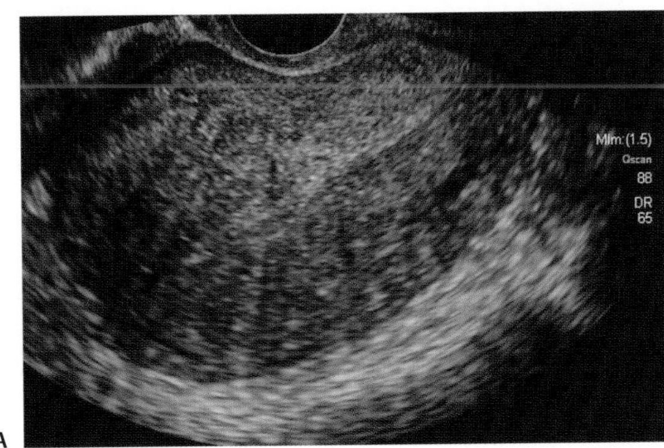

A

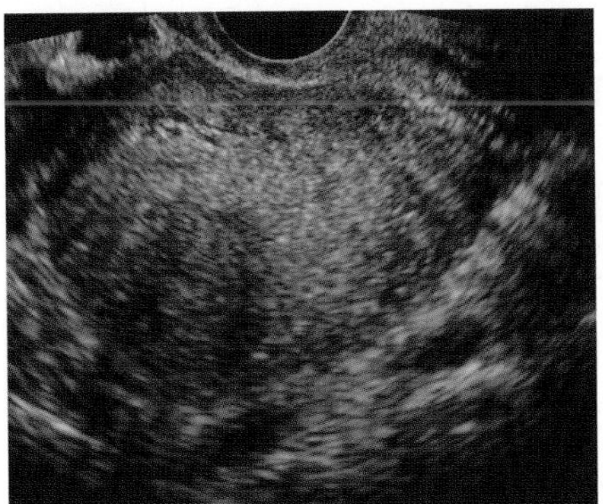

B

■ Clinical Presentation

A 40-year-old woman presents for evaluation of menorrhagia.

■ Further Work-up

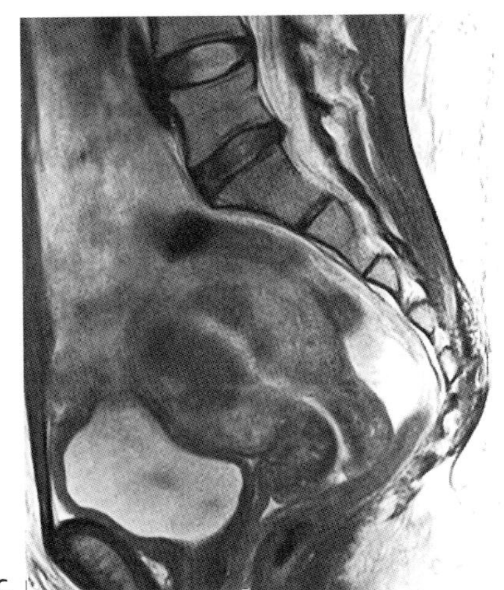

C

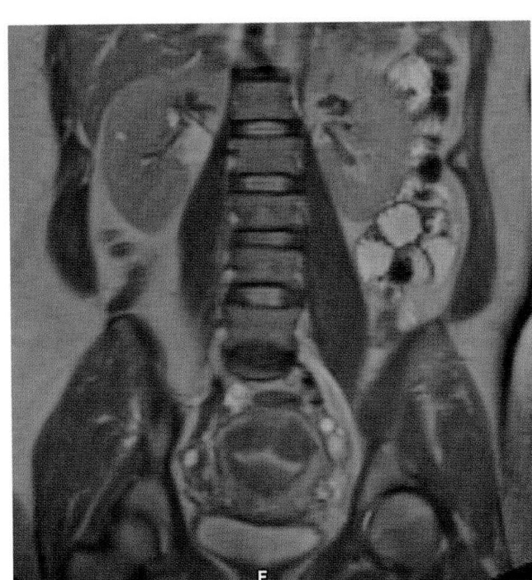

D

Imaging Findings

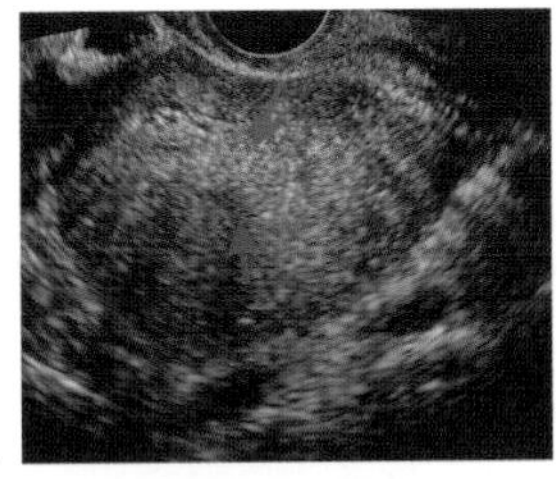

A

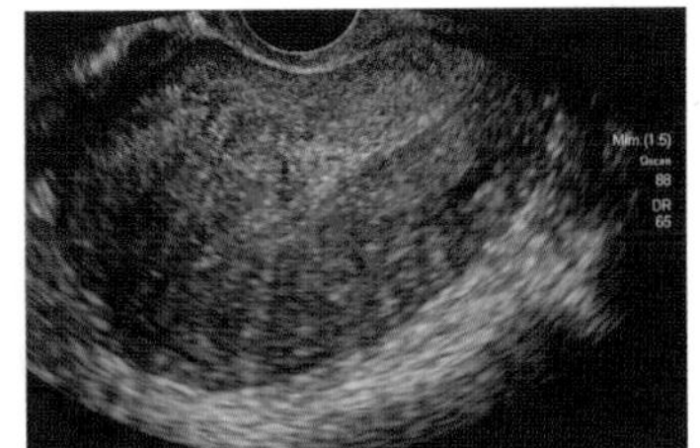

B

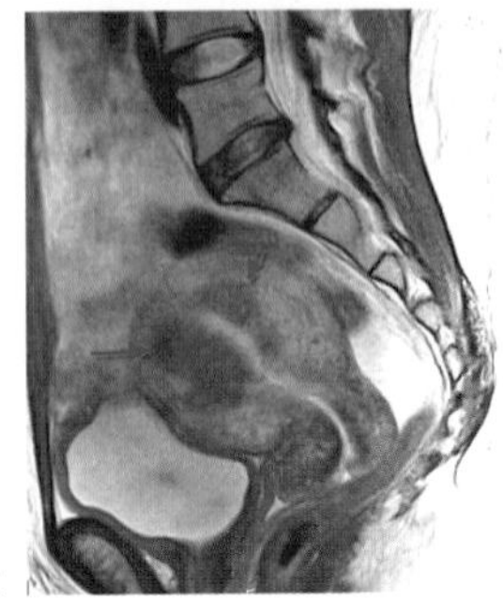

C

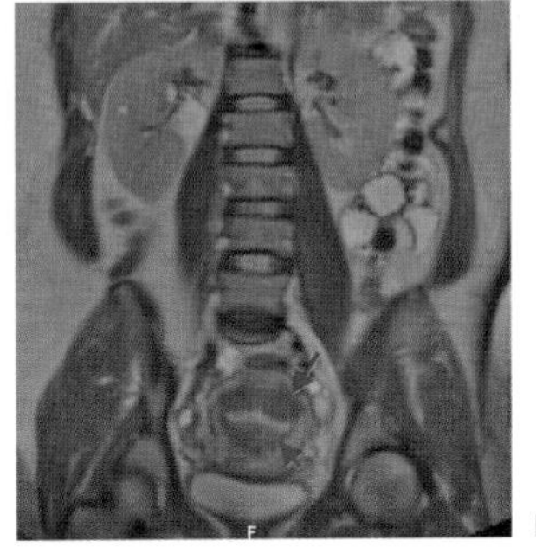

D

(A, B) Transvaginal ultrasound of the pelvis demonstrates normal thickness of the endometrium (*green arrows*). The relation between the endometrium and myometrium is poorly defined on the current examination (*red arrows*). No definite evidence of endometrial fluid is present on the current examination. **(C, D)** Magnetic resonance imaging (MRI) evaluation of the pelvis using T2-weighted images demonstrates marked thickening of the junctional zone (*red arrows*) with irregular margins. This appears to be focally thickened predominantly in the superior aspect of the endometrium anteriorly. No definite evidence of myometrial lesion is seen.

Differential Diagnosis

- ***Adenomyosis:*** Represents abnormal location of the endometrial gland within the myometrium. The sonographic appearance is nonspecific and includes diffuse uterine enlargement, heterogeneous myometrium, poorly defined junctional zone, and focal tenderness during transvaginal ultrasound.
- *Diffuse leiomyomas:* Most common neoplasm of the uterus, present in ~ 30% of women over the age of 30. Fibroids are classified as intramural, submucosal, and/or subserosal. Sonographically, the most common presentation is hypoechoic mass lesion. In case of multiple small fibroids, only heterogeneous appearance of the myometrium is noted on transvaginal ultrasound. Contour irregularity of the endometrium and/or myometrium could be the only sign of fibroids.
- *Endometrial polyp:* Most commonly seen in perimenopausal and postmenopausal women. Patients present with uterine bleeding and/or could be asymptomatic. On transvaginal ultrasound, polyps appear as nonspecific echogenic endometrial thickening that could be diffuse and/or focal. Presence of endometrial fluid clearly defined the margin of polyps. Vascular pedicle occasionally visualized on Doppler ultrasound defining the polyp stalk and vascular supply.

Essential Facts

- Pathologically represents endometrial gland and stroma within the myometrium.
- Associated myometrial hypertrophy is present.
- More commonly visualized within the posterior wall of the uterus.
- The endometrial glands arise from the basilar layer and are resistant to hormonal changes.
- Adenomyosis can be diffuse and/or nodular.
- Sonographically, adenomyosis could be visualized as uterine enlargement with heterogeneous myometrium.
- Inhomogeneous junctional zone could be seen sonographically.
- Poorly defined endometrial/myometrial borders.
- Adenomyosis is easily diagnosed on MRI imaging demonstrating irregular thickening of the junctional zone clearly visualized on T2-weighted images.
- The local form could be seen as an inhomogeneous, circumscribed area within the myometrium with poorly defined margins. They are difficult to distinguish from fibroid.

✓ Pearls & × Pitfalls

✓ The sonographic appearance of adenomyosis is nonspecific and diagnosis should not be made based on ultrasound findings. An accurate diagnosis could be obtained by MRI.

× Myometrial cyst could be the only manifestation of adenomyosis on transvaginal ultrasound; this could be misinterpreted as myometrial cyst (congenital in origin) and/or degenerating fibroids.

Case 80

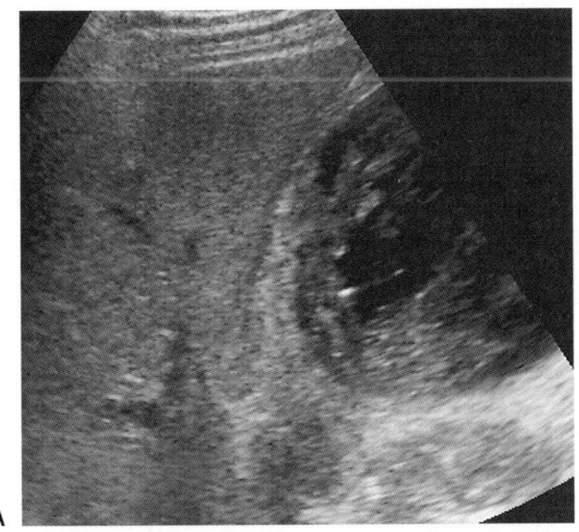
A

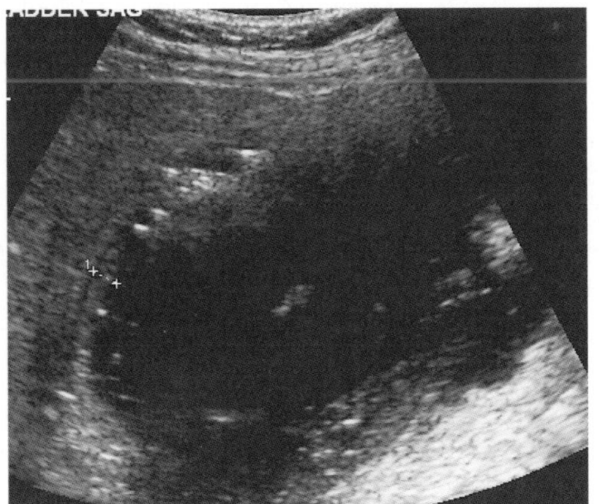

C

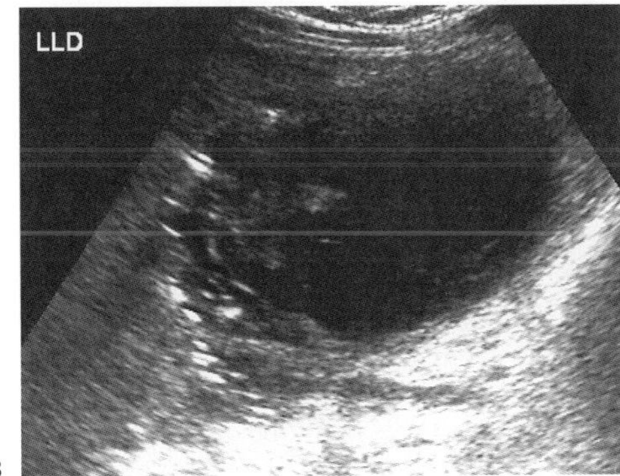

B

Clinical Presentation

A 72-year-old diabetic man with abdominal pain, nausea, and vomiting.

Further Work-up

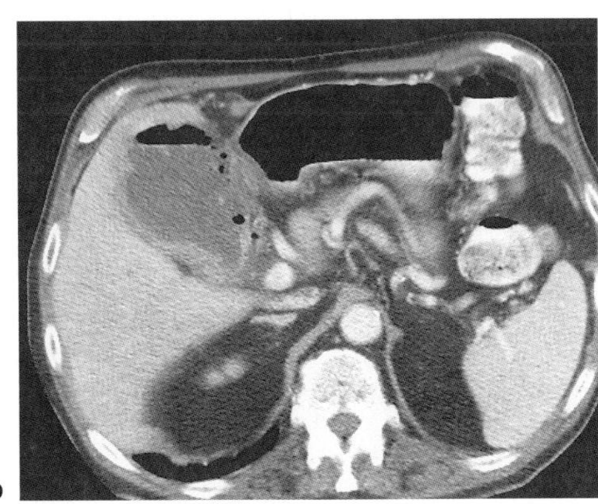
D

Imaging Findings

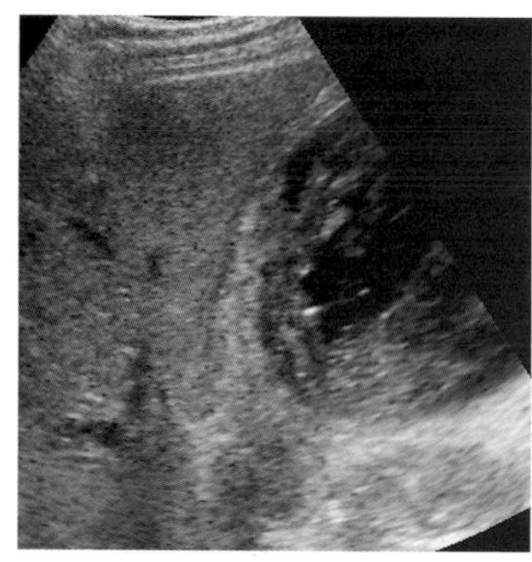

A

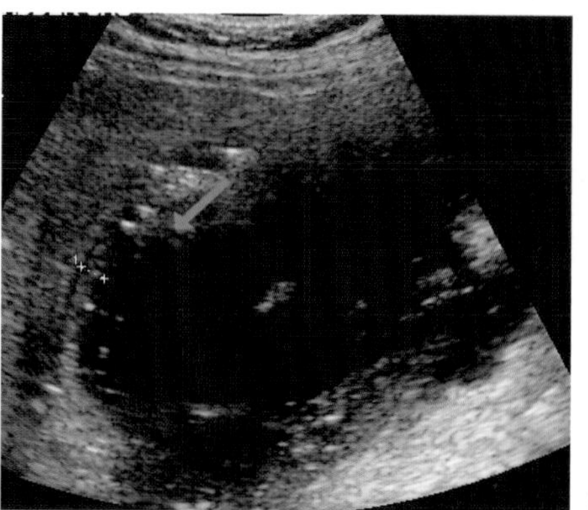

B

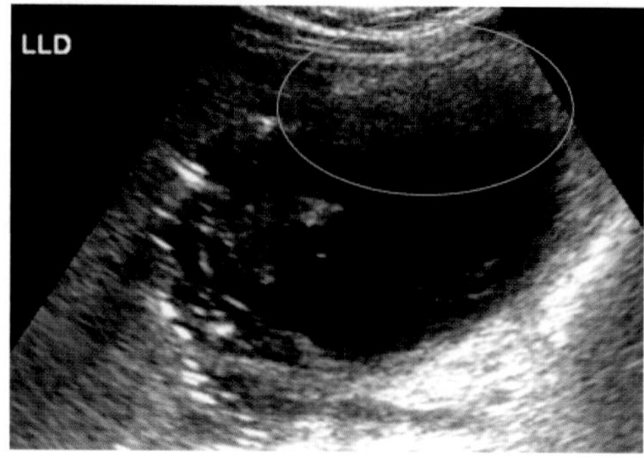

C

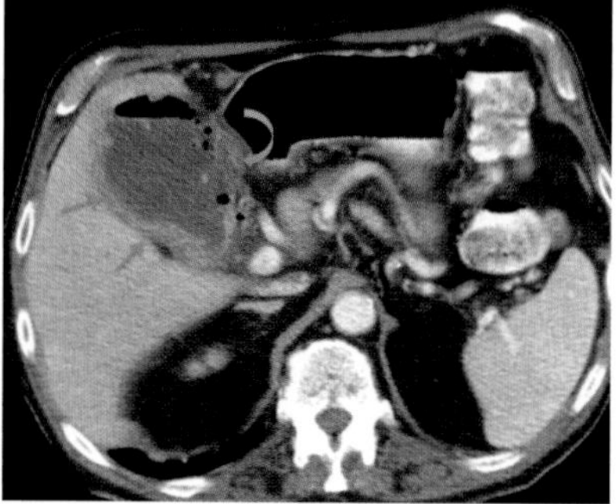

D

(A) Longitudinal and transverse images reveal a gallbladder wall that is thickened and heterogeneous. A large amount of debris is present in the gallbladder. Note the rounded configuration of the gallbladder indicating distension. Linear echoes adjacent to the gallbladder wall likely sloughed membranes. **(B)** Echogenic foci are present in the anterior wall of the gallbladder. These cause ring down artifact (*arrow*). **(C)** The anterior wall of the gallbladder near the fundus is not seen. Rather ring down artifact obscures the fundus (*circled*) the result of intraluminal gas. **(D)** The gallbladder wall is thickened and enhancing laterally (*arrows*). Medially, the wall appears disrupted with surrounding inflammatory changes (*curved arrow*). Gas is present within the gallbladder lumen and wall.

Differential Diagnosis

- ***Emphysematous cholecystitis:*** Gas within the lumen or wall of a thickened distended gallbladder is consistent with emphysematous cholecystitis.
- *Acalculous cholecystitis (AC):* The amount of debris in the gallbladder as well as the degree of wall thickening is not typical of AC. Gas is not seen with AC.
- *Gallbladder adenocarcinoma:* The sloughed membranes and debris in complicated cholecystitis (CC) can mimic a mass. Color Doppler would demonstrate flow in the solid components in a gallbladder mass.

Essential Facts

- Complicated cholecystitis (CC) includes emphysematous, gangrenous, hemorrhagic, and/or perforated cholecystitis.
- CC occurs with prolonged or inadequately treated acute cholecystitis. Patients are often elderly and diabetic.
- Computed tomography should be performed in the setting of CC to assess the extent of disease and to guide therapy. Percutaneous cholecystostomy is frequently the treatment of choice.
- Sonographic features include wall thickening, wall disruption (perforation), pericholecystic fluid, and intraluminal membranes from sloughed mucosa or strands of fibrinous exudate.
- Emphysematous cholecystitis (EC) occurs with gas-forming organisms including *Escherichia coli* or *Clostridium perfringens*.
- Gas in EC can be in the lumen, gallbladder wall, or pericholecystic.

✓ Pearls & × Pitfalls

✓ Color Doppler evaluation of material in an around the gallbladder is imperative to distinguish gallbladder malignancy from CC.

✓ Although complicated cholecystitis can mimic malignancy sonographically, the clinical presentation will be very different.

✓ Gallstones may not be present or not visible in the setting of CC.

× Gallstones are often seen with gallbladder carcinoma.

× It can be difficult to distinguish EC from a porcelain gallbladder.

✓ Intraluminal gas in the gallbladder may redistribute with patient repositioning.

× Pericholecystic fluid can be due to pancreatitis, duodenitis, and peptic ulcer disease.

× Intraluminal gas in the gallbladder can mimic near field artifact.

Case 81

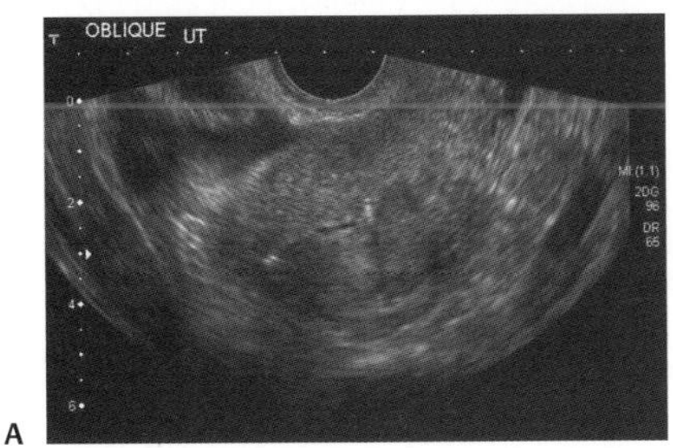

A

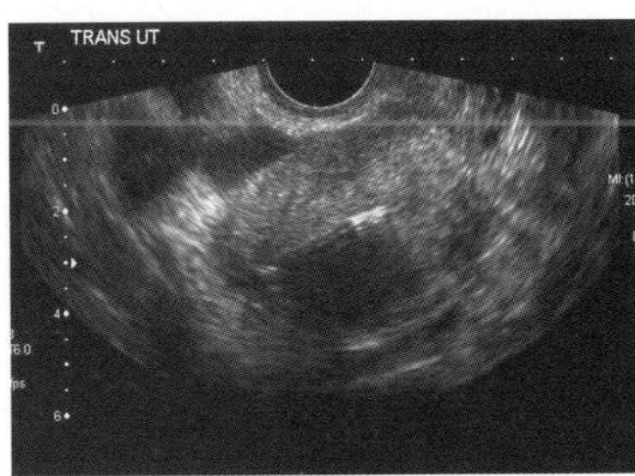

B

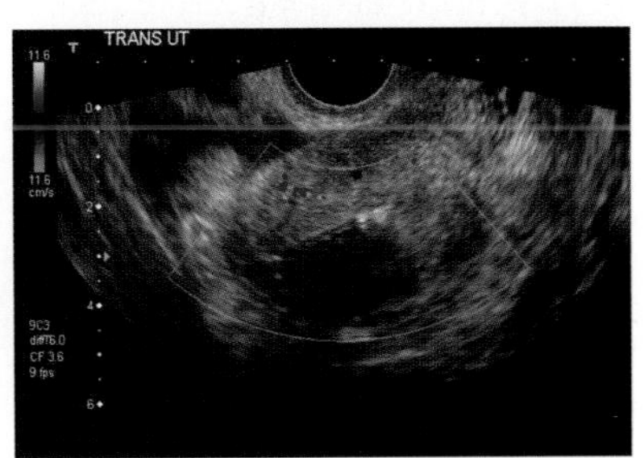

C

Clinical Presentation

A 35-year-old woman (G3, P3) presents for evaluation of intrauterine device (IUD); referring physician was unable to visualize the string.

Further Work-up

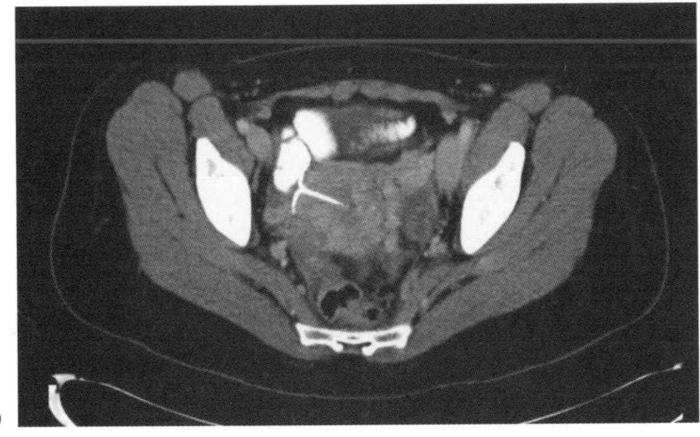
D

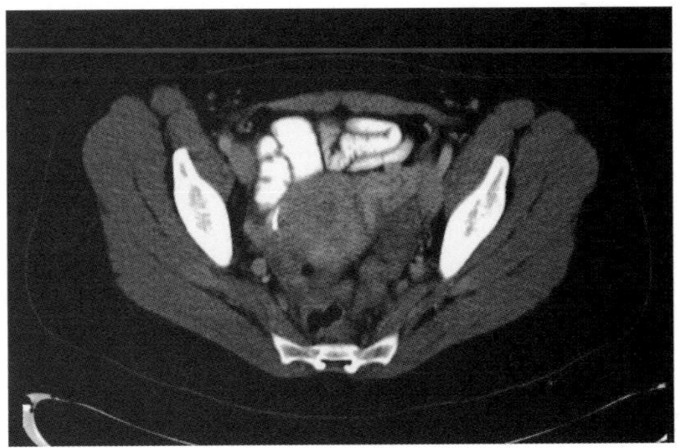
E

Imaging Finding

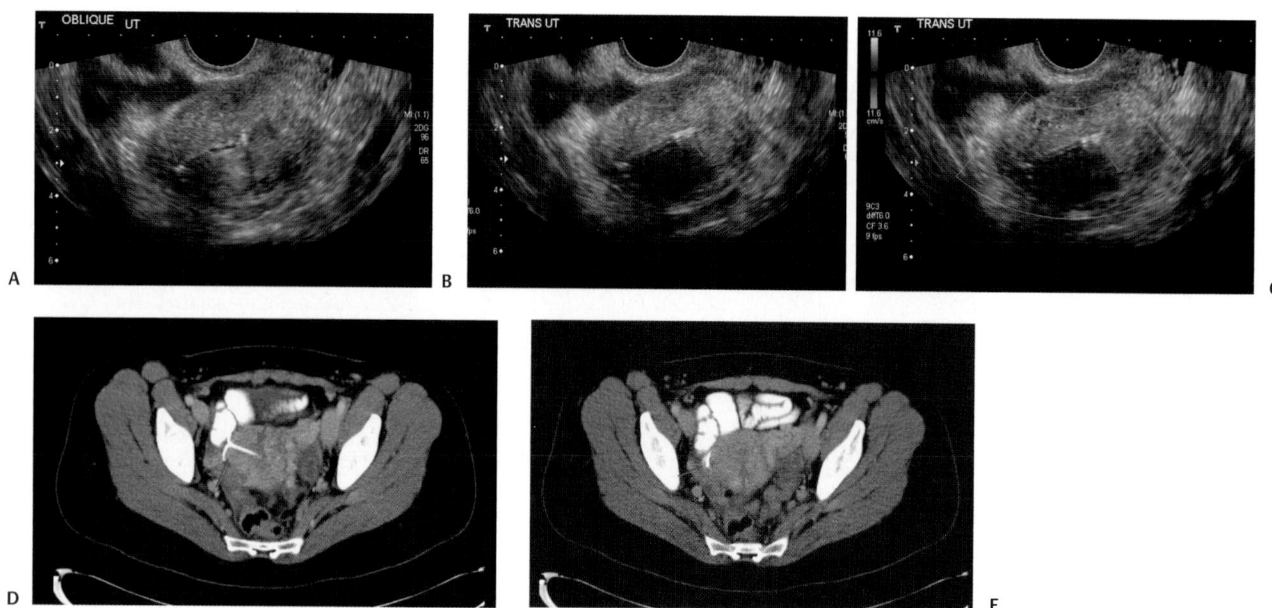

(A–C) Pelvic ultrasound using transvaginal approach demonstrates an IUD located to the right of the endometrium, probably within the myometrium (*red arrows*). No shadowing is appreciated within the endometrium (*green arrows*). Trace amount of endometrial fluid is present on the pelvic ultrasound. **(D, E)** Further evaluation using computed tomography of the pelvis demonstrates a T-shaped IUD (*red arrows*), which appears to be extrinsic to the endometrium (*green arrows*). The IUD is probably penetrating the right wall of the uterus with one side of the device; it is extrauterine in location.

Differential Diagnosis

- ***Perforating IUD:*** The IUD is visualized penetrating the myometrium. It may be partial, or complete. The distal shadowing from the IUD appears to be extrinsic to the endometrium. Transvaginal ultrasound would be helpful to delineate the extent and location of the IUD in relation to the endometrium.
- *Extrauterine location of an IUD:* The IUD is visualized in an extrauterine location. The perforation is usually associated with fluid collection and possible abscess formation. Although it may be difficult to visualize with ultrasound, bowel, bladder, and/or ovarian perforation may be present with possible fistula formation.
- *Normal location of an IUD:* The IUD is within the endometrium, visualized regardless of the uterine position or endometrial echogenicity. The string is also visualized sonographically as a thin longitudinal echo in the cervical canal. The presence of distal shadowing clearly defines the IUD and helps to differentiate it from echogenic endometrium.

Essential Facts

- Uterine perforation is one of the most serious complications of IUD.
- Other complications include infection, ectopic pregnancy, spontaneous abortion, premature delivery, and maternal death.
- The patient presents with pain and menorrhagia.
- Uterine perforation occurs at the time of the insertion; however, it is identified later.
- Patients are usually asymptomatic; however, abdominal pain is present later.
- Initial removal is crucial to avoid further complications such as bowel perforation, bladder perforation, and/or fistula formation.
- A missing string on physical exam after insertion should raise the suspicion of aberrant location.
- Plain films and/or computed tomography scan should be performed if the IUD is not visualized on ultrasound.
- If the IUD is visualized within the endometrium, no further imaging is required.
- In case of IUD perforation of the myometrium, the site and amount of perforation should be quantified.

✓ Pearls & × Pitfalls

✓ When the uterus is not midline in location, a sagittal oblique view would be helpful to determine the location of the IUD in relation to the endometrium.

× When the patient is in the secretory phase of the cycle, the endometrium is echogenic and thick, limiting appropriate evaluation of IUD.

Case 82

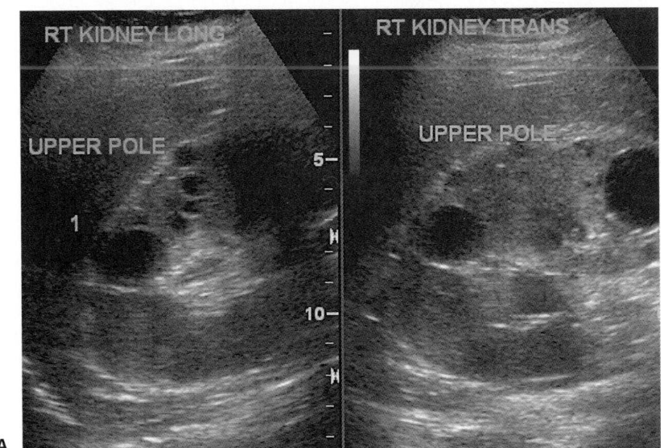

A

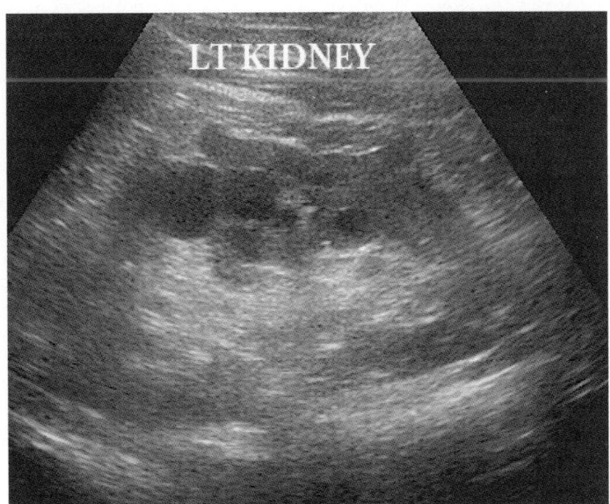

B

Clinical Presentation

A 28-year-old woman presents with hypertension and hematuria.

Imaging Findings

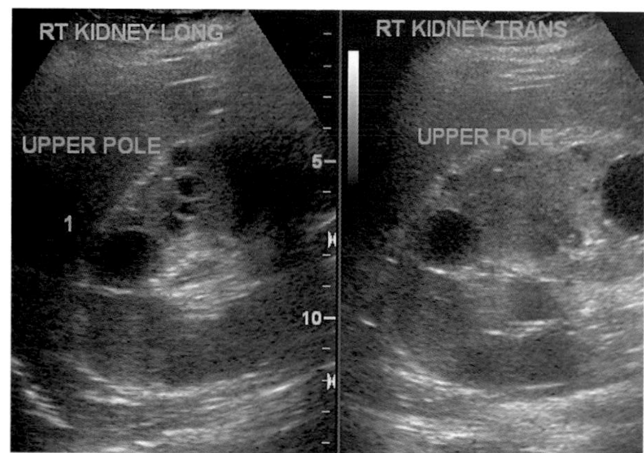

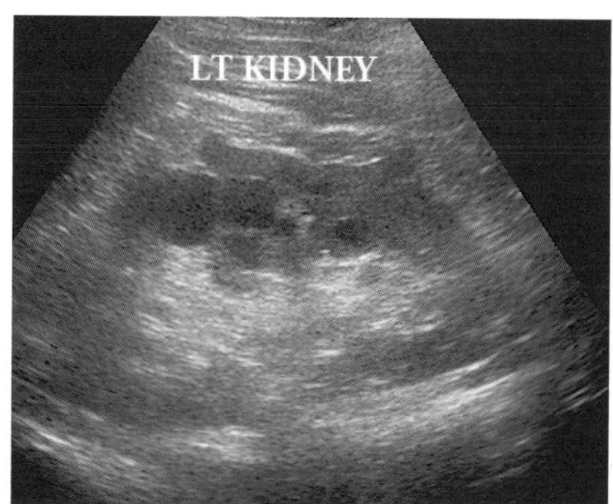

Several small cortical cysts of varying sizes are present in both the right **(A)** and left **(B)** kidneys. The sonographic window of the liver allows for much better visualization of the right kidney than the left.

Differential Diagnosis

- ***Early ADPKD:*** Several small cysts in each kidney in a patient of this age is consistent with ADPKD.
- *Multicystic dysplastic kidneys (MCDK):* Not usually bilateral. Significant renal cortex would not be present. By this age, MCDK are usually very small.
- *Tuberous sclerosis (TS):* Multiple renal cysts can be seen with TS, but renal AMLs would also be present.

Essential Facts

- Renal cysts are extremely common and the incidence of renal cysts increases with age, beginning in middle age. Renal cysts should not be present in a patient of this age.
- Patients with ADPKD present with hypertension, hematuria, urinary tract infection, or palpable masses.
- Only half of patients who are diagnosed with ADPKD have a family history. Others occur from spontaneous mutation.
- ADPKD usually presents in the fourth and fifth decades of life but can be picked up much earlier with screening ultrasound.
- If screened early with ultrasound, 50% of patients with a family history of ADPKD who go on to develop the disease will have cysts in the first decade of life.
- Complications of ADPKD (cyst rupture, hemorrhage, and infection) are suspected with findings of debris or thickened walls of a cyst. Stones are a common complication and cause of hematuria and pain.
- The kidneys get larger over time due to an increase in the size and number of cysts.

✓ Pearls & × Pitfalls

✓ In ADPKD, cysts occur in the liver (60%), spleen (5%), and pancreas (10%).

✓ If the diagnosis of ADPKD is suspected clinically, scanning should also be performed of the other solid organs.

× In early ADPKD, the kidneys can be normal in size and echogenicity with just a few small cysts, as in this case.

✓ Cysts can be seen in infancy, even in utero. If a fetal survey reveals a renal cyst, the mother should be screened for ADPKD.

✓ ADPKD is associated with berry aneurysms.

Case 83

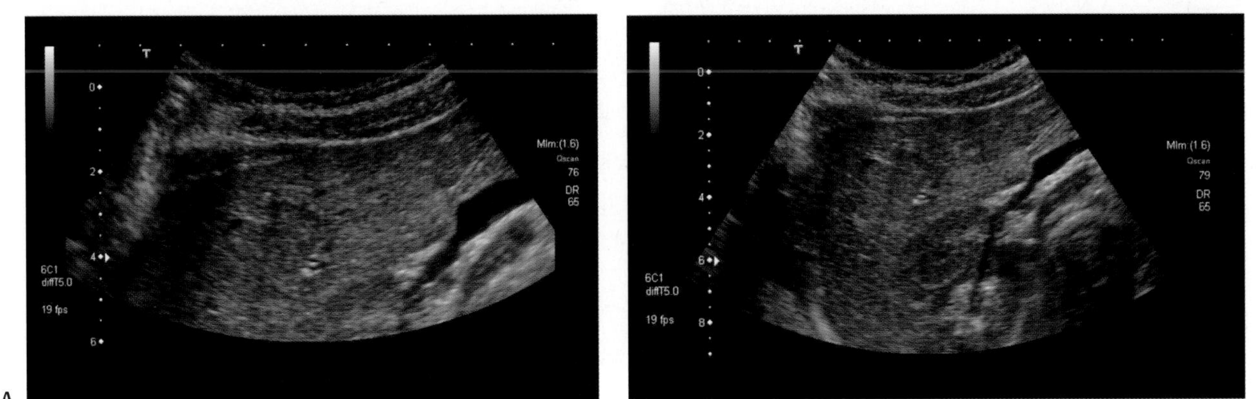

Clinical presentation

A 35-year-old woman presents with history of right upper quadrant pain.

Further Work-up

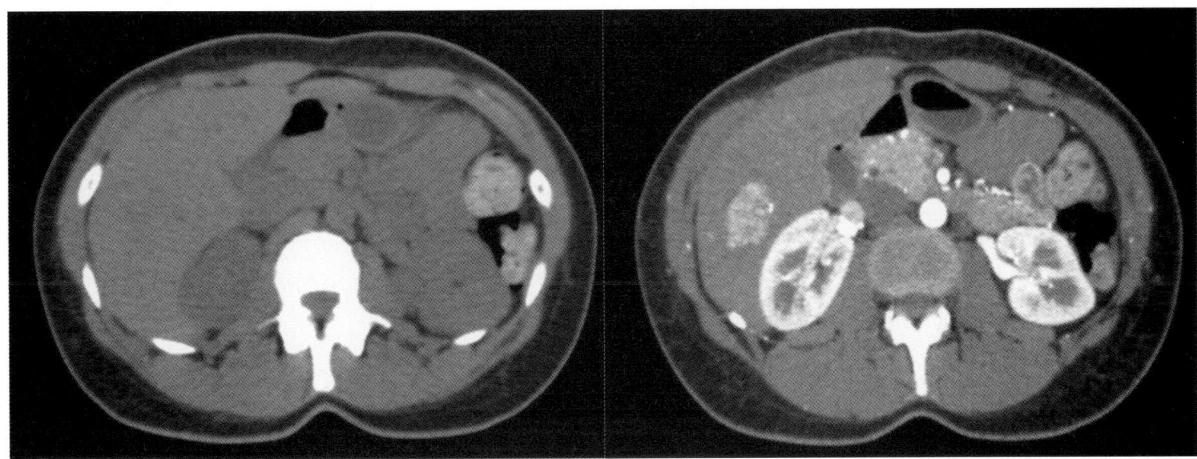

Imaging Findings

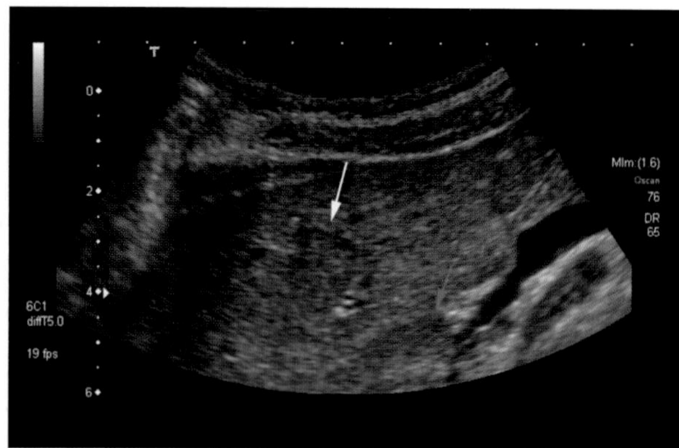

A

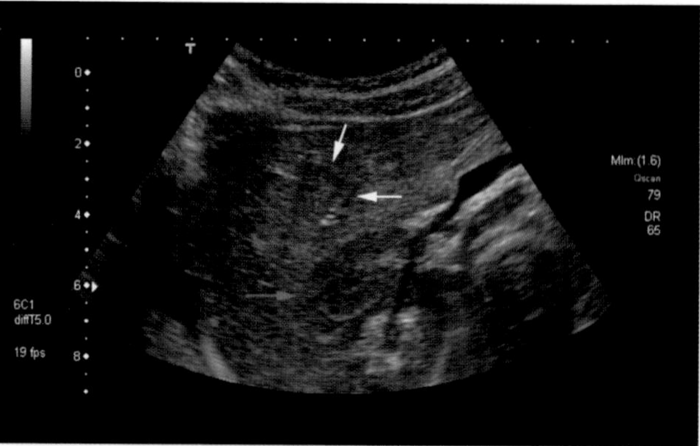

B

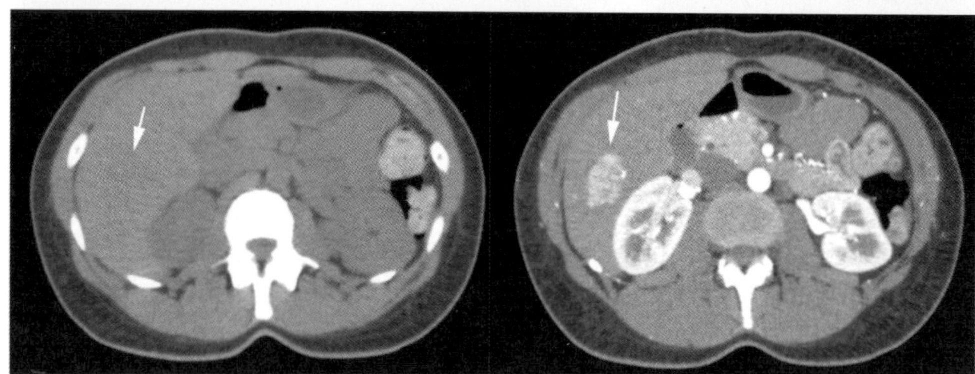

C

(A, B) Ultrasound images of the right upper quadrant show a hypoechoic geographic lesion in the inferior aspect of the right lobe of the liver (*white arrows*). The lesion is located inferiorly, adjacent to the right kidney (*red arrow*). **(C)** Follow-up CT shows intense enhancement on the arterial phase image (*white arrows*); the lesion is isodense on the precontrasted image.

Differential Diagnosis

- ***Focal nodular hyperplasia:*** Appears as isoechoic/hypoechoic and or echogenic lesion to the liver parenchyma; in 18%, central scar can be seen.
- *Hepatic adenoma:* Could have similar appearance, usually larger in size. More common in young women with oral contraceptive usage (more than 2 years).
- *Fibrolamellar hepatocellular carcinoma:* Occurs in younger patients without underlying liver disease. On ultrasound they usually appear as a large mass with heterogenous echotexture, echogenic central scar, and/or calcifications.

Essential Facts

- Second most common benign tumor in the liver after hemangioma.
- More common in females (85–90%).
- Usually seen as incidental finding.
- The classic appearance is abnormal nodular architecture, malformed vessels, and cholangiolar proliferation.
- Ultrasound appearance is nonspecific; the most common is subtle hepatic mass difficult to differentiate from normal parenchyma.
- Subtle contour abnormality and displacement of vessels could help in visualizing the lesion.
- On cross-sectional studies, the lesion is best seen on the arterial phase images. The lesion becomes isointense on the portovenous phase images.
- Delayed enhancement of central scar is suggestive of the diagnosis.

✓ Pearls & × Pitfalls

× Giving the isoechoic appearance of focal nodular hyperplasia, the lesions are not easily recognized on ultrasound. Close attention to contour abnormality and vessel displacement is critical.

✓ The presence of well-developed central and peripheral blood vessels is suggestive of the diagnosis on Doppler imaging.

Case 84

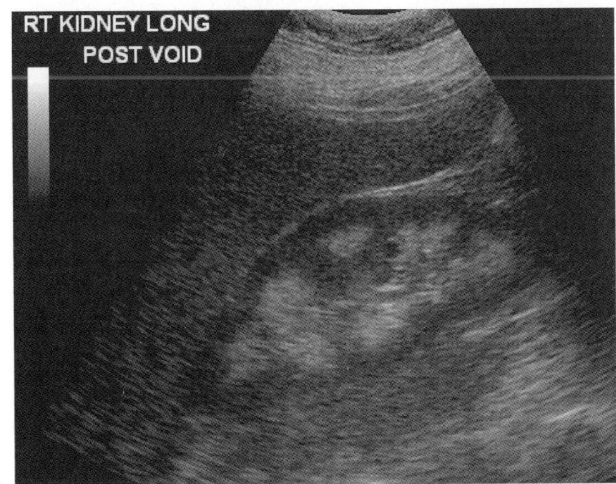

A

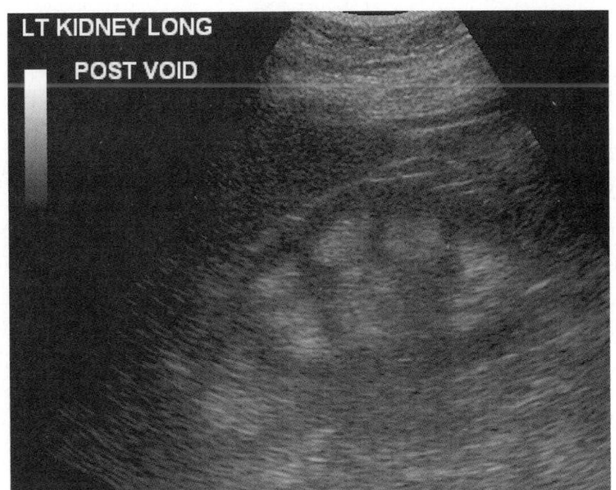

B

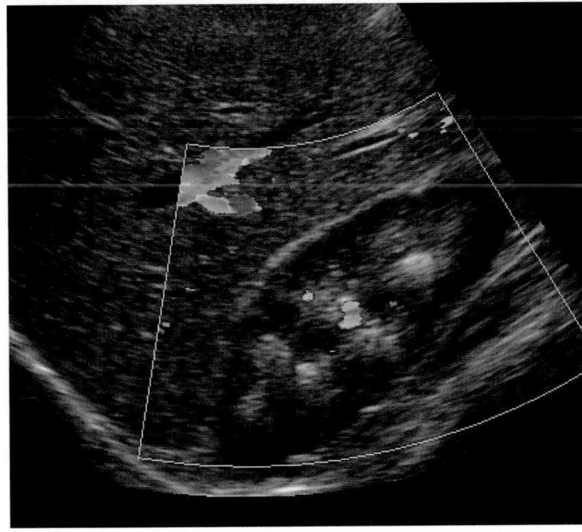
C

Clinical Presentation

A 45-year-old woman with hematuria.

Further Work-up

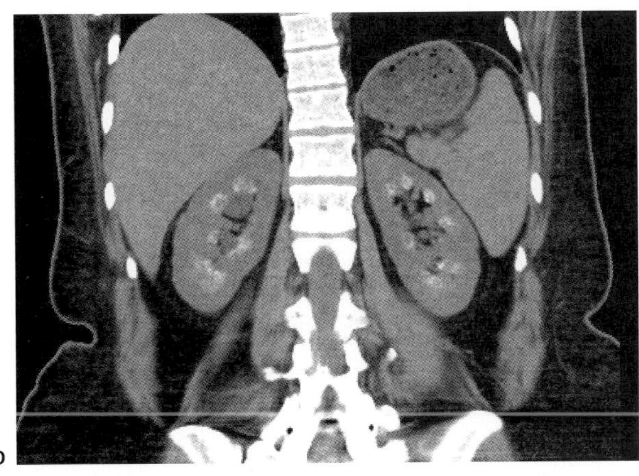
D

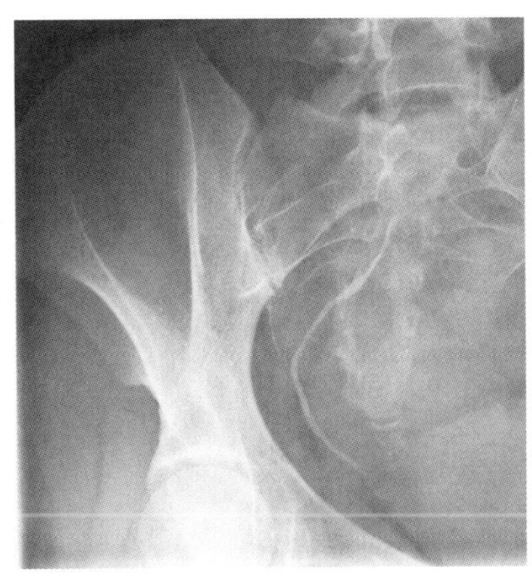
E

Imaging Findings

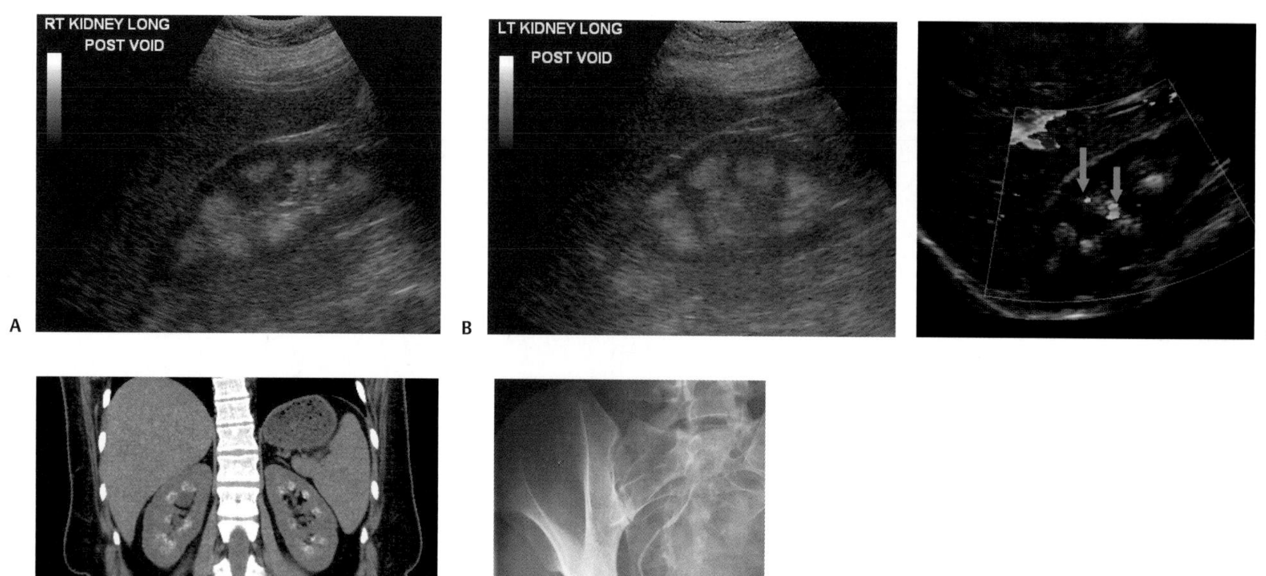

Very echogenic medullary pyramids (MP) are present in both the right **(A)** and left **(B)** kidneys. They are indistinguishable from the renal sinus fat. **(C)** With color Doppler imaging, twinkling artifact (*arrows*) is present in multiple locations within the medullary pyramids (MP). **(D)** Coronal reformatted non contrast CT confirms numerous tiny calcifications within the MP bilaterally consistent with medullary calcinosis. **(E)** IVP image from the excretory phase reveals the *paintbursh* appearance resulting from contrast in dilated tubules in the MP.

Differential Diagnosis

- ***Medullary sponge kidney (MSK):*** Echogenic medullary pyramids with or without medullary nephrocalcinosis in otherwise normal-appearing kidneys is consistent with MSK.
- *Staghorn calculus:* Large stones in the collecting system can conform to the calices and renal pelvis. They would be denser and central to the medullary pyramids.
- *Autosomal recessive polycystic kidney disease (ARPKD):* Diagnosed in infancy or childhood, kidneys in ARPKD are enlarged and diffusely echogenic. Macrocysts may be present.

Essential Facts

- MSK, also know as Lenarduzzi-Cacchi-Ricci disease, is a developmental abnormality resulting in ectasia and cystic dilation of the collecting ducts in the medullary pyramids.
- Most patients with MSK are asymptomatic. Historically they were diagnosed with IVP revealing the classic paintbrush appearance or papillary blush due to contrast in the dilated ducts.
- Clinically patients present third to fifth decade with recurrent stone disease. Up to 20% of patients with recurrent stones have MSK. It is rare in the general population.
- Inheritance is sporadic. Familial cases with AD inheritance also have been described. Clinical course is variable and can be asymptomatic.
- On ultrasound the dilated tubules result in very echogenic medullary pyramids. Calcification within the tubules (medullary nephrocalcinosis) adds to the increased echogenicity.

✓ Pearls & × Pitfalls

✓ Medullary nephrocalcinosis is common in MSK but not always present.

× Medullary calcifications can be missed in a background of echogenic pyramids.

✓ The twinkle artifact improves sensitivity for detection of medullary nephrocalcinosis.

× MSK is usually diffuse and bilateral but can be unilateral or focal.

× CT and ultrasound are less sensitive than IVP for the detection of MDK. Therefore as IVP becomes obsolete, the incidence of MSK will decrease.

Case 85

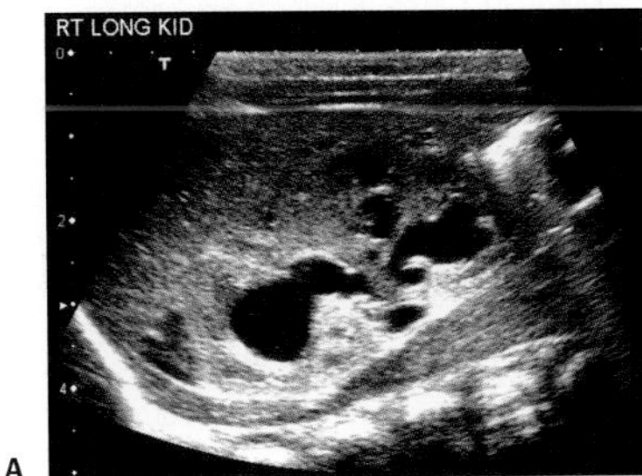

A

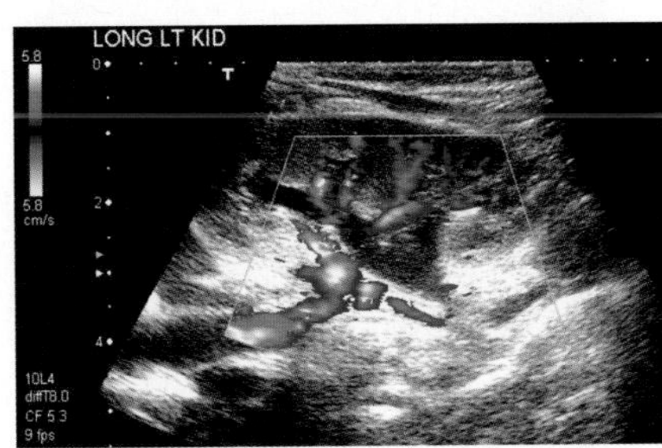

B

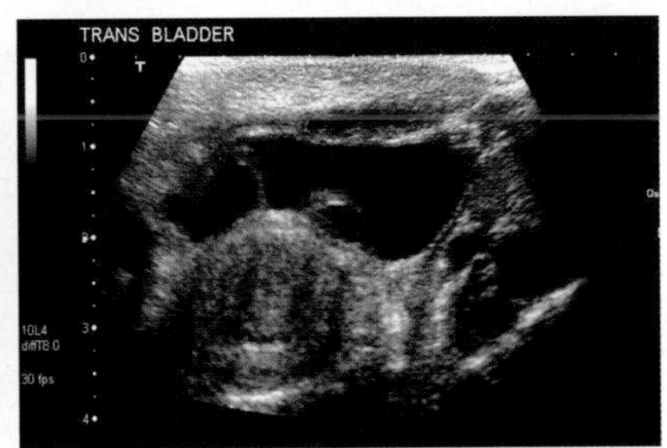

C

Clinical Indication

A one-year-old girl presents with a history of urinary tract infection.

Further Work-up

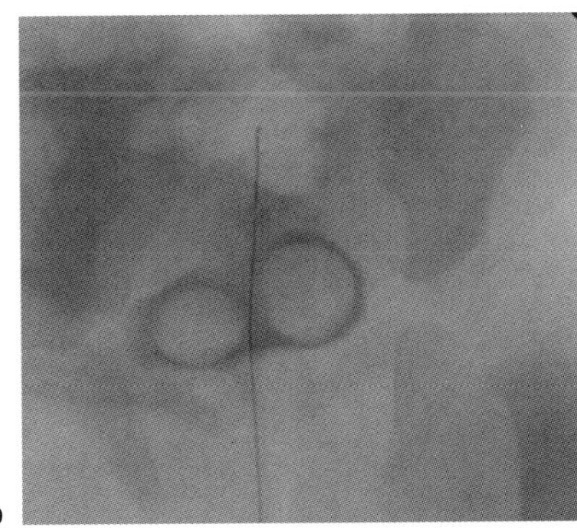
D

Imaging Findings

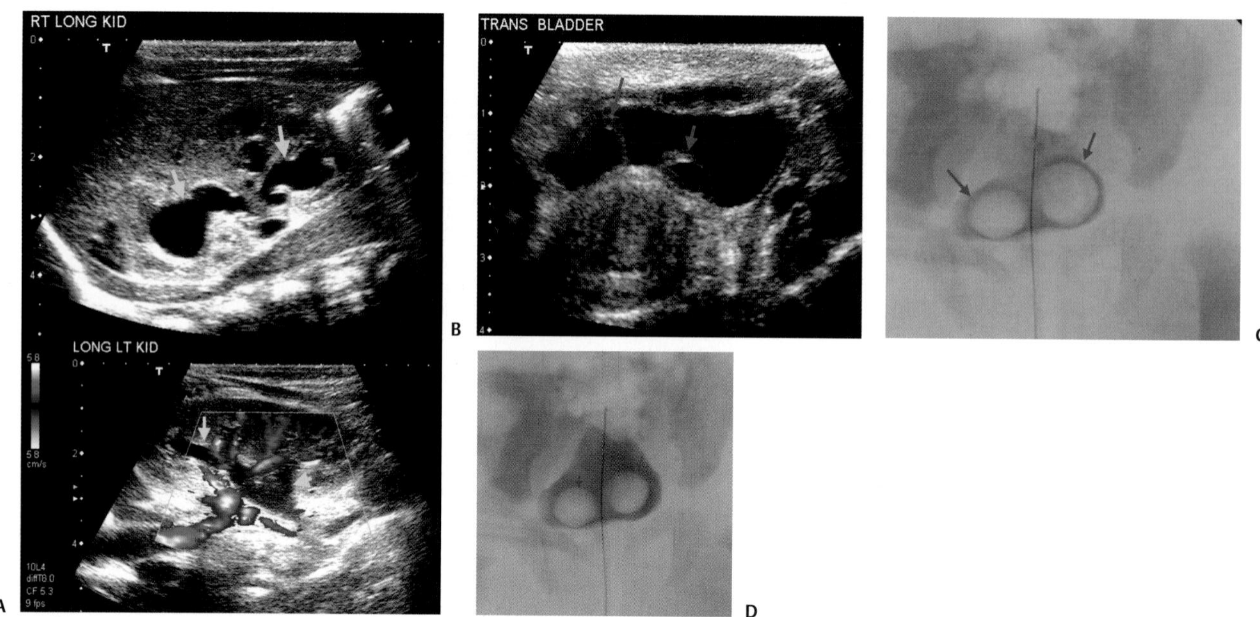

(A, B) Ultrasound evaluation of the kidneys demonstrates mild degree of hydronephrosis bilaterally—slightly more pronounced in the right kidney when compared to the left (*yellow arrows*). Further evaluation of the bladder demonstrates two thin-walled, cystic lesions located within the posterior wall of the bladder (*red arrows*). The visualized uterus demonstrates no gross finding. **(C, D)** Further evaluation with a voiding cystourethrogram demonstrates two well-defined filling defects within the bladder posteriorly, which corresponds to the findings on ultrasound (*red arrows*).

Differential Diagnosis

- ***Bilateral ureterocele:*** Is a thin wall cystic lesion within the bladder, which could be asymptomatic and or present with signs of obstruction. It is bilateral in approximately 15% of cases. Sonographically, a thin-walled cystic lesion is noted in the region of the trigon of the bladder. Associated signs of obstruction may be seen.
- *Dilatation of the ureter:* Could be pathologic secondary to reflux disease/obstruction and/or secondary to megaureter. A chronically dilated ureter would have a tortuous appearance that is more easily visualized posterior to the bladder. A multiloculated cystic mass may be visualized posterior to the bladder secondary to chronically dilated tortuous ureter. The multiloculated cystic mass is extraluminal in location.
- *Pseudoureterocele:* Could be related to urinary lower tract obstruction with subsequent dilatation of the intravesical segment of the ureter. Also, could be related to obstruction of the ureterovesical junction, with subsequent mucosa herniated into the bladder lumen, secondary to vigorous peristalsis. The pseudoureterocele appears as a ureterocele/cystic lesion within the bladder during sonographic evaluation.

Essential Facts

- The incidence is 1 in 4,000 children, more commonly in females.
- Ureterocele represents a thin-walled dilatation of the distal end of the ureter, with subsequent protrusion into the bladder lumen.
- Ureterocele may occur in one ureter or may be duplicated in approximately 15% of cases.
- Ureterocele can be associated with duplication of the ureter.
- Ureterocele may be asymptomatic and noted as incidental finding on subsequent images.
- Ureteroceles become symptomatic when stenosis of the ureterovesical junction occurs with subsequent development of hydronephrosis.
- Large ureteroceles may cause bladder outlet obstruction.
- Sonographically, a thin-walled cystic lesion is noted within the bladder, usually round in appearance.
- The shape of the ureterocele changes based on the bladder filling.
- Associated dilatation of the ureter and occasionally hydronephrosis might be seen.

✓ Pearls & ✗ Pitfalls

✗ When the urinary bladder is distended, ureterocele may invert, giving the sonographic appearance of bladder diverticulum.

✓ Doppler ultrasound will help in localizing the ureter insertion into the bladder by visualizing jet phenomena.

Case 86

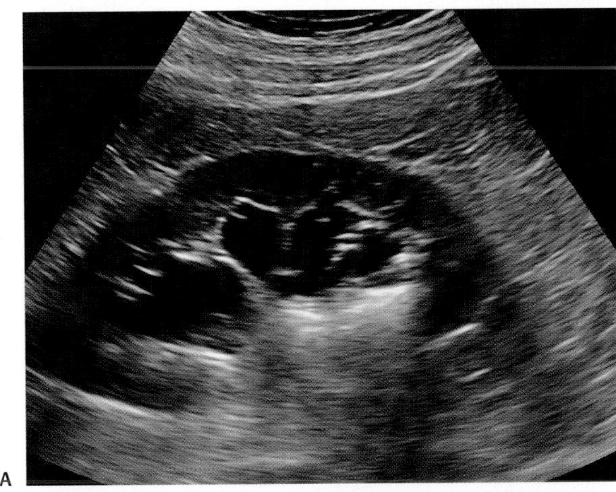
A

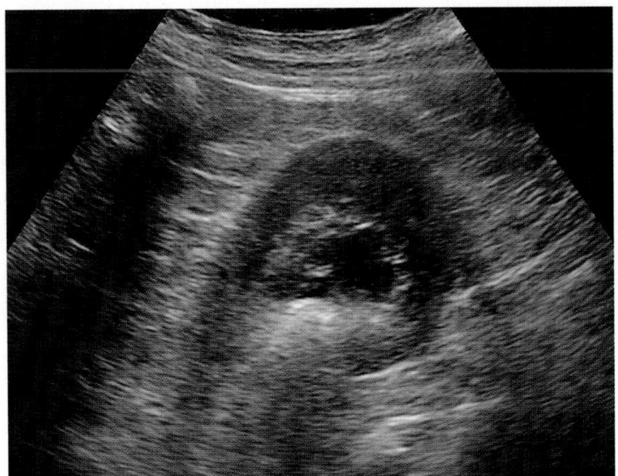
B

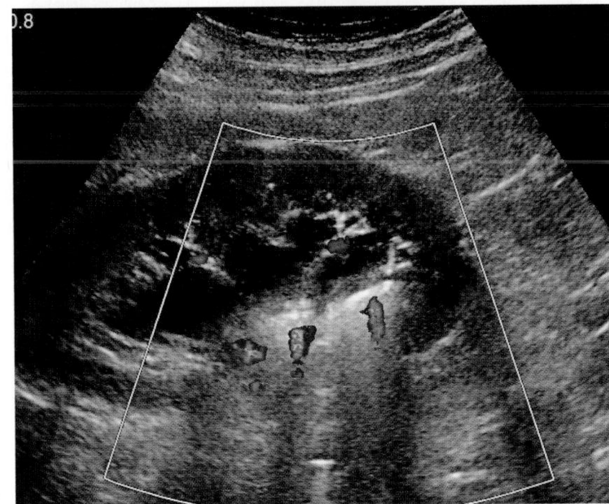
C

Clinical Presentation

A 50-year-old woman with recurrent urinary tract infections (UTIs).

Further Work-up

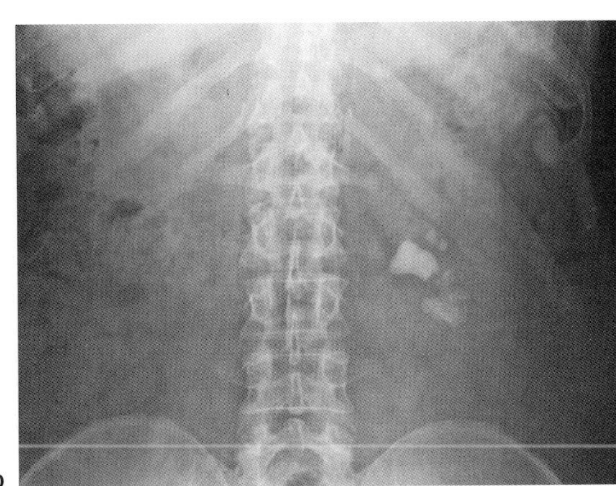
D

Imaging Findings

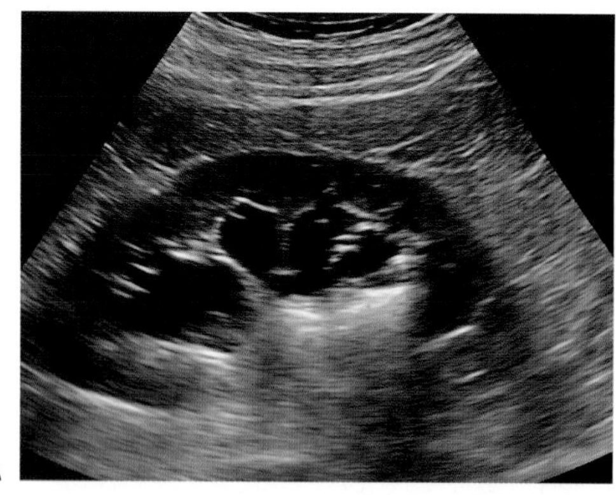

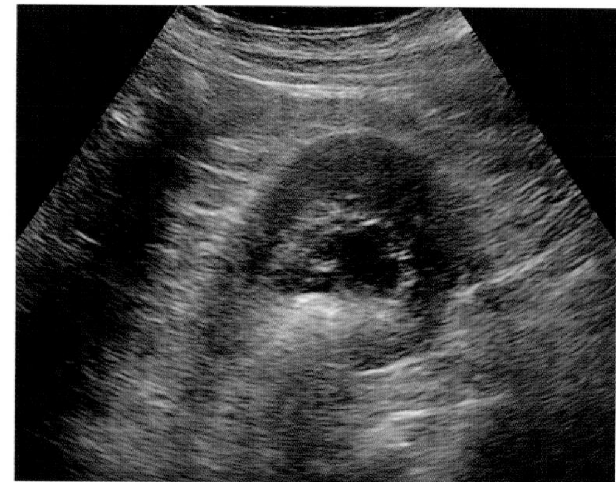

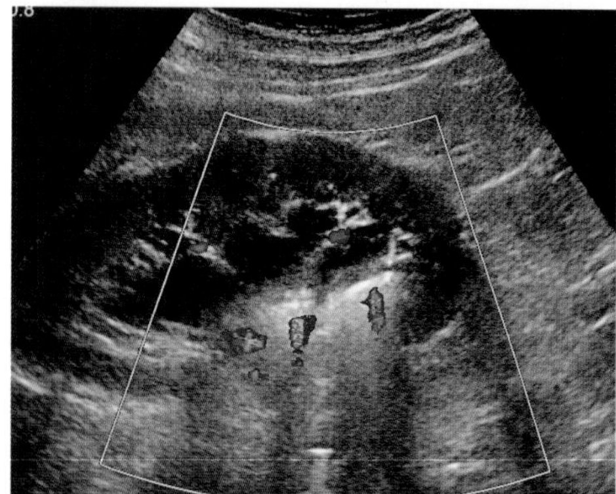

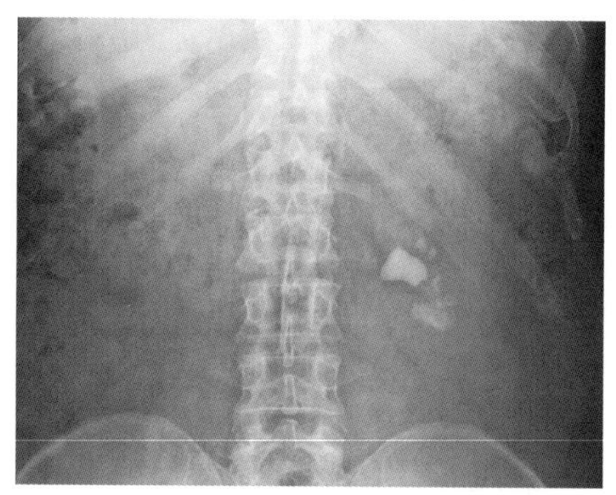

(A, B) Longitudinal and transverse images of the left kidney reveal dilated calyces and a large central area with increased echogenicity with shadowing. The right kidney (not shown) was normal. **(C)** Areas of twinkle artifact are present within the echogenic area centrally. **(D)** Abdominal radiograph reveals a large calcification partially filling the left renal pelvis and calyces particularly in the lower pole.

Differential Diagnosis

- ***Staghorn calculus:*** A large calcification filling or partially filling the calyces and renal pelvis with normal-appearing renal parenchyma is consistent with a staghorn calculus.
- *Xanthogranulomatous pyelonephritis (XGP):* Staghorn calculi and hydronephrosis are often present in XGP. The kidney would be enlarged and heterogeneous due to inflammation in XGP.
- *Emphysematous pyelonephritis:* Occurs in older, immunocompromised patients (usually those with diabetes). Gas can be located in the cortex and/or in the nondependent portion of the collecting system.

Essential Facts

- Stones that fill the greater part of the collecting system are called staghorn because they resemble the antlers of a male deer. There are complete and partial staghorn calculi.
- Classic staghorn calculi are struvite stones and form in the presence of urease-splitting bacteria (*Proteus*, *Klebsiella*, and others). Stones of other compositions can assume a staghorn configuration.
- They are referred to as infectious stones. They are large and develop rapidly in weeks to months.
- They are more common in women, as UTIs are more common in women.
- Untreated staghorn calculi result in renal dysfunction or failure.
- Treatments include lithotripsy, percutaneous nephrolithotomy, and surgery. Dissolution therapy is often used in poor surgical candidates.
- XGP usually occurs in the setting of a staghorn calculus and hydronephrosis. It is a chronic granulomatous process induced by recurrent bacterial UTIs. The kidney becomes enlarged with loss of the normal architecture.

✓ Pearls & × Pitfalls

✓ Patients with staghorn calculi do not typically present with renal colic.

✓ The term *staghorn* describes the configuration of a large stone, not the composition.

✓ Staghorn calculi are usually unilateral because they are infectious.

✓ Most patients with XGP have a staghorn calculus. Few patients with a staghorn calculus have XGP.

✓ Unlike a staghorn calculus, gas in the collecting system will change with repositioning the patient.

Case 87

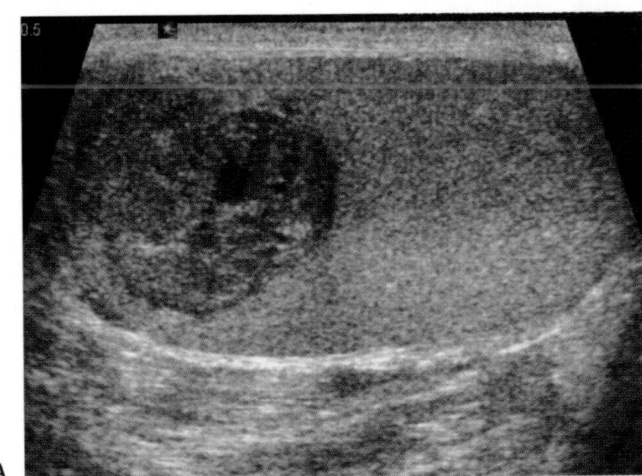
A

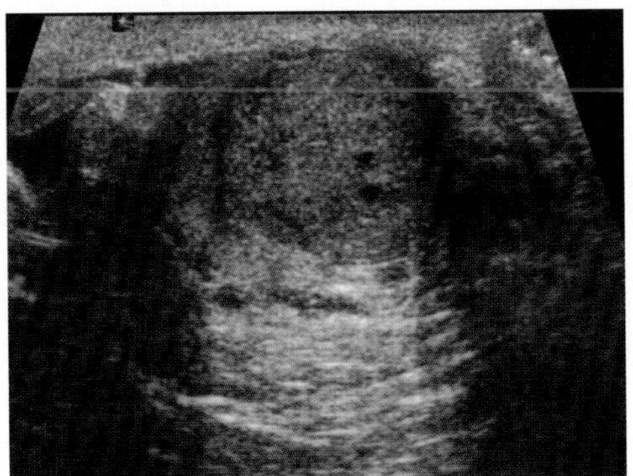
B

Clinical Presentation

A 35-year-old man presents with history of left testicular fullness.

Further Work-up

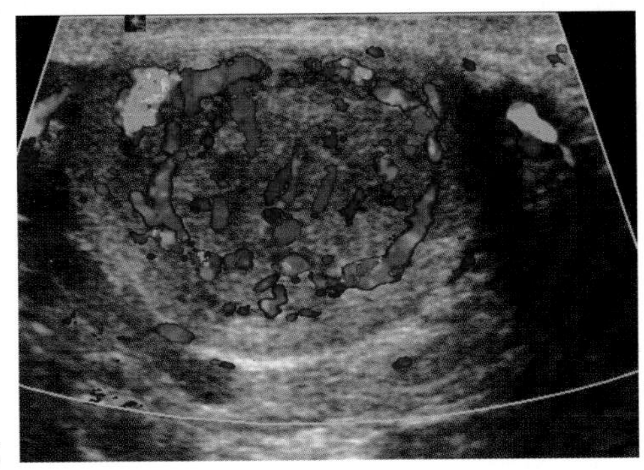
C

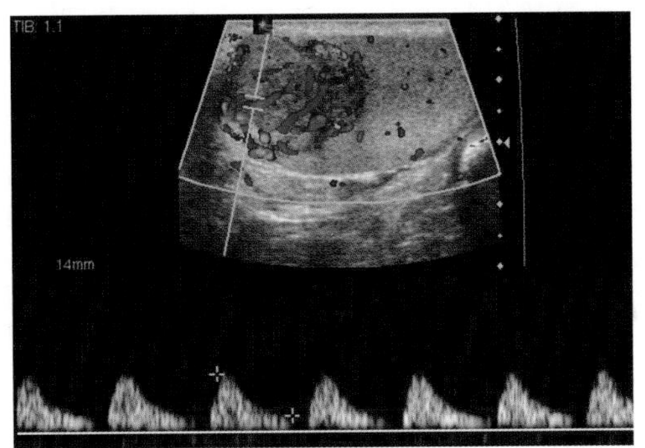

D

Imaging Finding

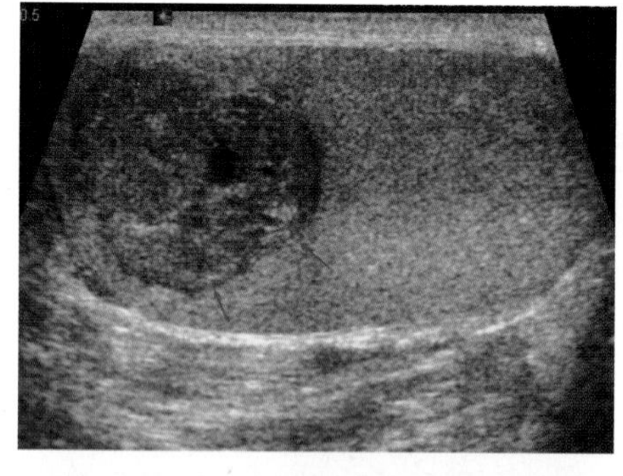
A

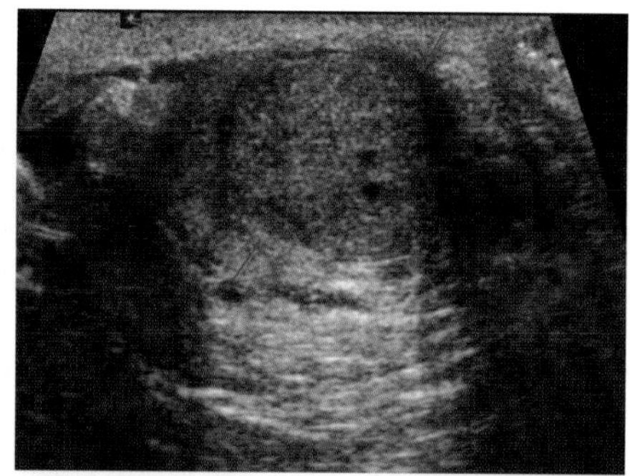
B

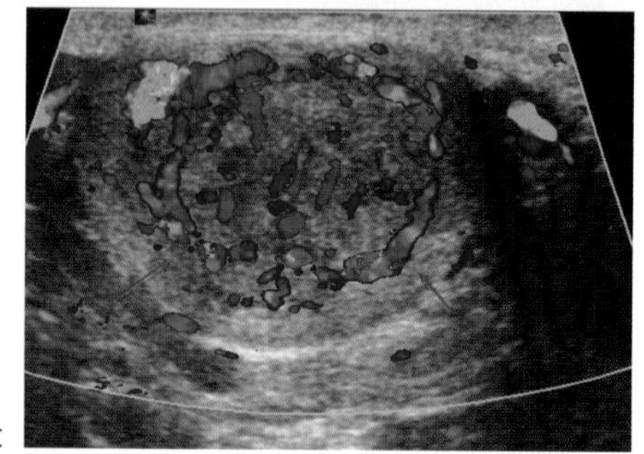
C

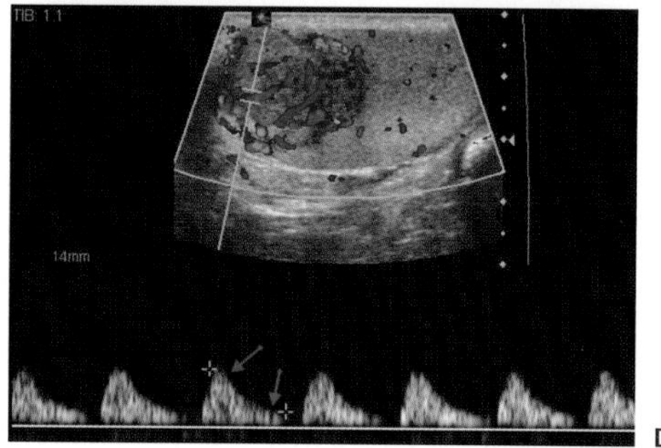
D

(A, B) Gray scale images of the left testicle demonstrate a heterogeneous lesion within the upper portion of the left testicle (*red arrows*). Small cystic component within this lesion are noted. **(C, D)** Color Doppler ultrasound demonstrates vascularity within the described lesion; the lesion appears hypervascular when compared with the left testicle. Pulse Doppler ultrasound demonstrates low-resistance waveform within the described lesion (*green arrows*).

Differential Diagnosis

- ***Germ cell tumors:*** Is the most common type of testicular tumor in adults. The sonographic appearance depends on the type of tumor; seminoma appears as well-defined hypoechoic intratesticular mass lesion. In embryonal cell carcinoma, a heterogeneous appearance is noted with occasional cystic changes. The lesions are usually vascular on Doppler ultrasound.
- *Teratoma:* Constitute ~5 to 10% of testicular neoplasm. They are divided into mature, immature, and teratoma with malignant transformation. Sonographically, appears as well-defined markedly heterogeneous mass with cystic and solid areas. Calcifications are also visualized.
- *Testicular abscess:* Usually related to hemorrhagic or ischemic necrosis, secondary to severe epididymo-orchitis. Sonographically, it appears as a complex cystic lesion. Testicular abscess potentially can rupture through the tunica albuginea into the scrotal sac leading to scrotal abscess. The treatment is surgical.

Essential Facts

- Testicular neoplasm accounts for 1 to 2% of all malignant neoplasm in men.
- The most common presentation is painless unilateral testicular mass.
- Occasionally, patient presents with diffuse metastatic disease.
- The vast majority (90 to 95%) of malignant testicular tumors are germ cell in origin.
- Sixty percent of germ cell tumors are of a single histologic type; the remaining contain two or more histologic types.
- Seminoma is the most common type of testicular tumor in adults.
- The peak incidence is the fourth and fifth decades of life.
- Sonographically appears as a uniform, hypoechoic mass without calcification or cystic changes.
- Embryonal cell carcinoma is the second testicular germ cell neoplasm; accounts for 20% of all germ cell tumors.
- It occurs in younger age group compared with seminoma.
- Sonographically, appearance as inhomogeneous, poorly defined mass with occasional invasion of the tunica albuginea.

✓ Pearls & × Pitfalls

✓ Color Doppler is helpful in characterizing focal testicular lesions. The presence of hypervascularity within the lesion is suggestive of malignancy. Decreased flow is present with focal orchitis and/or ischemic processes

× In patients with human immunodeficiency virus infection, differentiation of abscess from neoplastic process in the testicle is difficult sonographically, and orchiectomy might be needed to obtain histologic diagnosis.

Case 88

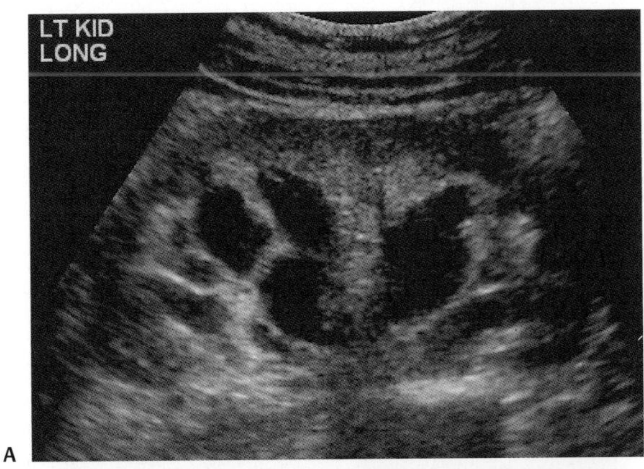

A

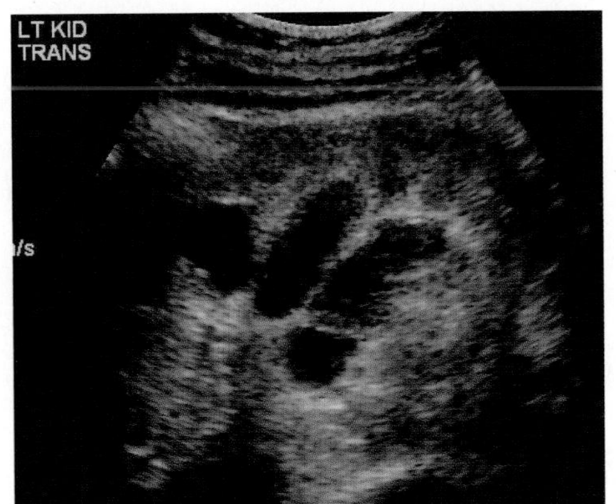

B

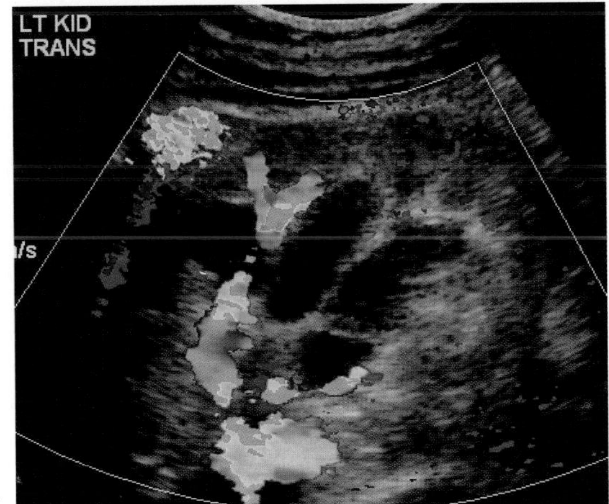

C

Clinical Presentation

A 71-year-old woman with right upper quadrant pain.

Further Work-up

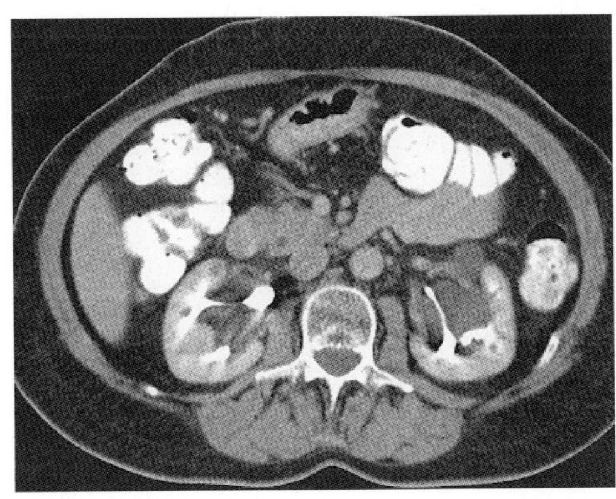

D

Imaging Findings

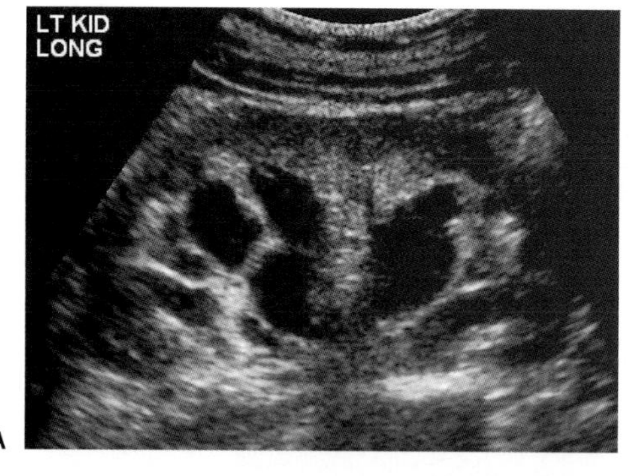

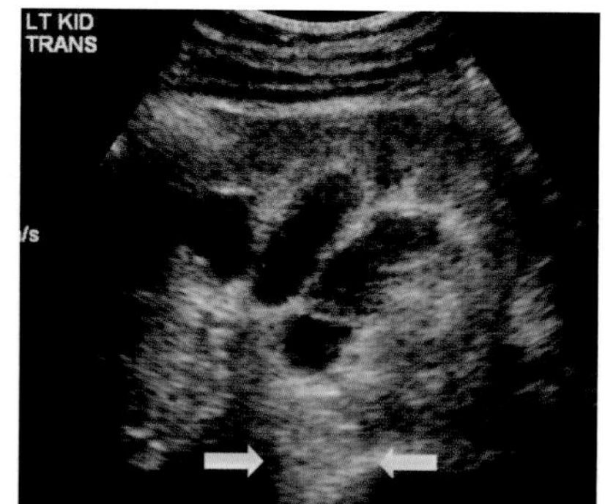

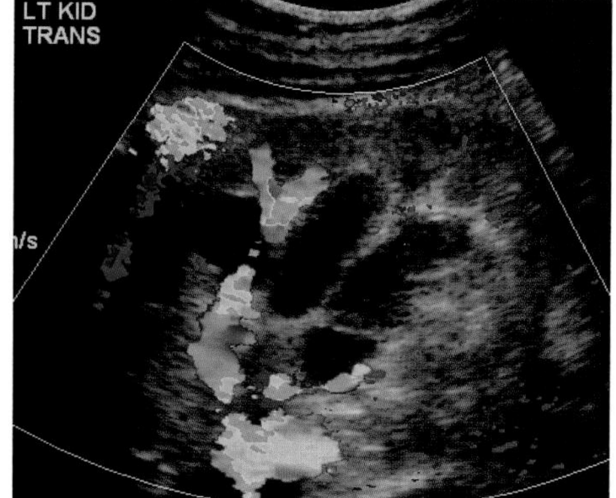

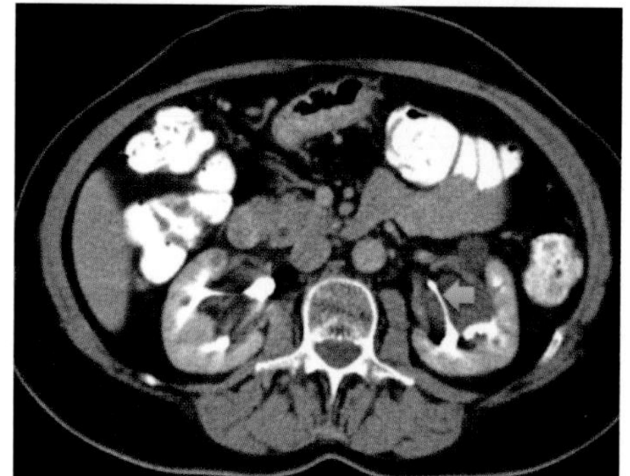

(A) Longitudinal and **(B)** transverse views of the left kidney reveal multiple cystic structures within the sinus fat. They are directed centrally but do not communicate. Acoustic enhancement is seen in **B** (*arrows*). Similar findings were present in the right kidney (not shown). **(C)** The vessels are diverted around the lesions with color Doppler imaging. **(D)** Delayed post contrast CT reveals compressed collecting systems (*arrow on Left Kidney*) surrounded by cystic structures.

Differential Diagnosis

- ***Renal sinus cysts mimicking hydronephrosis:*** Multiple noncommunicating cysts located in the renal sinus can mimic hydronephrosis, as seen in this case.
- *Hydronephrosis:* Dilated calyces connect with a dilated renal pelvis in the setting of hydronephrosis. The renal pelvis would be larger than the calyces.
- *Multicystic dysplastic kidney (MSD):* Normal remaining renal cortex would not be present with a MSD.

Essential Facts

- Renal sinus cysts occur in 1 to 2% of the population and include parapelvic and peripelvic cysts. Their sonographic appearance is similar.
- Peripelvic cysts are lymphatic in origin and are rarely symptomatic. They are often multiple and bilateral, and they can mimic hydronephrosis.
- Parapelvic cysts originate in the renal parenchyma and protrude into the renal sinus. They can compress the collecting system if large.
- The sonographic features of renal sinus cysts are those of all cysts: anechoic, sharp back wall, and enhanced sound transmission.
- Computed tomography can distinguish renal sinus cysts from hydronephrosis. On delayed images, the cysts will be distinguishable from the collecting system, which will be filled with contrast.

Other Imaging Findings

- On magnetic resonance imaging, renal sinus cysts exhibit signal characteristics of simple cysts.

✓ Pearls & × Pitfalls

× Even in experienced hands, computed tomography may be needed to distinguish hydronephrosis from renal sinus cysts.

✓ Real-time imaging is helpful to determine if the cystic structures are interconnected (hydronephrosis) or not (sinus cysts).

× Small cysts may not appear entirely anechoic.

✓ Cortical and parapelvic cysts tend to be larger than peripelvic cysts.

✓ In the setting of what appears to be asymptomatic hydronephrosis, think about peripelvic cysts.

Case 89

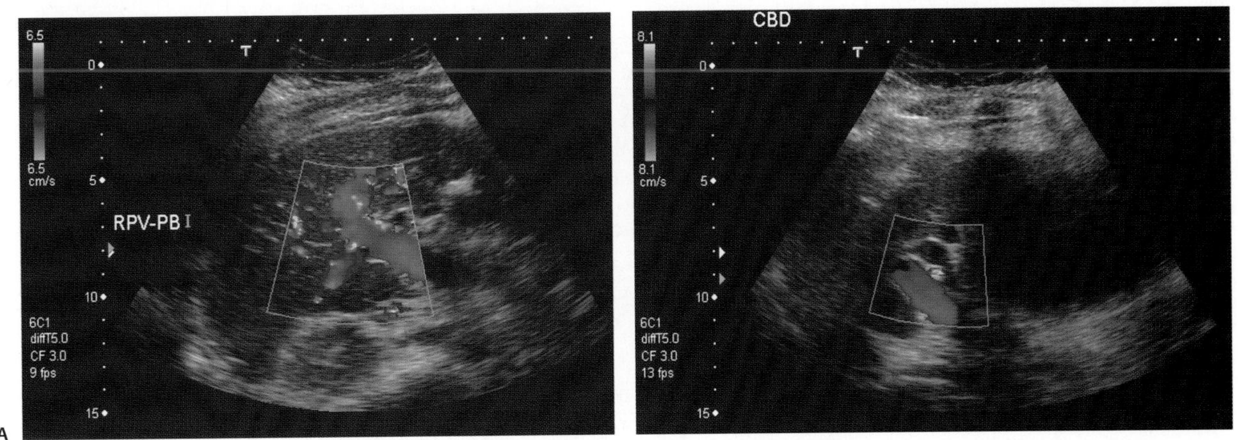

Clinical Presentation

A 52-year-old man with a history of hepatitis C presents for Doppler evaluation.

Further Work-up

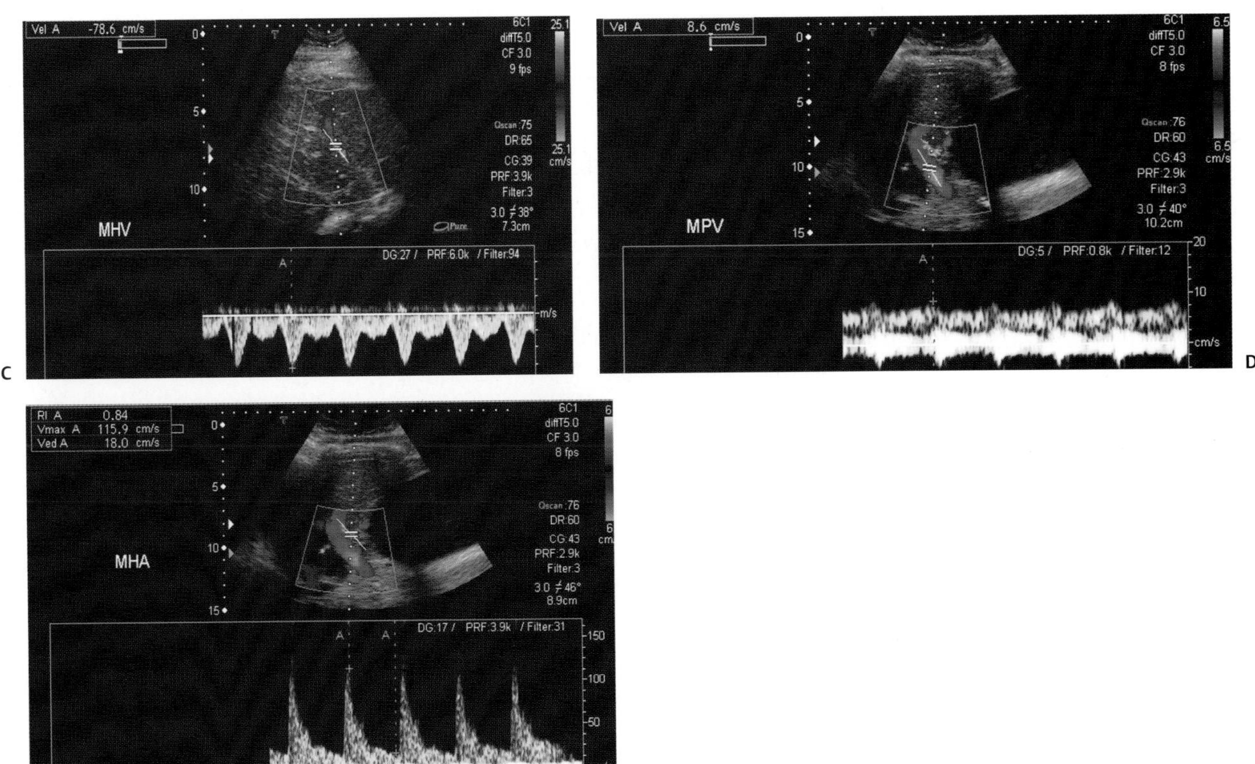

Imaging Findings

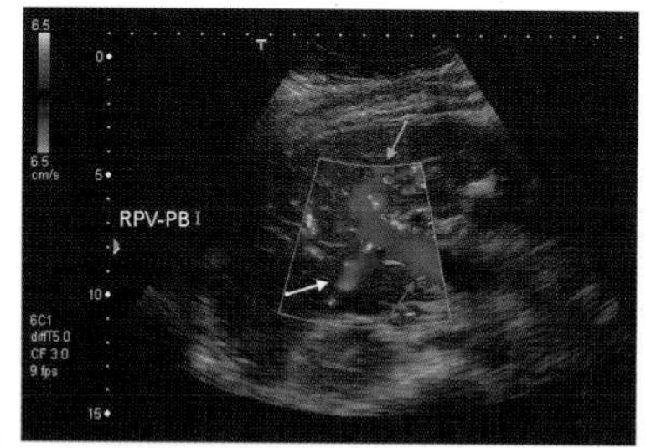

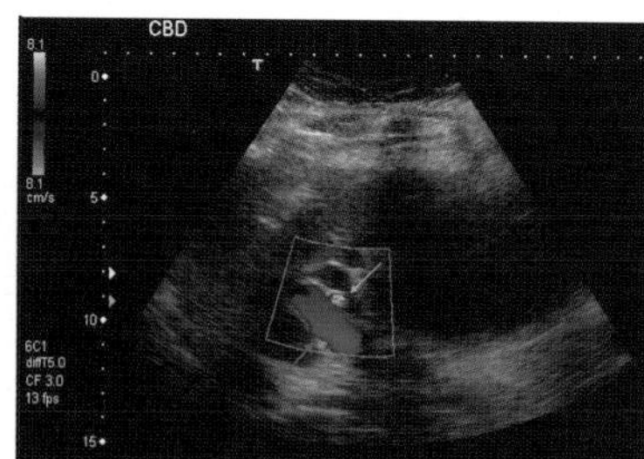

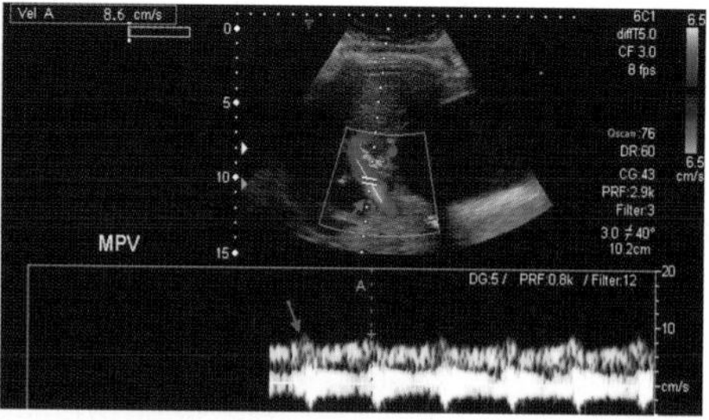

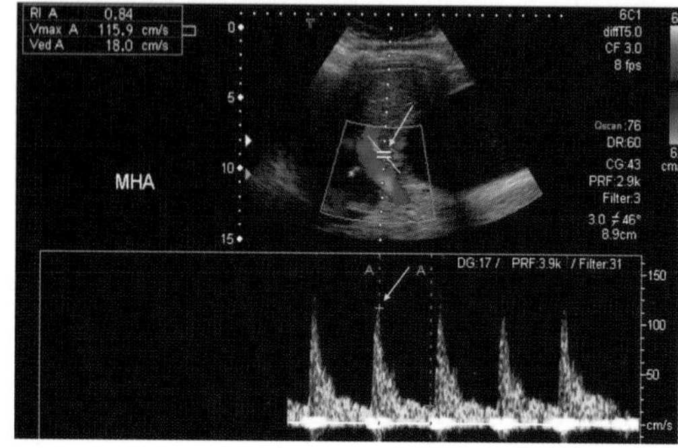

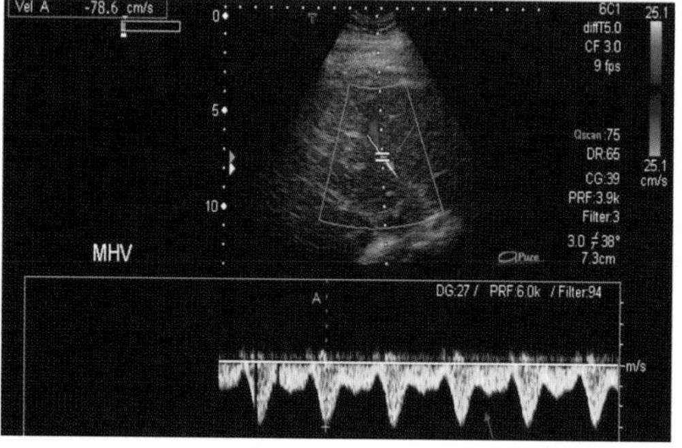

(A, B) Color Doppler ultrasound evaluation demonstrates normal direction of flow within the right portal vein (*green arrow*) and the anterior (*green*) and posterior (*white*) branches. The direction of flow within the main portal vein remains antegrade (*green arrow*). **(C–E)** Further evaluation with pulse Doppler demonstrates normal direction of flow within the main portal vein; however, the velocity is decreased to 8 cm/sec (*green arrow*). The waveform remains normal. Dominant flow within the main hepatic artery is noted (*orange arrow*). Persistent visualization of normal triphasic waveform within the hepatic veins (*red arrow*).

Differential Diagnosis

- ***Slow flow in the portal veins secondary to portal hypertension:*** In early portal hypertension, the flow velocity within the portal vein decreases with loss of respiratory variations. This will progress to pulsatile wave form. Other signs of hypertension might be visualized.
- *Normal Doppler evaluation of the liver:* Normal waveform flow pattern within the portal vein is hepatopetal throughout the cardiac cycle, with an average velocity of 15 to 30 cm/sec. Slight respiratory variations within the portal vein are noted. Triphasic waveform within the hepatic veins and low-resistance arterial flow in the artery is noted. Other signs of portal hypertension are not visualized sonographically.
- *Slow flow within the portal system secondary to Budd-Chiari syndrome*: Sonographically, thrombus within the hepatic vein with occasional extension into the inferior vena cava is visualized. Budd-Chiari is usually segmental in the liver. The flow pattern could be normal in one segment and abnormal in other hepatic segments. The velocity within the portal vein is reduced and/or reversed depending on the extension of hepatic veins occlusion.

Essential Facts

- Portal hypertension is defined as a portal vein pressure > 10 mm Hg.
- The pressure gradient between the hepatic veins and the portal vein exceeds 5 mm Hg.
- Etiologies could be prehepatic, intrahepatic, and suprahepatic.
- The portal vein diameter is enlarged, exceeding 16 mm.
- In the early stages of portal hypertension, sluggish flow within the portal vein (< 10 cm/sec) is noted.
- Subsequently, pulsatile flow within the portal vein is noted. A bidirectional flow is noted later.
- In advanced stages, hepatofugal flow is present.
- Loss of hepatic vein phasicity secondary to increased hepatic stiffness is noted on Doppler evaluation of the hepatic veins.
- With increased hepatic stiffness, more dominant arterial flow is noted in the liver. An arterioportal shunting might be seen.

✓ Pearls & ✗ Pitfalls

✓ The sonographic diagnosis of portal hypertension should be based on a constellation of findings on grayscale and Doppler imaging.

✗ When portosystemic collaterals are formed, the flow pattern within the portal vein would become normal.

Case 90

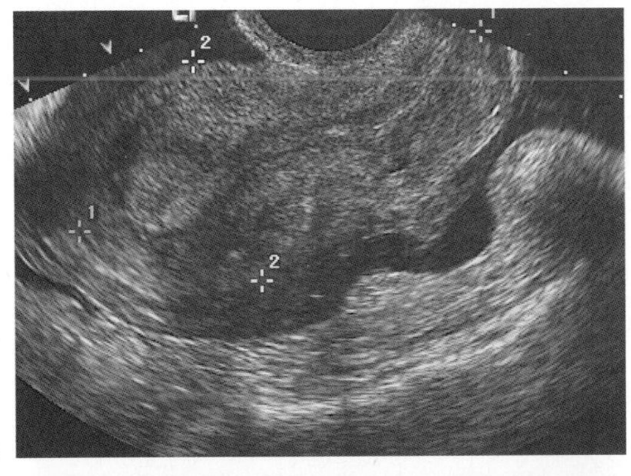
A

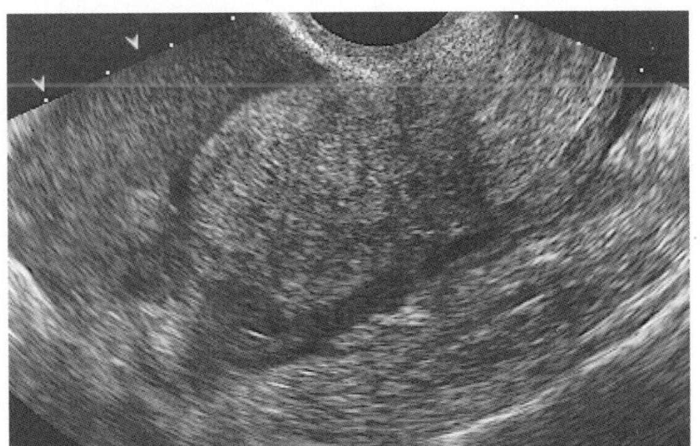
B

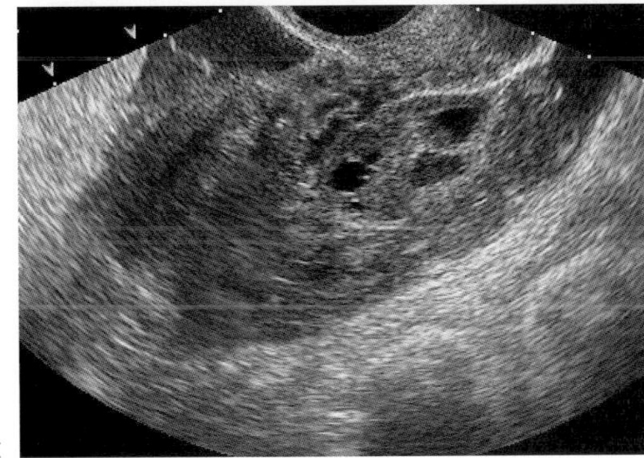
C

■ Clinical Presentation

An 18-year-old, not sexually active woman.

■ Further Work-up

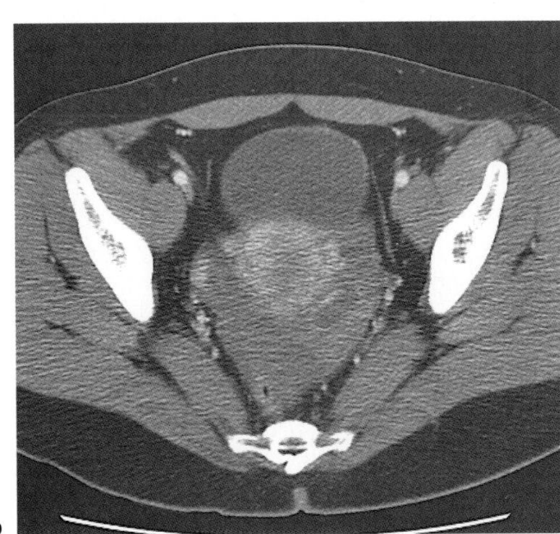
D

Imaging Findings

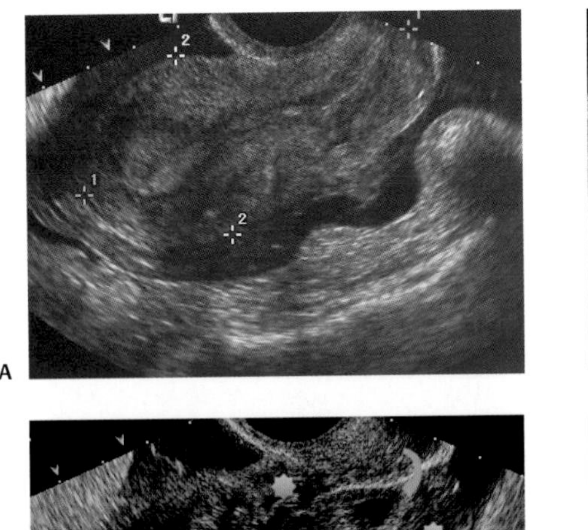
A

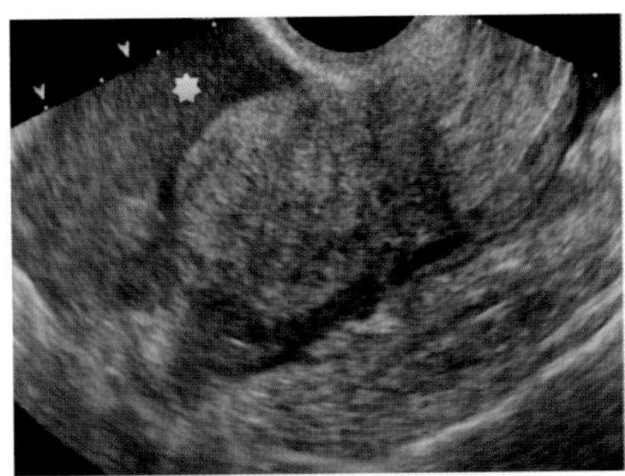
B

C

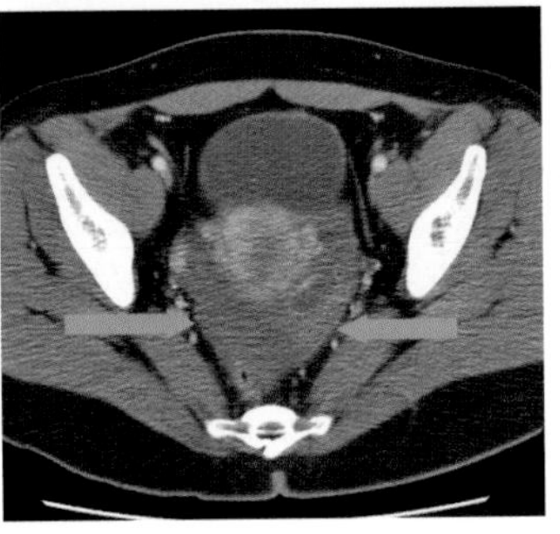
D

(A) Transvaginal longitudinal view of the pelvis reveals a normal uterus (measured with calipers). **(B)** Surrounding the uterus is complex free fluid. This is most pronounced in the anterior cul-de-sac (*asterisk*). **(C)** The right ovary is completely surrounded by complex fluid (*asterisks*). The ovary can be identified due to the presence of follicles (*curved arrow*). **(D)** On CT high density free fluid is present in the pelvis predominantly in the posterior cul-de-sac on this image (*arrows*).

Differential Diagnosis

- ***Hemoperitoneum:*** Complex free fluid in the pelvis that is high density on computed tomography in this clinical setting is most commonly due to blood from cyst rupture.
- *Ruptured ectopic:* Rupture of an ectopic pregnancy can result in hemoperitoneum. Despite the stated history, a pregnancy test should be performed to exclude ectopic pregnancy in the setting of hemoperitoneum.
- *Pus or enteric contents in the pelvis:* Complex free fluid in the pelvis can represent enteric contents from a ruptured viscous or pus from an infection such as appendicitis. Such patients would have symptoms of infection (fever or elevated white count) and usually a more prolonged illness.

Essential Facts

- Hemoperitoneum on ultrasound appears as complex fluid usually with low- to medium-level echoes. The more acute the hemorrhage, the more echogenic the fluid. The most common cause for hemoperitoneum in a nonpregnant patient is rupture of a physiologic cyst (follicle or corpus luteum).
- In the setting of hemoperitoneum, always scan up in in the right upper quadrant. Morrison's pouch is the most dependent portion of the peritoneum and may indicate a larger volume hemorrhage.
- The ruptured cyst may be irregular in contour. It may not be identifiable with ultrasound.
- A blood clot can mimic a solid adnexal mass. Blood can obscure visualization of an ovary.
- The finding of hemoperitoneum should be reported immediately, as intraperitoneal bleeding can be life threatening. Patients should be taken directly to the emergency department.

Other Imaging Findings

- Hemoperitoneum on computed tomography appears as high-density ascites.

✓ Pearls & × Pitfalls

× Hemoperitoneum can be difficult to distinguish from other complex fluid collections in the pelvis, such as a ruptured appendicitis.

× In an acute bleed, hemoperitoneum can be isoechoic to the uterus (as in our case) and therefore difficult to recognize.

× When evaluating the pelvis with ultrasound, we are so focused on the uterus and ovaries we forget to look outside these structures. We are used to ignoring the heterogeneous echogenicity of bowel and the pelvic fat seen in every pelvic ultrasound.

Case 91

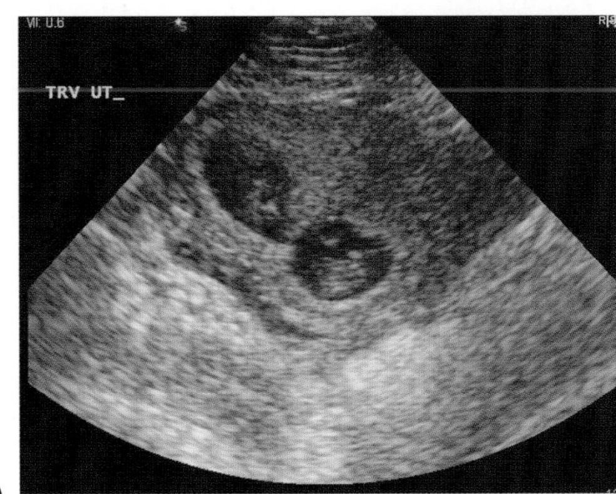

A

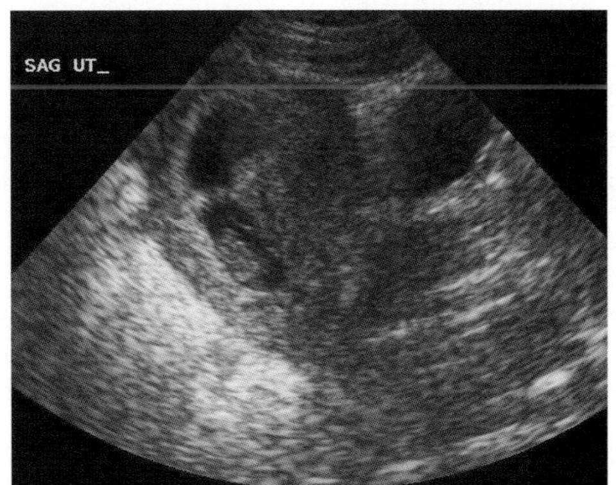

B

Clinical Presentation

A 22-year-old woman presents for dating ultrasound.

Further Work-up

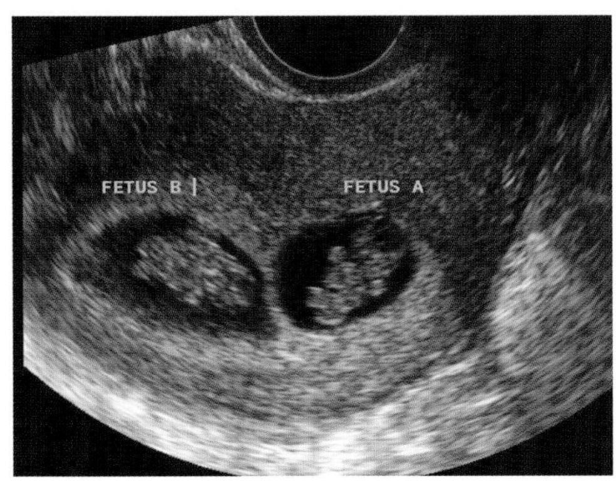

C

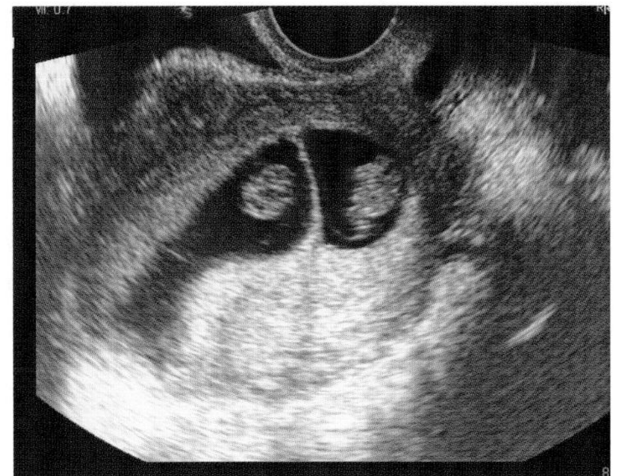

D

Imaging Findings

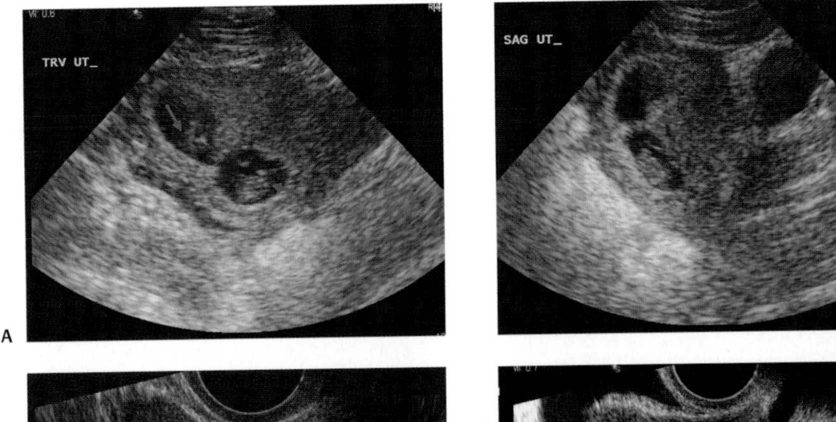

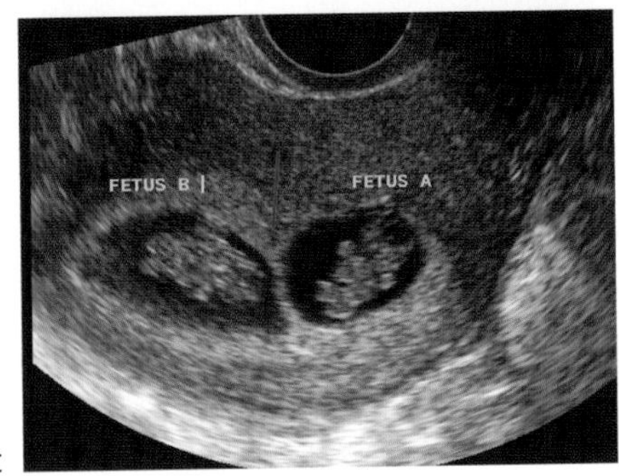

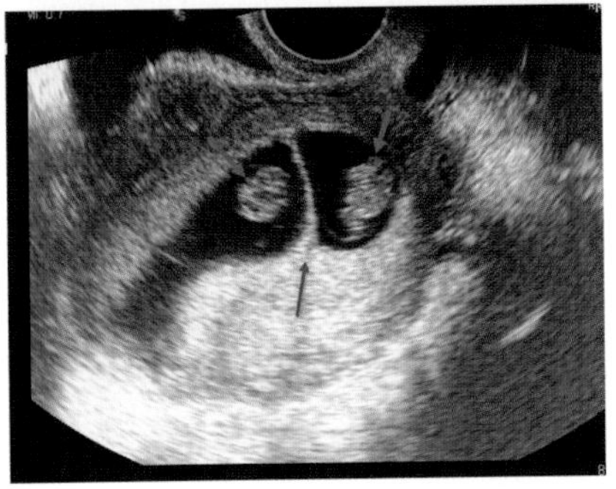

(A, B) Transabdominal ultrasound images of the pelvis demonstrate twin pregnancy (*green arrows*). Two gestational sacs are noted. The gestational sacs appear to be separated by a thick septation (*red arrow*). **(C, D)** Further evaluation with transvaginal ultrasound demonstrates thick separation of the gestations, with possible visualization of twin peak sign (*red arrow*).

Differential Diagnosis

- ***Dichorionic diamniotic twins:*** Divisions occurs ~ 3 days postconception (in monozygotic) with subsequent formation of two embryos, two amnions, two chorions, and two yolk sacs. Dichorionic diamnionic twin pregnancy could be dizygotic and/or monozygotic.
- *Monochorionic diamniotic twins:* Most common type of monozygotic twin pregnancy. Division of the embryonic disc occurs 4 to 8 days postconception. Sonographically, two embryos, two amnions, and two yolk sacs would be formed within a single chorion. The twins will have a single placenta.
- *Monochorionic monoamniotic twin pregnancy:* Division of embryos occurs 8 days postconception. Two embryos within a single amnion and a single chorion is formed (single sac). A single yolk sac is visualized. Monochorionic monoamniotic pregnancy represents ~ 4% of monozygotic twins. Complications related to separation, such as conjoined twins, might be present.

Essential Facts

- The incidence of twin pregnancy is ~ 1 to 1.5% of live birth.
- Could be monozygotic and/or dizygotic in origin.
- Dizygotic twin pregnancy increases with maternal age, parity, and hereditary.
- Increased incidence with ovulation-inducing agents
- Chronicity and amnionicity have important prognostic value.
- The higher mortality rate is in monochorionic diamniotic twin pregnancies.
- In dichorionic diamniotic twins, two separate placentas are present.
- A diagnosis of chorionicity and amnionicity is more accurate in the first trimester.
- In dichorionic twins, there is a thick septum between the sacs.
- In early pregnancies, the amnion could be visualized as a thin member surrounding each embryo.
- Two yolk sacs are visualized.
- The presence of thin membrane between the embryos indicates a monochorionic diamniotic twin pregnancy
- The presence of two placentas indicates dichorionic diamniotic twins.

✓ Pearls & × Pitfalls

✓ The presence of twin peak sign between the two gestations is diagnostic of dichorionic diamniotic twin pregnancy.

× In dichorionic diamniotic pregnancy, the two placentas may fuse and appear as a single placenta; this could be misinterpreted as monochorionic diamniotic twin pregnancy.

Case 92

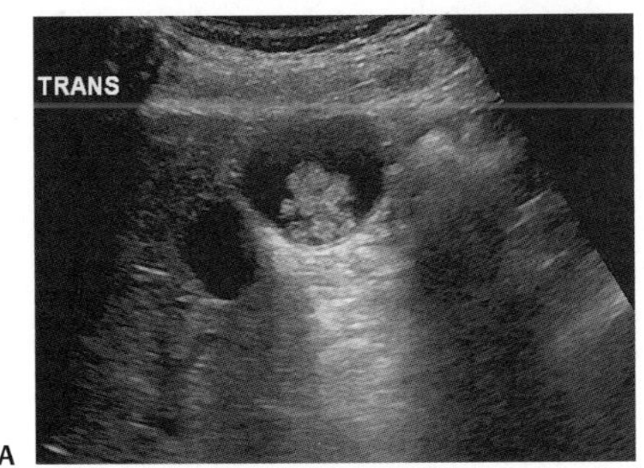

A

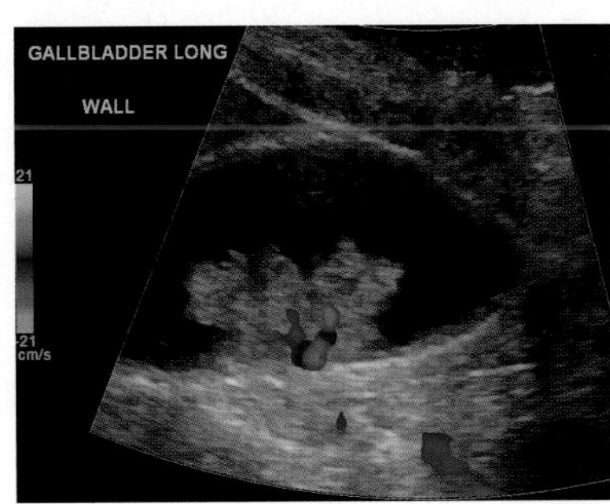

B

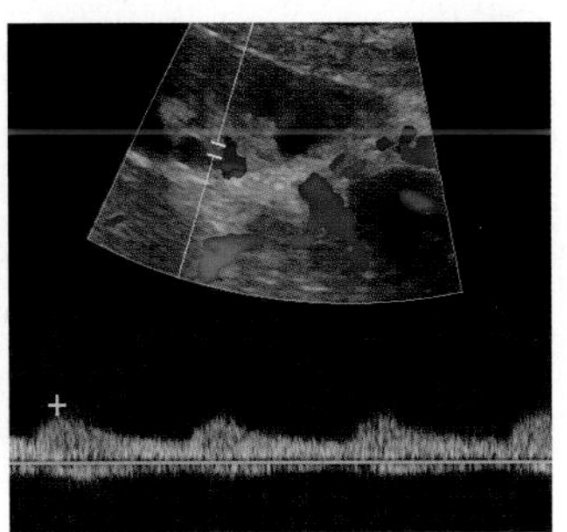
C

Clinical Presentation

A 52-year-old woman with right upper quadrant pain.

Further Work-up

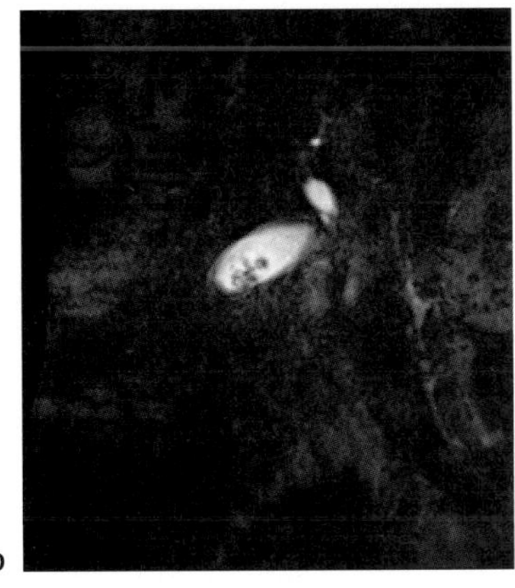
D

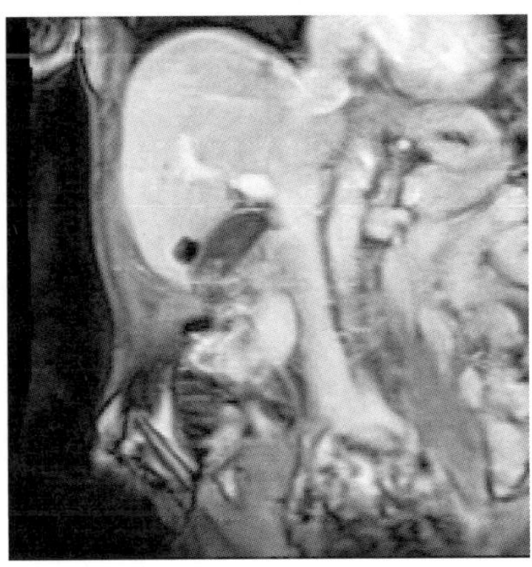
E

Imaging Findings

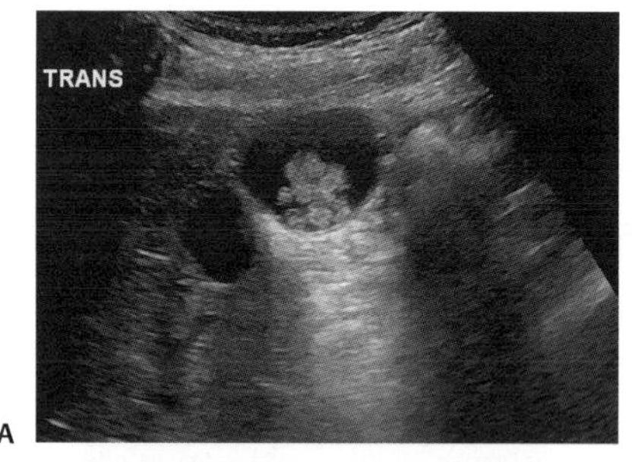

A

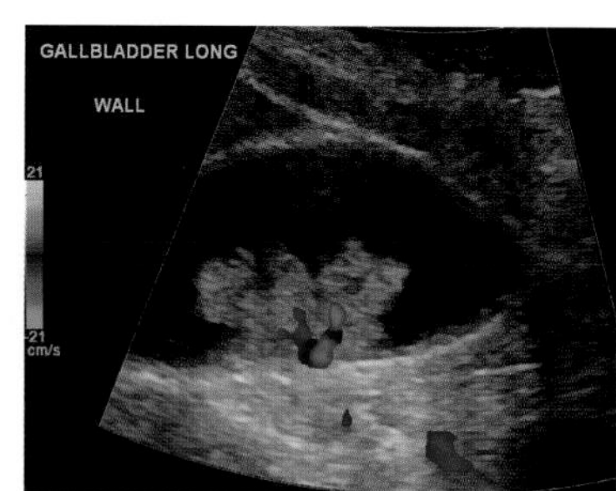

B

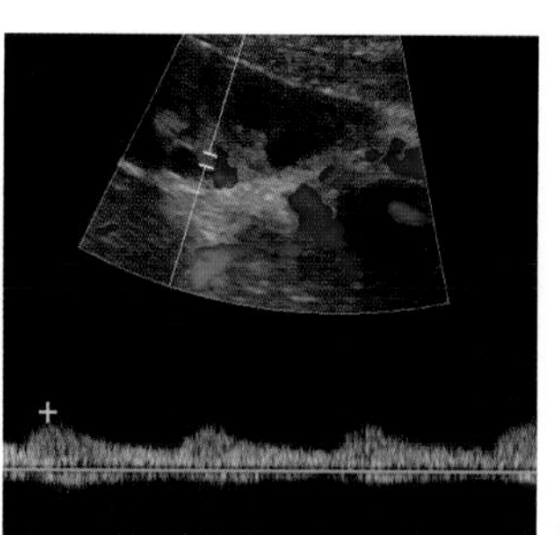
C

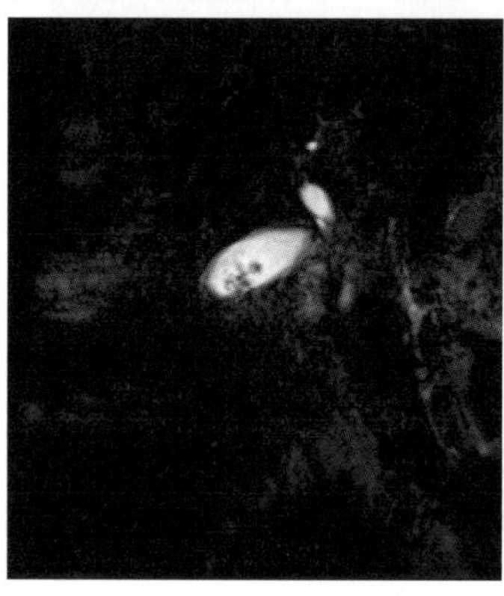
D

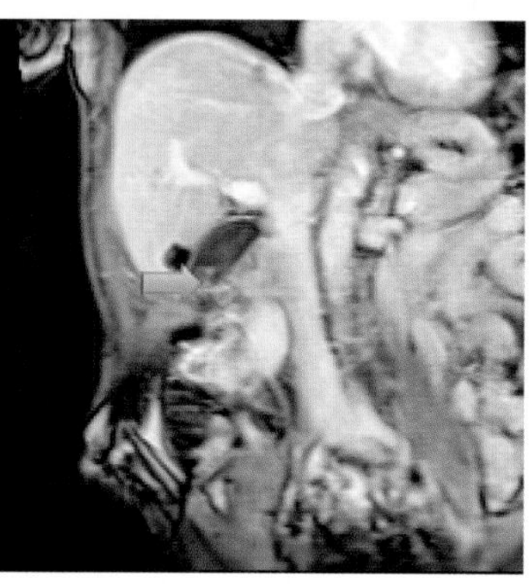
E

Transverse **(A)** and longitudinal images reveal a broad-based polypoid lesion that demonstrates internal vascularity with color **(B)** and spectral **(C)** Doppler. MRCP **(D)** confirms a persistent intraluminal fungating lesion. Post contrast coronal MR image **(E)** demonstrates enhancement of the lesion (*arrow*).

Differential Diagnosis

- ***Gallbladder polyp:*** Intraluminal gallbladder lesion with an intact underlying wall is most consistent with a polyp. Although most polyps are small, they can be up to 2 to 3 cm. Rarely, polyps are tubular or papillary as in this case. A lesion this size is considered surgical.
- *Gallbladder carcinoma:* Gallbladder cancer is rare and usually presents with a large mass obliterating the gallbladder or invading the gallbladder wall eccentrically. Flow is often visible in a gallbladder carcinoma.
- *Sludge ball or tumefactive sludge:* This would be gravity dependent and should move with changing patient position. It would not demonstrate vascularity.

Essential Facts

- Gallbladder polyps are quite common and usually seen on a daily basis in an ultrasound department.
- Polyps measuring < 7 mm require no follow-up. Polyps measuring 7 to 9 mm should be followed annually. Polyps > 12 mm deserve surgical consultation.
- Prevalence of gallbladder polyps ranges from 4 to 7%. Incidence in females is greater than or equal to males (F > M or F = M).
- Originate from the mucosal surface of the gallbladder. Polyps are usually pedunculated but can be sessile in this case. Polyps may be single, multiple, or carpeted as in cholesterolosis.
- Most polyps are hyperplastic cholesterol polyps and therefore echogenic, often with a ring down artifact or v-shaped artifact deep to the polyp.
- Twinkle artifact with color Doppler can occur in polyps due to crystalline deposits in cholesterol polyps and should not be confused with vascular flow.

✓ Pearls & × Pitfalls

✓ Polyps are usually only a few millimeters; most measure < 10 mm. Rarely they can measure up to 2 to 3 cm.

× The stalk of pedunculated polyps may not be visible so the polyp appears separate from the wall of the gallbladder.

× Both gallstones and polyps can cause the twinkle artifact with color Doppler.

✓ Adenomatous polyps are rare, usually larger, considered premalignant, and are associated with Peutz-Jeghers syndrome.

✓ Metastases to the gallbladder are rare but classically occur in the setting of melanoma.

Case 93

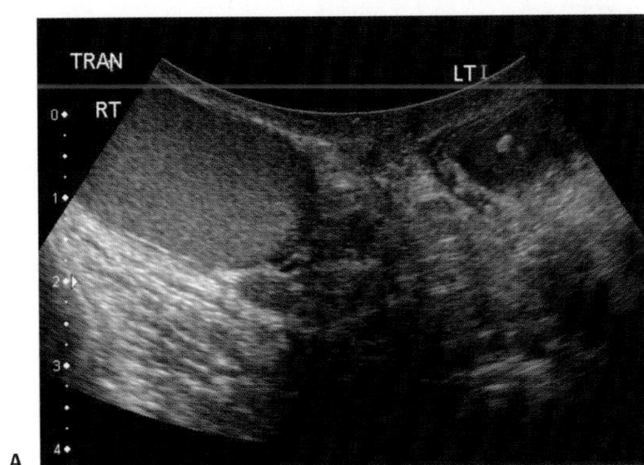

A

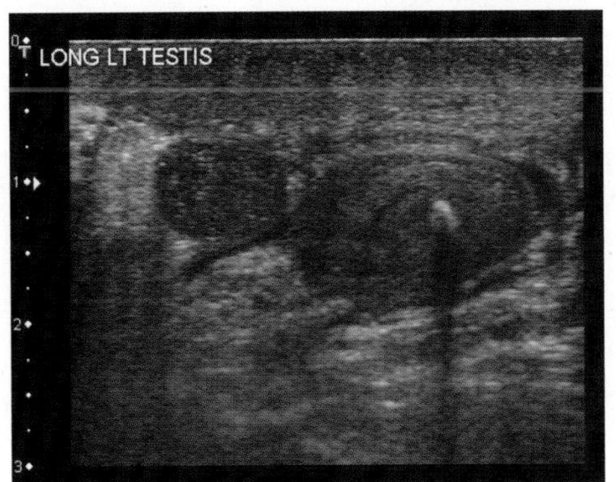

B

Clinical Presentation

A 35-year-old man presents with a history of chronic left-sided scrotal pain.

Further Work-up

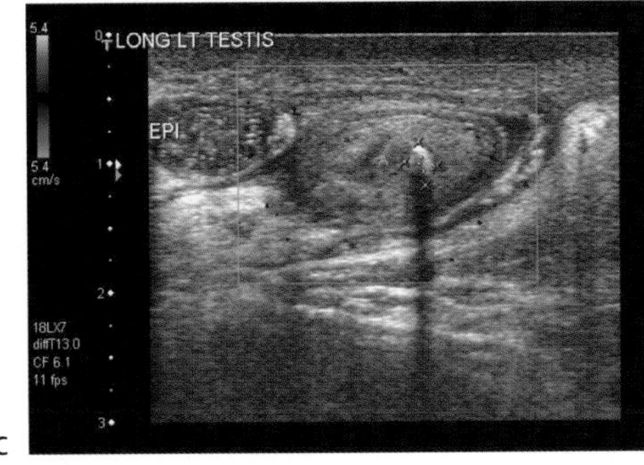

C

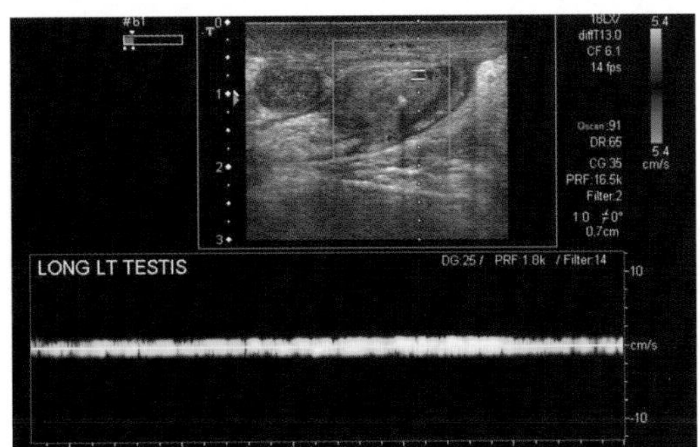

D

Imaging Findings

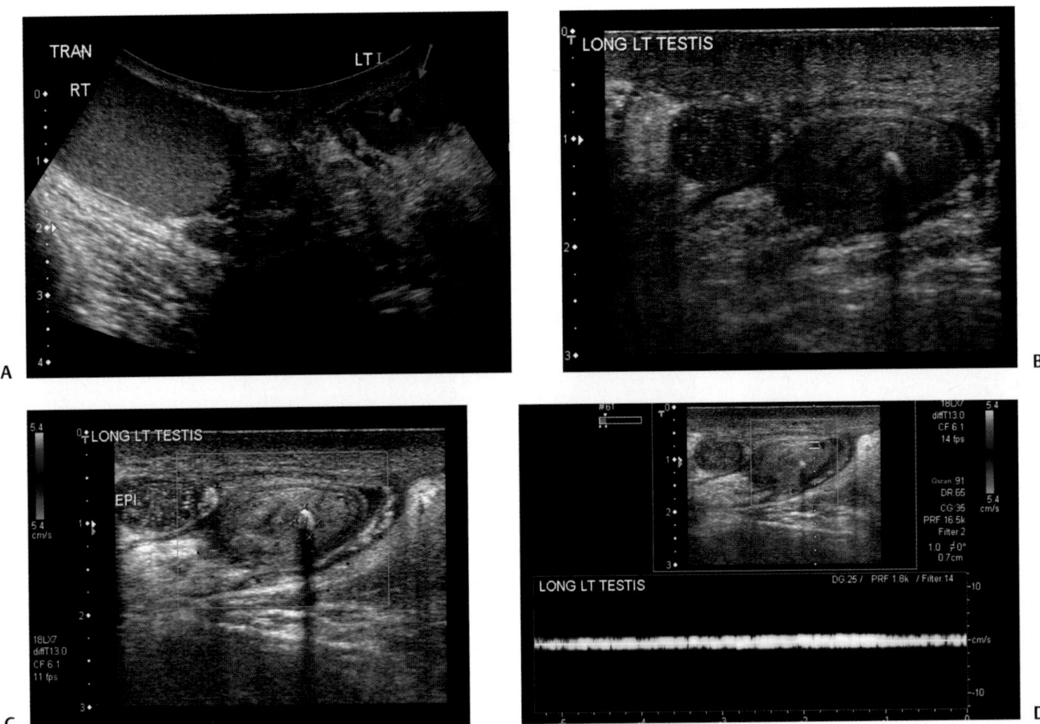

(A, B) Gray scale images of the right and left testicle demonstrate atrophic left testicle (*green arrow*). Focal dense calcification within the center of the left testicle is also noted (*red arrow*). **(C, D)** Further evaluation with color Doppler imaging demonstrates no evidence of flow within the left testicle. Minimal flow within the capsule of the left testicle is noted. Dense calcification within the left testicle is also noted (*red arrow*).

Differential Diagnosis

- ***Missed testicular torsion:*** Defined as torsion exceeding 24 hours since onset of symptoms. Testicle becomes nonviable and cannot be surgically salvaged. The sonographic appearance depends on the stage of torsion; heterogeneous large testicle is present early with subsequent development of small, atrophic testicle in delayed torsion. Calcifications could be seen on ultrasound.
- *Intratesticular mass:* Dense intratesticular calcifications could be seen within intratesticular masses like teratoma. Sonographically, mixed echogenicity mass with dense calcification is present. The testicle is larger when compared with the normal side.
- *Testicular tuberculosis:* Usually related to homogenous spread, the testicle appears heterogeneous on sonography in early stages. Epididymal involvement favors inflammatory process rather then intratesticular mass. Dense calcification or fistula formation may develop on follow-up imaging.

Essential Facts

- Missed torsion is defined as torsion exceeding 24 hours since the onset of symptoms.
- The testicle becomes nonviable and cannot be salvaged surgically.
- In early stages, the testicle appears to be enlarged with mixed echogenicity.
- Hemorrhage within the testicle may be present sonographically.
- A reactive hydrocele and enlargement of the epididymis could also be present.
- In delayed missed torsion, the testicle appears hypoechoic and atrophic.
- Intratesticular dense calcification may be seen in chronic missed torsion, presumably a sequela of hemorrhagic infarcts.
- On Doppler ultrasound, no evidence of intratesticular flow is noted on power and/or Doppler imaging.
- Peripheral flow does not exclude the diagnosis.

✓ Pearls & × Pitfalls

✓ Documentation of flow within the intratesticular arteries not into the capsule arteries should be obtained to exclude torsion.

× Flow within the tunica vaginalis can be mistaken for flow within the capsular artery with subsequent delaying in the diagnosis.

Case 94

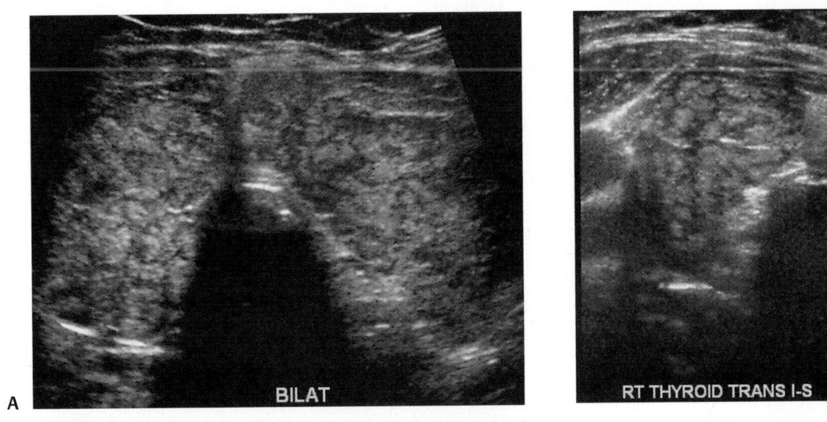

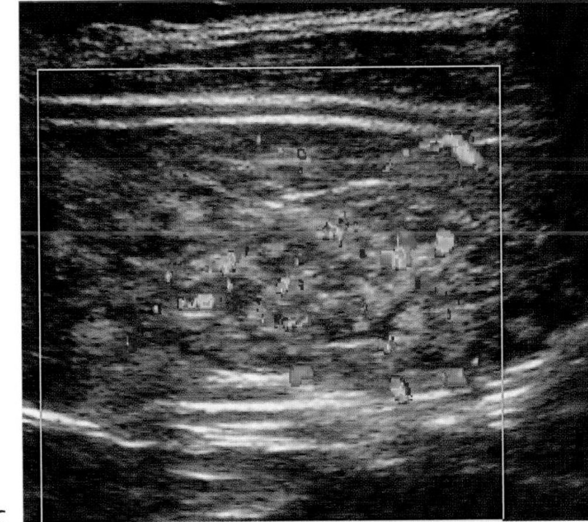

■ Clinical Presentation

A 40-year-old woman with a painless enlarged thyroid on exam, found to be hypothyroid.

Imaging Findings

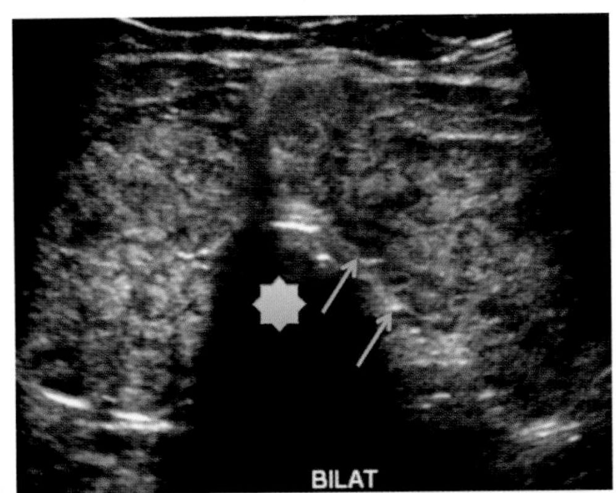

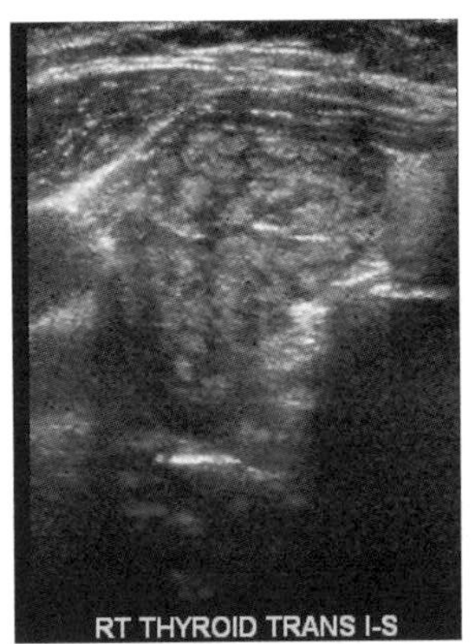

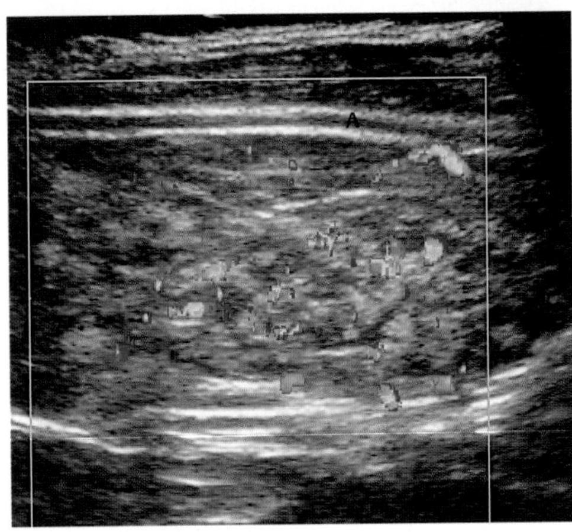

(A) Transverse image demonstrates an enlarged heterogeneous thyroid. The *asterisk* denotes the trachea. The gland is nodular in contour (*arrows*). **(B)** Transverse image of the right lobe reveals hypoechoic curved lines alternating between echogenic areas resulting in a *giraffe pattern*. **(C)** With color Doppler imaging, the gland is not hypervascular.

Differential Diagnosis

- ***Hashimoto's thyroiditis (HT):*** A diffusely heterogenous gland with a giraffe-like pattern and a lobular contour is classic for HT.
- *Multinodular goiter:* In a multinodular goiter, the nodules will be larger and of varying echogenicity. Nodules would be more discrete. The gland may be asymmetric.
- *Acute thyroiditis:* In acute thyroiditis, the thyroid gland will be hypervascular and tender.

Essential Facts

- HT, also known as *chronic lymphocytic thyroiditis*, is the most common cause of hypothyroidism.
- It is an autoimmune disease with antibodies to thyroglobulin and thyroid peroxidase.
- It is very common, occurring in 4% of women. Four times more common in women than men. Typically, patients are over 40.
- Patients usually present with painless diffuse enlargement of the thyroid gland. Hypothyroidism is usually present.
- The sonographic appearance of HT is variable and may be related to stage of disease. There are a few classic appearances including
  - A giraffe-like pattern with round or ovoid areas of hyperechogenicity separated by thin linear areas of hypoechogenicity that appear similar to the two-tone blocklike coloring of a giraffe (as in this case)
  - Numerous hypoechoic rice-like nodules
  - Nodular form contour or inhomogenous echotexture
- Not all patients with HT demonstrate the classic appearance on ultrasound. The gland can demonstrate a coarsened or inhomogeneous echotexture.
- In HT, the thyroid can be normal in volume, small, or enlarged. End-stage disease appears as a small, scarred gland.

✓ Pearls & × Pitfalls

× Not all patients with HT demonstrate the classic appearance on ultrasound.

× The ultrasound findings in HT overlap with other causes of diffuse thyroid disease. However, the clinical presentations and biochemical profiles are different.

✓ Perithyroidal lymph nodes may be present in HT including the Delphian node just cephalad to the isthmus.

✓ HT has an increased risk of thyroid malignancies.

✓ The classic benign node seen in HT is very echogenic and referred to as a *white knight*.

Case 95

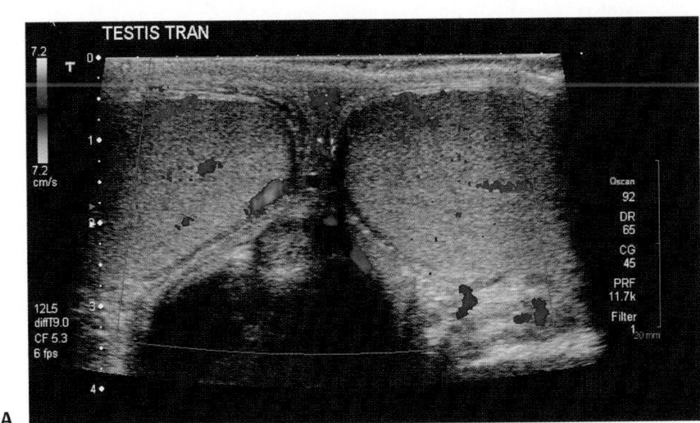

A

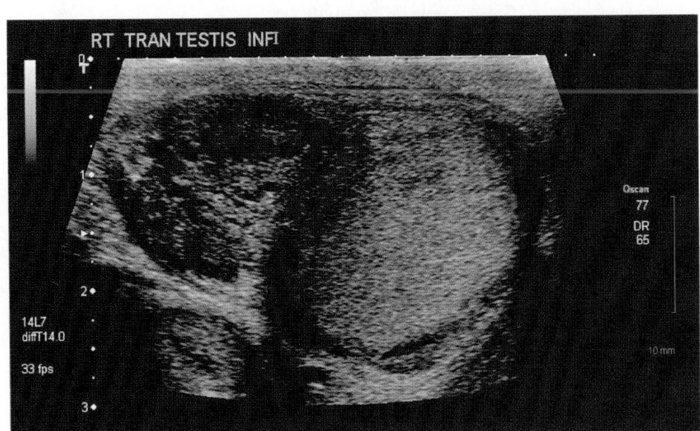

B

■ Clinical Presentation

A 23-year-old man presents with right-sided testicular pain for 2 days.

■ Further Work-up

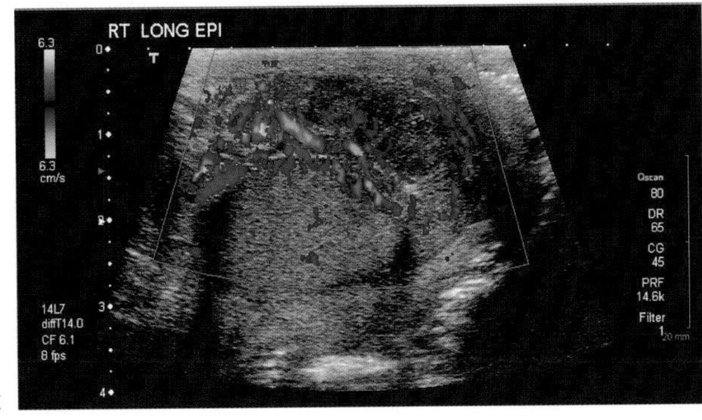

C

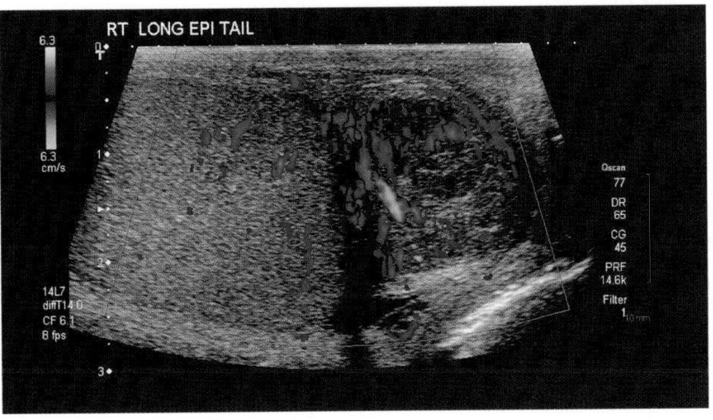

D

Imaging Findings

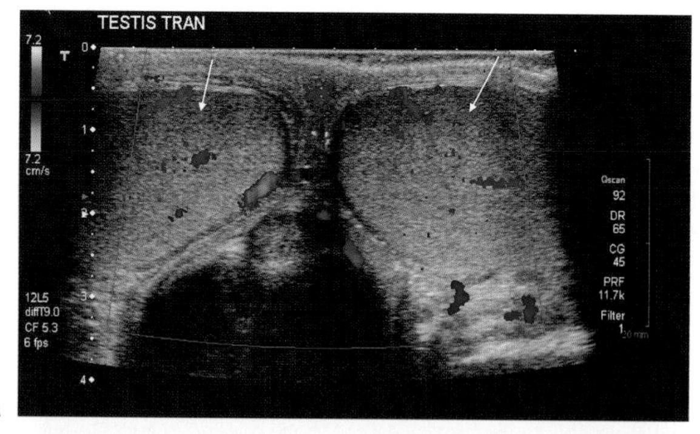

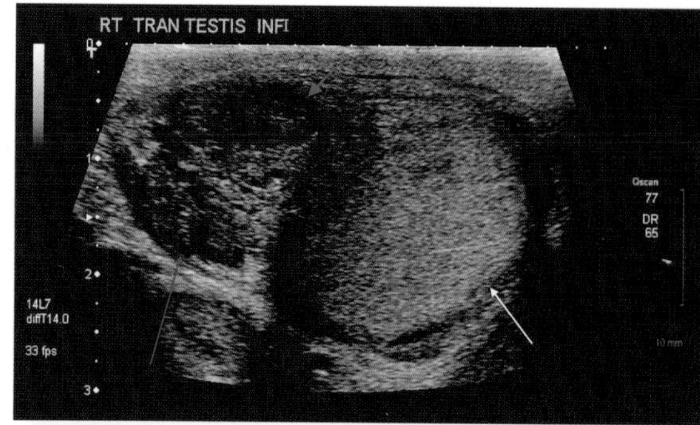

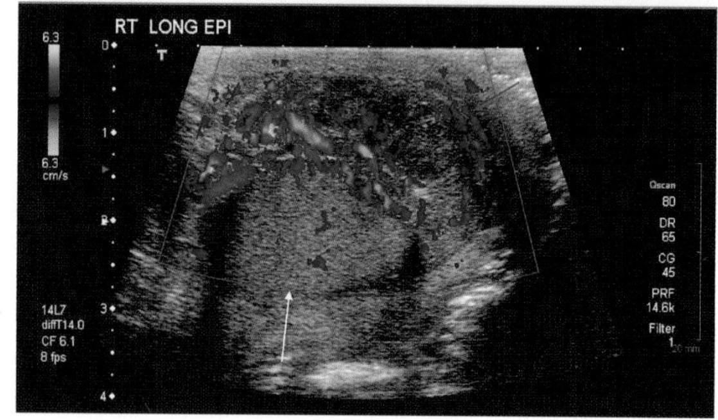

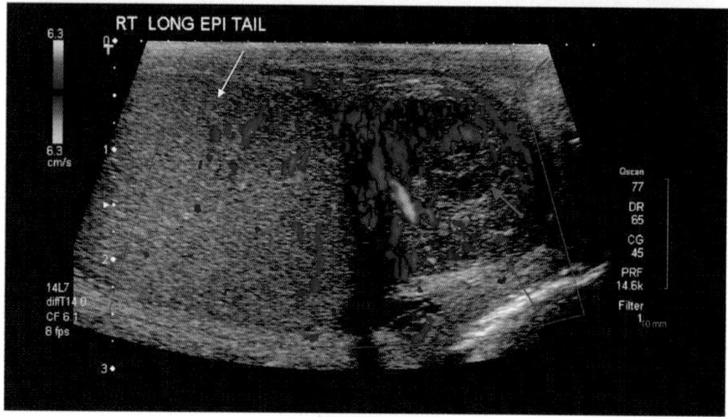

(A, B) Doppler evaluation of the right and left testicles demonstrates symmetric flow bilaterally (*white arrow*). Heterogeneous appearance of the right epididymis is noted (*red arrow*), with possible visualization of hypoechoic lesion within the epididymal body (*green arrow*). **(C, D)** Further Doppler evaluation of the right epididymis demonstrates marked hyperemia within the epididymis (*red arrow*) when compared with the adjacent testicle (*white arrow*). No significant flow is noted within the questionable hypoechoic area within the epididymal body (*green arrow*).

Differential Diagnosis

- ***Acute epididymitis:*** More commonly affects sexually active males. The patient presents with acute scrotal pain, pyuria, and fever. Ultrasound demonstrates focally and/or diffusely enlarged hypoechoic epididymis with increased Doppler flow. Reactive hydrocele may also be seen.
- *Tuberculous epididymitis:* The patient presents with chronic course; a large indurated mass is noted on physical examination. A heterogeneous mixed echogenicity, large epididymal lesion is noted on gray scale imaging. Doppler evaluation of the epididymis demonstrates predominantly peripheral flow; the epididymis is usually not hyperemic when compared with the testicle.
- *Epididymal mass:* The majority of epididymal masses are benign, with adenomatoid tumor as the most common tumor. The patient presents with nontender epididymal mass that is discovered incidentally. Gray scale ultrasound demonstrates focal epididymal lesion with hypoechoic and/or hyperechoic rim. Doppler ultrasound demonstrates predominantly hypovascular lesion with minimal number of vessels within the mass.

Essential Facts

- Epididymitis is the most common etiology of acute scrotal pain.
- Likely related to sexually transmitted infection and less likely related to hematogenous spread or trauma.
- The peak incidence is 14 to 50 years.
- The patient presents with pain, increasing over 1 to 2 days. Fever, dysuria, and urethral discharge may be present.
- Sonographically, thickening and enlargement of the epididymis is present, with decreased echogenicity.
- Epididymal involvement could be focal and/or diffuse.
- Reactive hydrocele could also be visualized sonographically. The hydrocele may appear complex.
- Doppler imaging demonstrates hyperemia of the epididymis when compared with the asymptomatic side.
- Phlegmon appears as a hypoechoic lesion with lack of flow centrally.
- Complications include testicular infarction, abscess formation, pyocele, and chronic pain.

✓ Pearls & × Pitfalls

✓ Pulse Doppler demonstrates low-resistance waveform within the inflamed epididymis; reversal of flow in diastole may indicate venous infarction.

× Relative hyperemia within the epididymis could be related to lack of or decreased flow in a torsed ipsilateral testicle; documentation of flow in the testicle should be performed in all patients with testicular pain.

Case 96

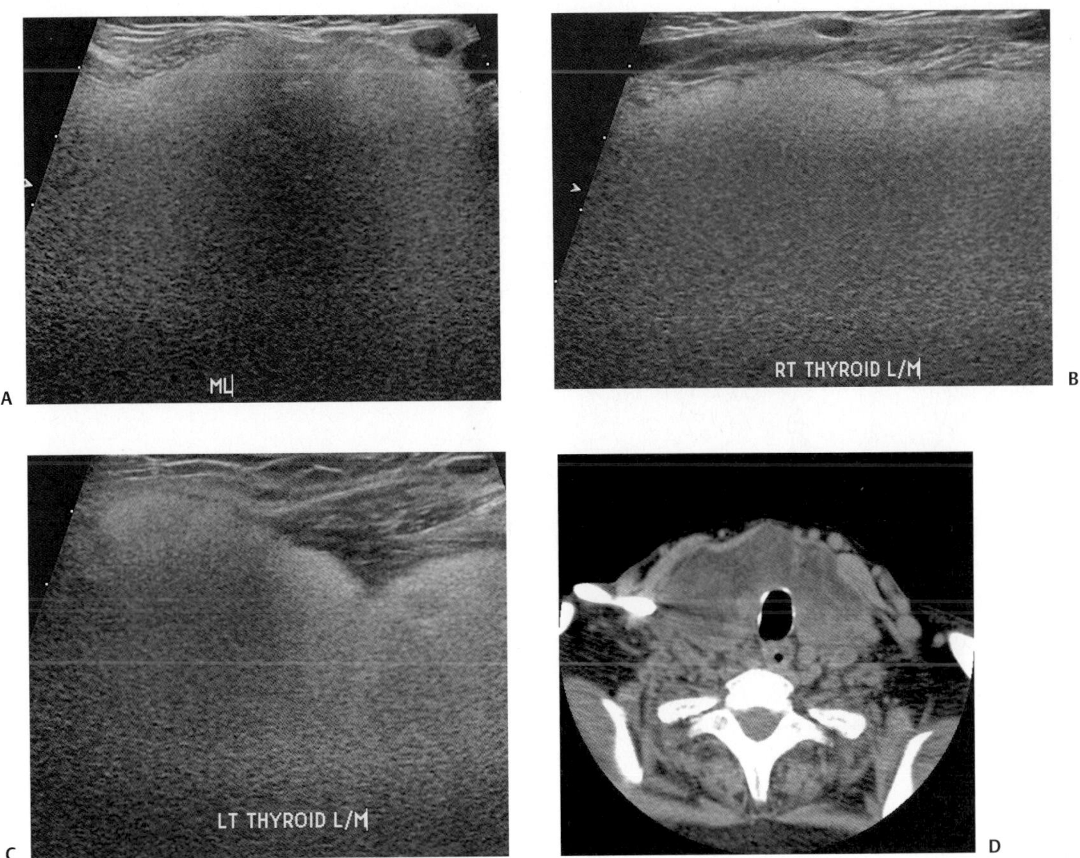

A B C D

Clinical Presentation

A 52-year-old euthyroid woman with long-standing thyroid enlargement and multiple medical problems.

Imaging Findings

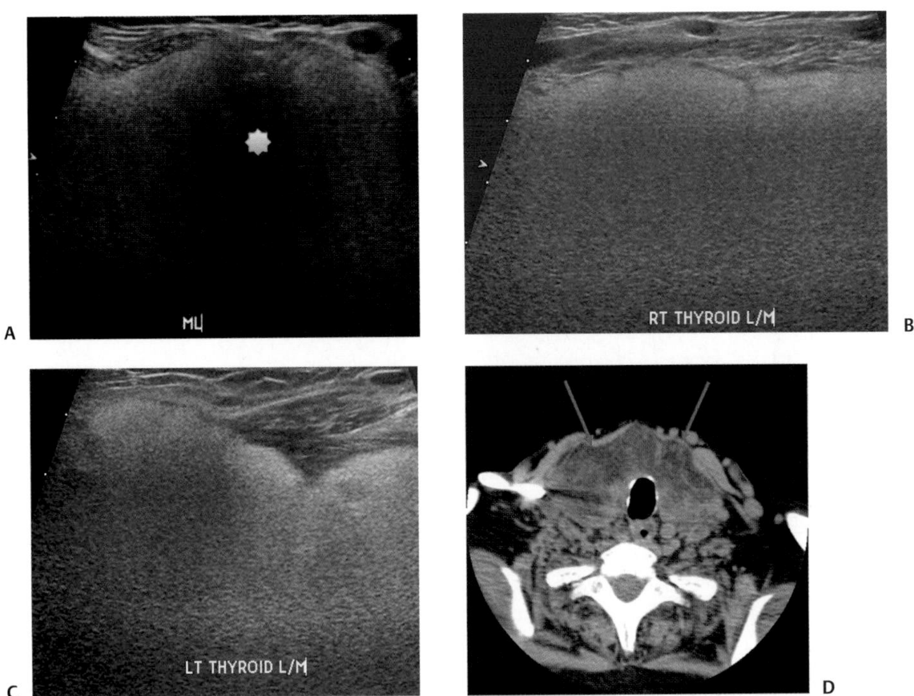

(A) Transverse image at the base of the neck reveals echogenic thyroid with marked absorption of sound in the far field. The trachea (*asterisk*) is barely discernible due to distortion of sound. **(B, C)** Longitudinal views of the right and left lobes reveal adequate detail of the near-field structures but absorption of sound by the thyroid and distortion of the image in the far field. **(D)** CT image through the lower neck demonstrates an enlarged diffusely fatty infiltrated thyroid gland (*arrows*).

Differential Diagnosis

- ***Diffuse lipomatosis of the thyroid gland:*** The finding of increased echogenicity with absorption and distortion of the sound beam resulting in dirty shadowing is diagnostic of a fatty structure. In this case, diffuse lipomatous infiltration of the thyroid gland.
- *Acute thyroiditis:* Would result in enlargement of the thyroid gland but the echotexture would be hypoechoic due to edema. Tenderness is often present in the setting of an acute thyroiditis.
- *Multinodular goiter (MNG):* The gland may be echogenic in the setting of a MNG if the nodules are echogenic. However, discrete nodules would be visible with a MNG.

Essential Facts

- Although fatty lesions in the thyroid are extremely rare, the classic appearance of fat on ultrasound allows for definitive identification of fat or fatty lesions in the thyroid gland.
- Because there are only a limited number of adipocytes in the normal thyroid gland, fatty lesions are extremely rare.
- Causes of fatty lesions in the thyroid include thyrolipoma, heterotopic fat rest, amyloid goiter, lymphocytic thyroiditis, or liposarcoma.
- A liposarcoma may have a similar appearance, although is usually found in the retroperitoneum or extremities. The history of long-term thyroid enlargement is not typical of malignancy.
- Fatty lesions are readily identified on CT due to the negative Hounsfield density measurements.
- Markedly enlarged thyroid glands, although usually a benign etiology, are often surgically removed to relieve the mass effect on the trachea.

✓ Pearls & ✗ Pitfalls

✓ Fatty tissue on ultrasound is very echogenic. It causes absorption and distortion of the ultrasound beam. Therefore, the far field may be obscured (tip of the iceberg sign of a dermoid).

✗ Distortion and absorption of sound can obscure structures (i.e., focal lesions in the setting of a fatty liver).

✗ Because the ultrasound beam does not travel through air (trachea), retropharyngeal extension of the thyroid gland is not usually visible with ultrasound.

✓ Hyperechoic fat is indicative of inflammation. An example is increased echogenicity of the surrounding fat in the setting of acute appendicitis.

Case 97

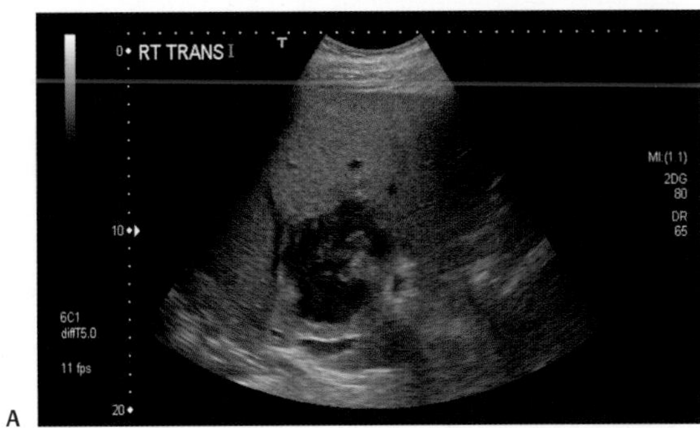

A

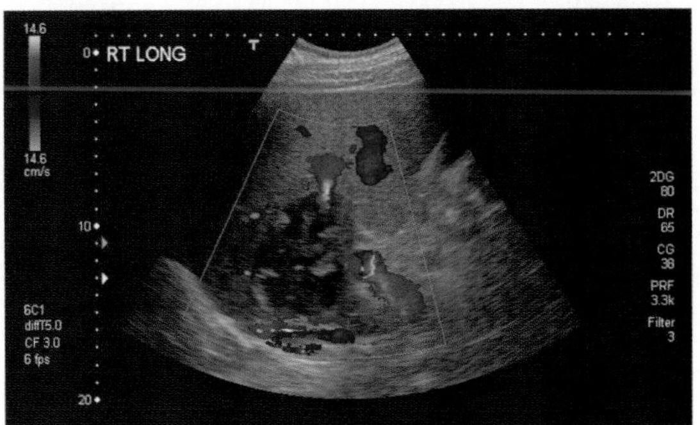

B

■ Clinical Presentation

A 55-year-old man presents with fever and shortness of breath.

■ Further Work-up

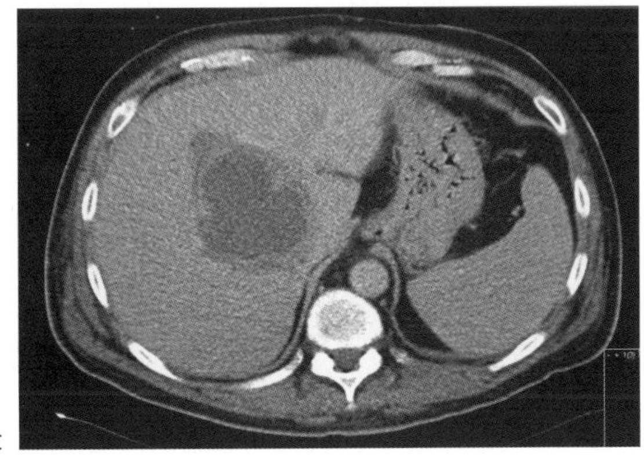
C

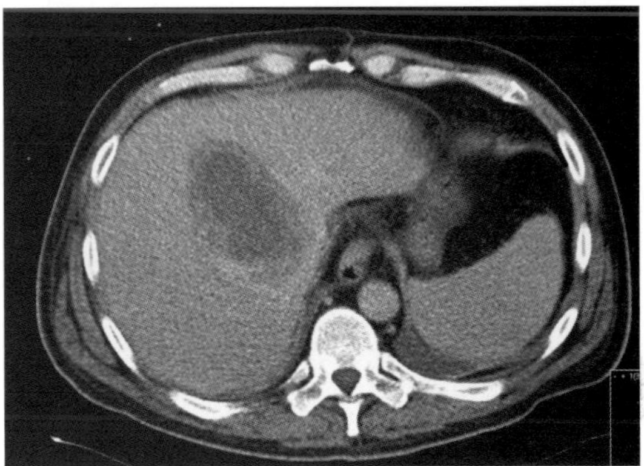
D

Imaging Findings

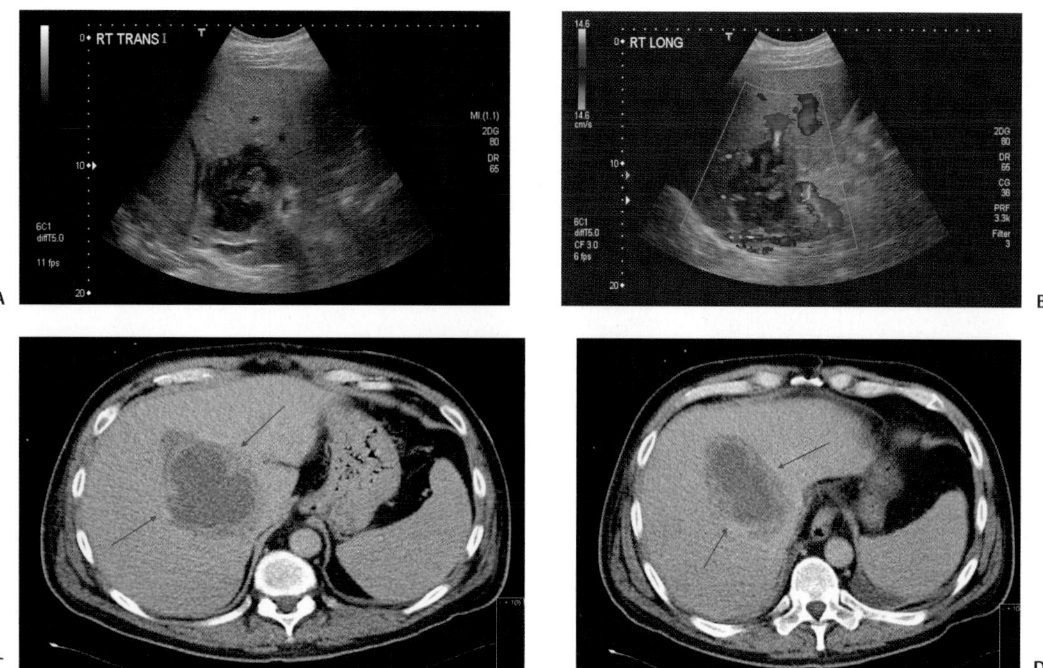

(A, B) Ultrasound images of the liver demonstrate a complex cystic lesion with irregular borders in the liver. Hyperechoic foci within the lesion are noted, as well as internal echoes with posterior acoustic enhancement. Color Doppler imaging reveals no evidence of flow within the lesion. **(C, D)** Follow-up computed tomography (CT) demonstrates a large hypodense lesion in the right hepatic lobe with irregular thickened walls (*red arrows*); thick reactive wall enhancement is noted on CT.

Differential Diagnosis

- ***Liver abscess:*** Bacterial or amebic abscesses appear sonographically as a well-defined mixed-echogenicity mass, round or oval, with low-level echoes and distal acoustic enhancement. Compared with pyogenic abscesses, amebic abscesses are more likely to have round or oval shape (82 versus 60%) and a hypoechoic appearance with fine, low-level internal echoes at high-gain settings (58 versus 36%).
- *Hydatid disease:* This entity is usually seen on ultrasound as a sharply defined anechoic cystic lesion with multiple daughter cysts. Sonographically, a floating undulating membrane known as the *water lily sign* may be appreciated as well. The presence of ringlike calcifications on CT and ultrasound is a common feature of hydatid cyst of the liver.
- *Hepatic cystadenoma and cystadenocarcinoma:* Presents as a large unilocular or multilocular cystic mass on ultrasound; Doppler ultrasound unlikely to show Doppler flow within the septations. CT angiography shows avascular lesion, though a small peripheral vascular blush may be seen. On magnetic resonance imaging, it appears as multiseptated, predominantly high signal on T2-weighted images and mixed or low signal on T1-weighted images.

Essential Facts

- No cause is found in 50% of patients.
- A direct extension from biliary tract (as in cholangitis and cholecystitis), via the portal system (as in diverticulitis and appendicitis), via the hepatic artery (as in pneumonitis) and in cases of traumatic penetrating injuries.
- Pyogenic liver abscess are more common in older patients.
- Ultrasound detects abscesses as small as 1.5 cm with a sensitivity of 75 to 90%.
- Ultrasound appearance is variable from a solid mass of any echogenicity to a complex, partially cystic, multiseptated mass with a cluster sign.
- Gas-producing organisms give rise to echogenic foci with reverberation and/or twinkle artifact.
- Pyogenic liver abscesses may occur in liver transplantation patients secondary to hepatic artery stenosis and/or thrombosis.
- Early lesions tend to be echogenic and poorly demarcated, progressing into well-demarcated nearly anechoic lesions.
- Contrast-enhanced sonography improves characterization of abscess lesions.

✓ Pearls & ✗ Pitfalls

✓ Ultrasound-guided aspiration is an easy-to-perform and accurate method of diagnosing liver abscess.

✗ Multifocal liver abscesses may mimic metastatic disease.

Case 98

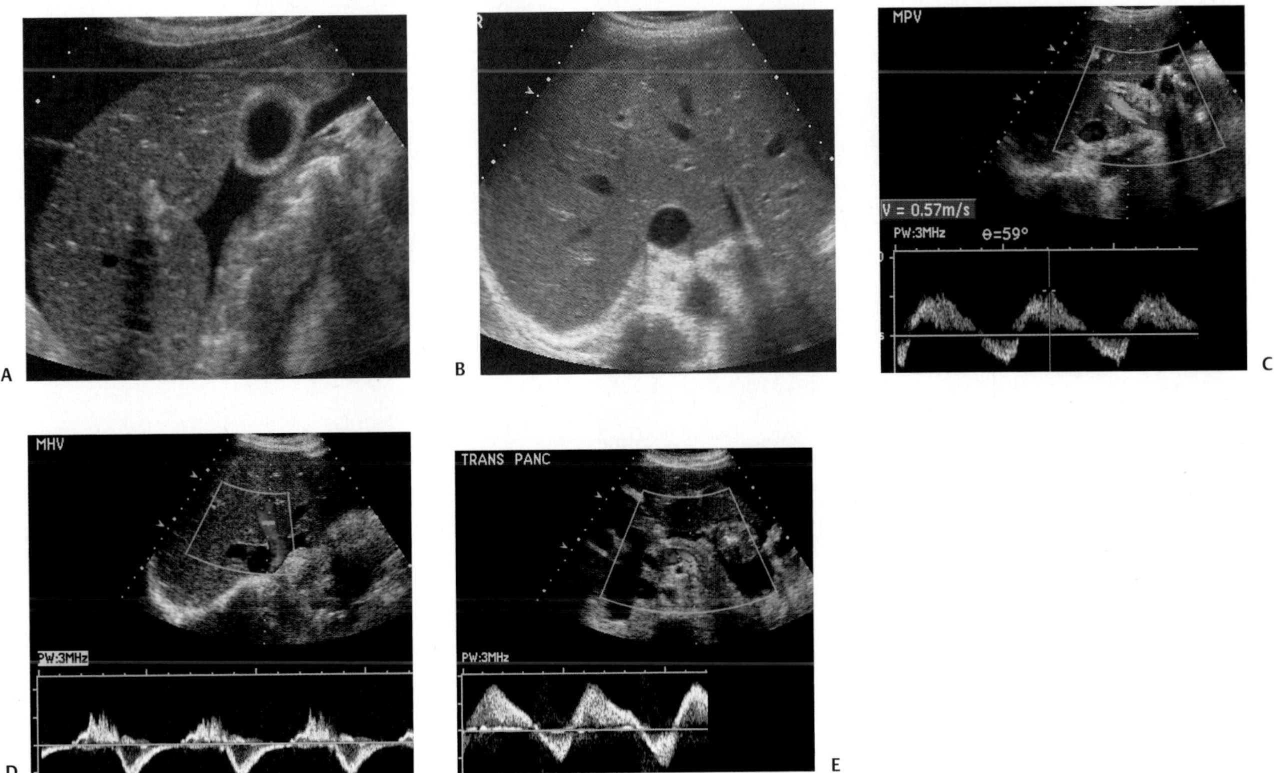

Clinical Presentation

A 67-year-old Haitian woman with a history of cardiac disease who presents with abdominal pain and distension.

Imaging Findings

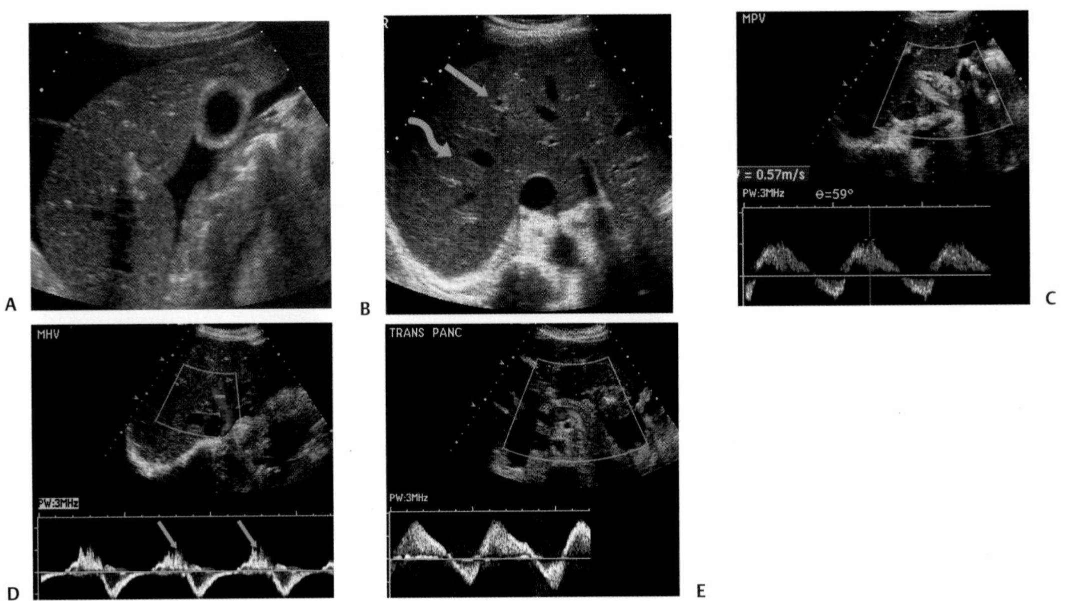

(A) The liver is normal in size and configuration but outlined by a large amount of ascites in this longitudinal view of the RUQ. Note the smooth contour of the liver. Gallbladder wall edema is present. **(B)** The hepatic veins (*curved arrow*) are much larger than the portal veins (*straight arrow*) in this transverse image of the liver. Hepatic veins have imperceptible walls, portal veins have echogenic walls from the portal triads. **(C)** Spectral Doppler tracing of the main portal vein demonstrates flow well above and below the baseline indicating forward and reversed rapid flow. **(D)** Transverse image through the confluence of hepatic veins with spectral tracing demonstrating a jet of reversed flow (*arrows*). **(E)** Spectral tracing in the splenic vein with to and fro flow similar to the MPV. The spleen (not shown) is not enlarged.

Differential Diagnosis

- ***Tricuspid insufficiency (TI):*** Fast forward and reversed flow in the portal vein is seen with TI. The reversed jet of flow in the hepatic veins results from TI.
- *Cirrhosis with portal hypertension:* In the setting of cirrhosis the contour of the liver would be nodular and the configuration of the liver would be altered with enlargement of the caudate lobe. The echotexture of the liver would be coarsened. The hepatic veins would demonstrate dampened flow. The spleen would be enlarged.
- *Right heart failure:* Right heart failure can result in altered flow in the hepatic and portal veins. It would be less severe than that seen with TI.

Essential Facts

- The normal hepatic venous waveform is pulsatile and reflects the changing pressure in the right atrium.
- Ordinarily only a small amount of retrograde flow is seen in the hepatic veins. It is due to atrial contraction and referred to as the A wave.
- Two waves of antegrade flow (toward the heart) are seen with atrial then ventricular filling. These are referred to as the S and D waves.
- In the setting of TI the reversed jet of flow in the hepatic veins is transmitted through the sinusoids of the liver and reflected in the portal vein. In this case it is demonstrated in the splenic vein as well.
- In the setting of TI the pulsatility of the hepatic veins is increased. In cirrhosis the pulsatility is dampened due to fibrosis compressing the hepatic veins and preventing pulsation.
- The hepatic venous waveform can be altered by several cardiac and pulmonary conditions, but TI is the most striking with a large amount of retrograde flow.

✓ Pearls & × Pitfalls

✓ In the setting of portal hypertension with impending reversed flow, to-and-fro flow can be seen in the portal vein. This would be very slow, much slower than normal or seen with the rapid reversed flow with TI.

✓ Even if you cannot remember the normal waves seen in the hepatic veins, the significant retrograde flow in the HV and reversed flow in the main portal vein (MPV) will allow you to make the diagnosis of TI.

✓ In the setting of portal hypertension, the hepatic artery is recruited to supply oxygen to the liver. Therefore the hepatic artery resistive index is decreased.

× The normal pulsatile hepatic waveform may be dampened due to deep inspiration or Valsalva maneuvering.

Case 99

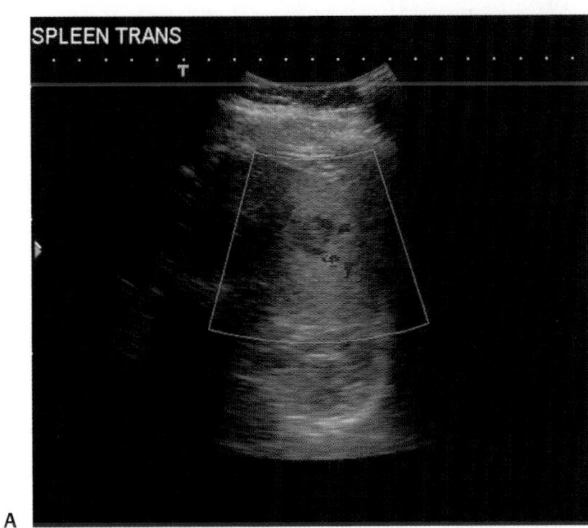

A

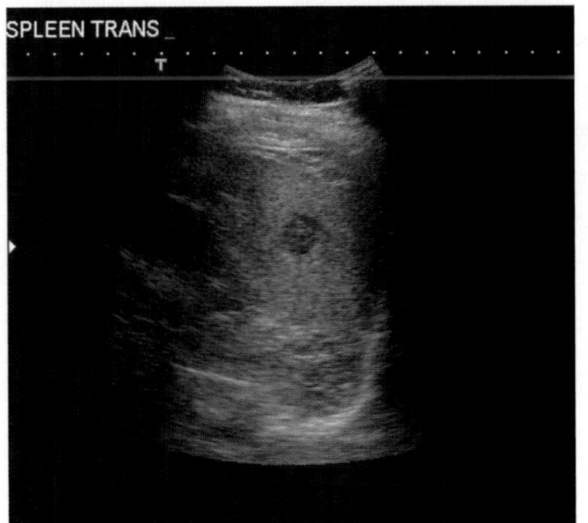

B

Clinical Presentation

A 61-year-old woman with history of malignancy presents for splenic lesion assessment.

Further Work-up

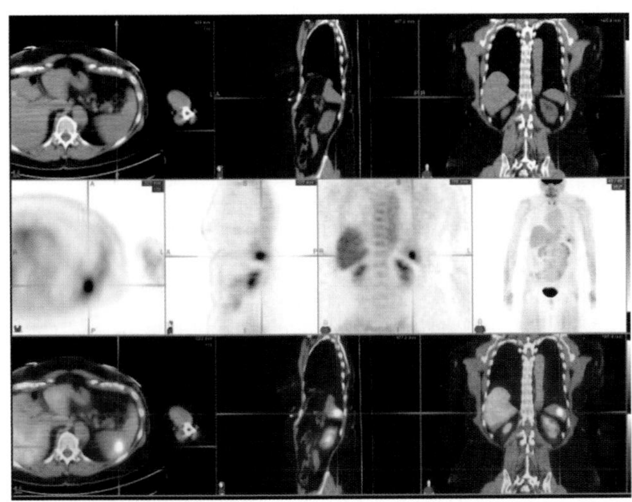
C

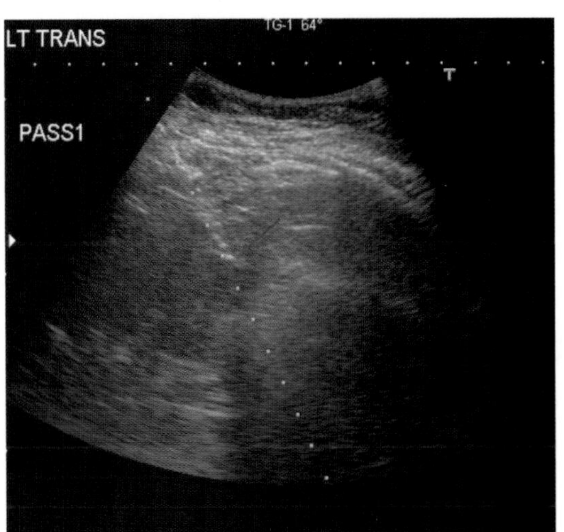

D

Imaging Findings

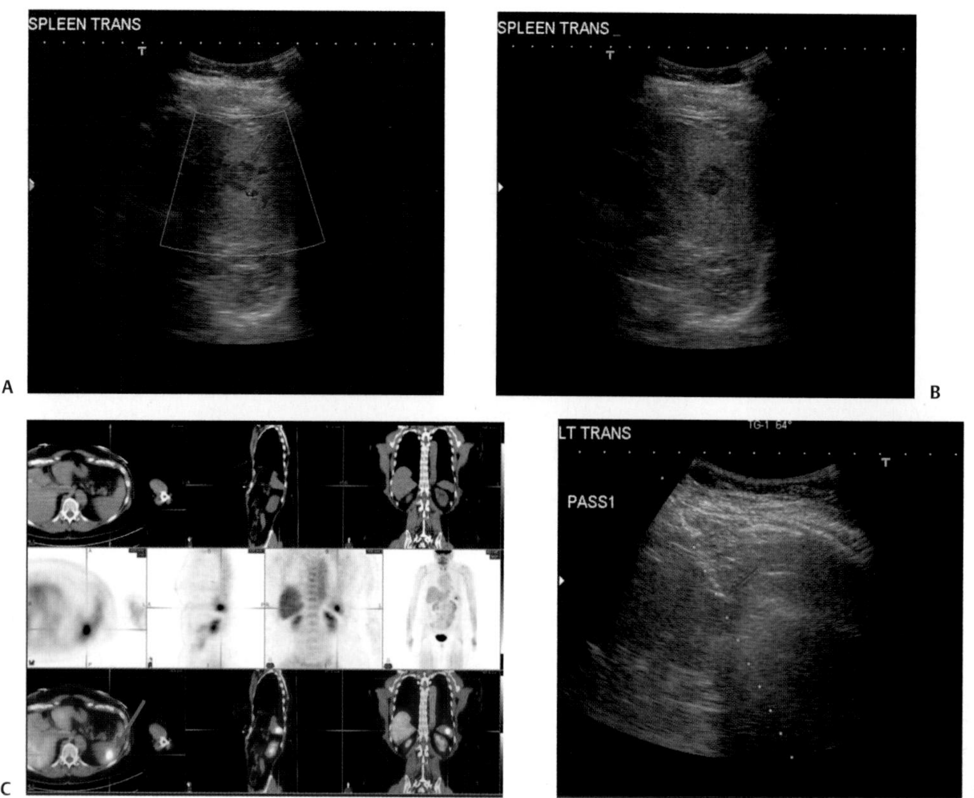

(A, B) Ultrasound images of the spleen with Doppler showing a small hypoechoic lesion (*red arrow*) in the spleen. No significant vascular flow is noted within the lesion. The spleen is not enlarged. **(C)** Follow-up positron emission tomography (PET) scan shows intense uptake of radiopharmaceutical (*green arrow*) within the questionable lesion. **(D)** Ultrasound-guided core biopsy of the spleen (*red arrow*) was used to obtain diagnostic tissue of the described lesion.

Differential Diagnosis

- ***Splenic lymphoma:*** The most common tumor of the spleen, the most common sonographic appearance is hypoechoic nodule/s. The presence of splenomegaly or additional lymphadenopathy is suggestive of the diagnosis.
- *Metastatic disease to the spleen:* Can be serosal or intrasplenic. The usual sonographic appearance is a hypoechoic mass, but a target lesion could be seen. The most common metastases to the spleen are melanoma, breast, and ovarian malignancies.
- *Pyogenic splenic abscess:* Single or multiple, more common in immunocompromised patients. Appear as irregular wall, cystic lesion with low-level echoes. Smaller lesion may be hard to visualize on gray scale images.

Essential Facts

- The most common primary malignant tumor of the spleen. Splenic involvement associated with lymphadenopathy is the most common presentation.
- Could present as diffuse enlargement, multisplenic lesions, and/or rarely as single lesion.
- The most common sonographic appearance is a hypoechoic nodule(s); occasionally, it could appear as anechoic nodule overlapping with splenic cyst.
- High-grade lymphoma usually presents as multiple large splenic lesions.
- Solitary enlargement of spleen without focal lesions is a rare presentation of lymphoma.
- Primary, solitary involvement of the spleen makes up $<$ 1% of non-Hodgkin's lymphoma.

✓ Pearls & × Pitfalls

✓ Small lesions in the spleen could appear as heterogeneously enlarged spleen on gray scale ultrasound. Doppler might be helpful to delineate the small lesions.

× Lymphoma of the spleen could be anechoic on ultrasound and misinterpreted as splenic cyst. Evaluation of enhanced through transmission helps to differentiate the two entities.

Case 100

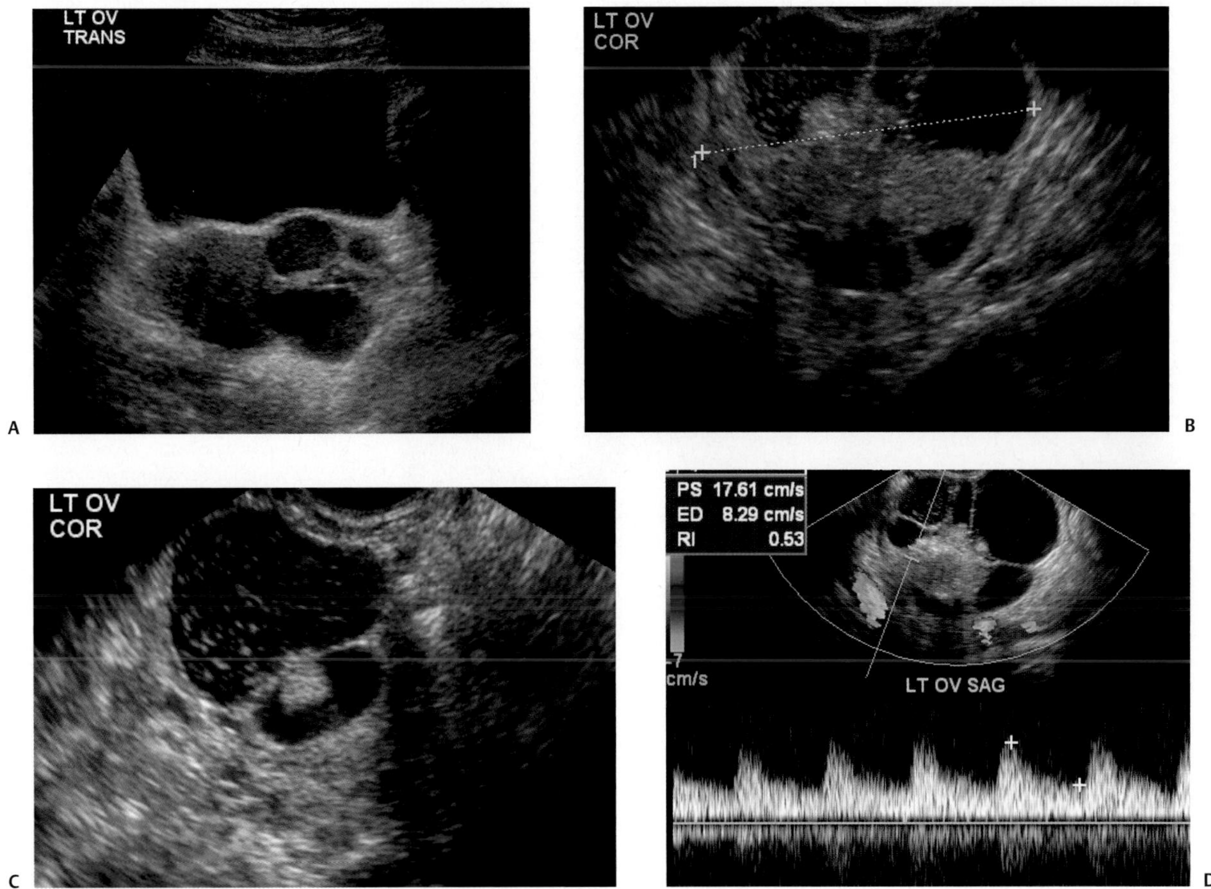

A B C D

■ Clinical Presentation

A 45-year-old woman with pelvic mass on exam.

Imaging Findings

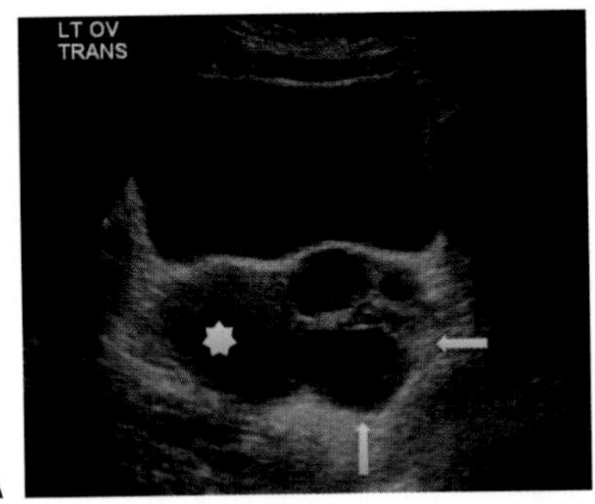

A

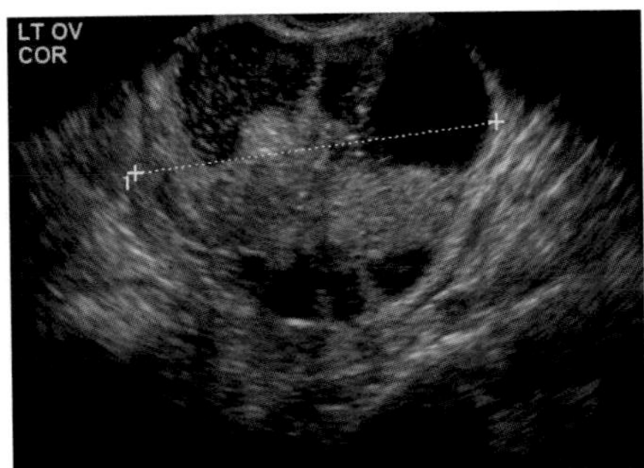

B

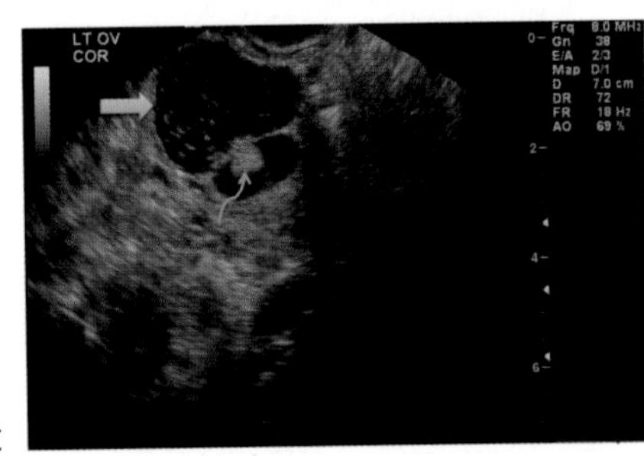

C

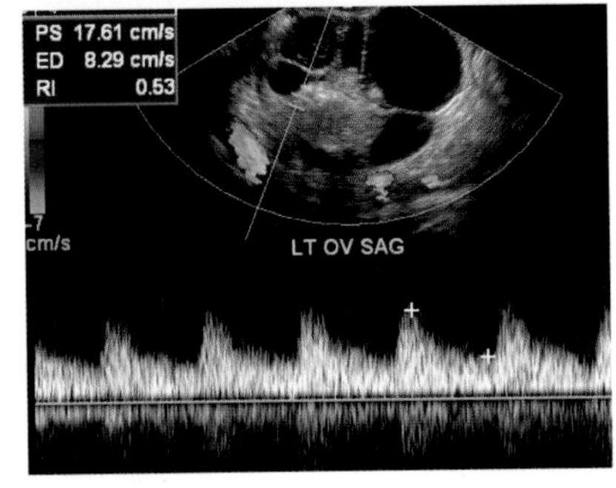

D

(A) Transabdominal image of the pelvis in the transverse plane reveals a complex cystic mass enlarging the left ovary (*arrows*). It is adjacent to a normal uterus (*asterisk*). **(B)** Transvaginal images of the lesion better define the multiple cystic loculations and septations. **(C)** A particularly complex loculation (*thick arrow*) is adjacent to a septation with a mural nodule (*curved arrow*). **(D)** Spectral Doppler analysis confirms the presence of flow within the solid components of the lesion. The flow is fairly low resistance, typical of neovascularity seen with malignancy.

Differential Diagnosis

- ***Ovarian malignancy:*** A complex lesion enlarging an ovary with vascularity in the solid components is seen with ovarian cancer. Thick nodular septations and mural nodules are suspicious for malignancy, regardless of the size of a lesion.
- *Dermoid tumors:* Dermoid tumors do not have internal vascularity. They may contain complex loculations and echogenic components such as this lesion, but no flow in the solid components. Dermoids often demonstrate shadowing from calcifications or dirty shadowing from fat not seen in this lesion.
- *Hemorrhagic cyst:* Hemorrhagic cysts may be complex with retracting clot that may mimic solid components. No internal vascularity would be seen in a clot or lesion. Retracting clots are often concave or contain straight lateral margins.

Essential Facts

- Cystic ovarian lesions containing solid elements that are vascular should be considered malignant until proven otherwise.
- Ovarian cancer is the fifth most common malignancy in women and the leading cause of death from gynecological malignancy.
- Eighty-five percent of ovarian cancers present in stage III or IV. Twenty-five percent of ovarian cancer is bilateral.
- Ninety percent of cases are sporadic. Ten percent are associated with hereditary syndromes including BRAC1 and BRAC2 mutation (risk of breast cancer) and Lynch syndrome II (colon cancer). Patients with endometriosis are at increased risk.
- Average age at presentation is 63. Risk of ovarian cancer increases with age and decreases with number of pregnancies. Oral contraceptives have a protective affect.
- Screening for ovarian cancer with pelvic ultrasound is not standard practice but is often performed for patients with significant family history.
- CA125 is a tumor marker for ovarian cancer. It is nonspecific and can be elevated due to benign entities, including fibroids and endometriosis.
- Other terms for solid elements are *mural nodules* or *papillary excrescences.*
- Screening for ovarian cancer with ultrasound has not been found to be effective and is not recommended.

✓ Pearls & × Pitfalls

✓ The presence of a solid component is the most useful feature for identifying ovarian malignancy.

✓ Regardless of the size of a lesion, solid elements, internal vascularity, and thick nodular components are signs of malignancy.

× Although ovarian malignancy is associated with larger masses, the sonographic morphology of a mass is a more useful predictor of malignancy than its size.

Further Readings

Case 1

Chawla Y, Dilawari JB, Katariya S. Gallbladder varices in portal vein thrombosis. AJR Am J Roentgenol 1994;162(3):643–645 PubMed

Case 2

Kwak JY, Kim EK, Son EJ, et al. Papillary thyroid carcinoma manifested solely as microcalcifications on sonography. AJR Am J Roentgenol 2007;189(1):227–231 PubMed

Case 3

Thurston W, Wilson SR. The urinary tract. In: Rumack CM, Wilson SR, Charboneau JW, Johnson J, eds. Diagnostic Ultrasound. 3rd ed. St. Louis: Elsevier; 2005:321–393

Case 4

Rao PK, Sabanegh ES. Genitourinary sarcoidosis. Rev Urol 2009;11(2):108–113 PubMed

Case 5

Jain KA. Endometrioma with calcification simulating a dermoid on sonography. J Ultrasound Med 2006;25(9):1237–1241 PubMed

Case 6

Langer JE, Oliver ER, Lev-Toaff AS, Coleman BG. Imaging of the female pelvis through the life cycle. Radiographics 2012;32(6):1575–1597 PubMed

Levine D, Brown DL, Andreotti RF, et al. Management of asymptomatic ovarian and other adnexal cysts imaged at US: Society of Radiologists in Ultrasound Consensus Conference Statement. Radiology 2010;256(3):943–954 PubMed

Case 7

Ching ASC, Ahuja AT. High-resolution sonography of the submandibular space: anatomy and abnormalities. AJR Am J Roentgenol 2002;179(3):703–708 PubMed

Case 8

Langer JE, Oliver ER, Lev-Toaff AS, Coleman BG. Imaging of the female pelvis through the life cycle. Radiographics 2012;32(6):1575–1597 PubMed

Levine D, Brown DL, Andreotti RF, et al. Management of asymptomatic ovarian and other adnexal cysts imaged at US: Society of Radiologists in Ultrasound Consensus Conference Statement. Radiology 2010;256(3):943–954 PubMed

Case 9

Chavhan GB. The cobra head sign. Radiology 2002;225(3):781–782 PubMed

Thornbury JR, Silver TM, Vinson RK. Ureteroceles vs. pseudoureteroceles in adults. Urographic diagnosis. Radiology 1977;122(1):81–84 PubMed

Case 10

Levine D1, Brown DL, Andreotti RF, et al. Management of Asymptomatic ovarian and other adnexal cysts imaged at US: Society of Radiologist in Ultrasound Consensus Conference Statement. Radiology 2010;256(3):943–954

Case 11

Glassberg KI. Renal dysgenesis and cystic disease of kidney. In: Wein AJ, Kavoussi LR, Novick AC, Partin AW, Peters CA, eds. Campbell-Walsh Urology. Vol 4. 9th ed. Philadelphia: Saunders; 2006:3354–3356

Kabala JE. The kidneys and ureter. In: Sutton D, ed. Textbook of Radiology and Imaging. Vol 2. 7th ed. London: Churchill Livingstone; 2003:951

Case 12

Langer JE, Oliver ER, Lev-Toaff AS, Coleman BG. Imaging of the female pelvis through the life cycle. Radiographics 2012;32(6):1575–1597 PubMed

Levine D, Brown DL, Andreotti RF, et al. Management of asymptomatic ovarian and other adnexal cysts imaged at US: Society of Radiologists in Ultrasound Consensus Conference Statement. Radiology 2010;256(3):943–954 PubMed

Case 13

Baxter GM. Imaging in renal transplantation. Ultrasound Q 2003;19(3):123–138 PubMed

Gao J, Ng A, Shih G, et al. Intrarenal color duplex ultrasonography: a window to vascular complications of renal transplants. J Ultrasound Med 2007;26(10):1403–1418 PubMed

Case 14

Balen AH, Laven JS, Tan SL, Dewailly D. Ultrasound assessment of the polycystic ovary: international consensus definitions. Hum Reprod Update 2003;9(6):505–514 PubMed

Case 15

Solbiati L, Charboneau JW, Osti V, James EM, Hay ID. The thyroid gland. In: Rumack CM, Wilson SR, Charboneau JW, Johnson J, eds. Diagnostic Ultrasound. 3rd ed. St. Louis: Elsevier; 2005:735–770

Case 16

Woodward PJ, Schwab CM, Sesterhenn IA. From the archives of the AFIP: extratesticular scrotal masses: radiologic-pathologic correlation. Radiographics 2003;23(1):215–240 PubMed

Case 17

Grant EG, Benson CB, Moneta GL, et al. Carotid artery stenosis: grayscale and Doppler ultrasound diagnosis - Society of Radiologist in Ultrasound Consensus Conference. Radiology 2003;229(2):340–346 PubMed

Case 18

Cast JE, Nelson WM, Early AS, et al. Testicular microlithiasis: prevalence and tumor risk in a population referred for scrotal sonography. AJR Am J Roentgenol 2000;175(6):1703–1706 PubMed

Case 19

Murray CP, Yoo SJ, Babyn PS. Congenital extrahepatic portosystemic shunts. Pediatr Radiol 2003;33(9):614–620 PubMed

Santamaría G, Pruna X, Serres X, Inaraja L, Zuasnabar A, Castellote A. Congenital intrahepatic portosystemic venous shunt: sonographic and magnetic resonance imaging. Eur Radiol 1996;6(1):76–78 PubMed

Case 20

Manning MA, Woodward PJ. Testicular epidermoid cysts: sonographic features with clinicopathologic correlation. J Ultrasound Med 2010;29(5):831–837

Loya AG, Said JW, Grant EG. Epidermoid cyst of the testis: radiologic-pathologic correlation. Radiographics 2004;24(Suppl 1):S243–S246 PubMed

Case 21

Atri M, Finnegan PW. The pancreas. In: Rumack CM, Wilson SR, Charboneau JW, Johnson J, eds. Diagnostic Ultrasound. 3rd ed. St. Louis: Elsevier; 2005:213–267

Silas AM, Morrin MM, Raptopoulos V, Keogan MT. Intraductal papillary mucinous tumors of the pancreas. AJR Am J Roentgenol 2001;176(1):179–185 PubMed

Case 22

Muradali D, Colgan T, Hayeems E, Burns PN, Wilson SR. Echogenic ovarian foci without shadowing: are they caused by psammomatous calcifications? Radiology 2002;224(2):429–435 PubMed

Case 23

Doubilet PM, Benson CB. Atlas of Ultrasound in Obstetric and Gynecology. Philadelphia: Lippincott Williams & Wilkins; 2003

George SM, Kumar P. Miscarriage. In: Arulkumaran S, Sivanesaratnam V, Chatterjee A, Kumar P, eds. Essentials of Obstetrics. New Dehli: Jaypee Brothers; 2004:80–87

Case 24

Levine D, Brown DL, Andreotti RF, et al. Management of asymptomatic ovarian and other adnexal cysts imaged at US: Society of Radiologists in Ultrasound Consensus Conference Statement. Radiology 2010;256(3):943–954 PubMed

Case 25

Ghersin E, Soudack M, Gaitini D. Twinkling artifact in gallbladder adenomyomatosis. J Ultrasound Med 2003;22(2):229–231 PubMed

Case 26

Chopra S, Lev-Toaff AS, Ors F, Bergin D. Adenomyosis:common and uncommon manifestations on sonography and magnetic resonance imaging. J Ultrasound Med 2006;25(5):617–627, quiz 629 PubMed

Case 27

Levy AD, Murakata LA, Rohrmann CA Jr. Gallbladder carcinoma: radiologic-pathologic correlation. Radiographics 2001;21(2): 295–314, 549–555 PubMed

Case 28

Fishman M, Boda M, Sheiner E, Rotmensch J, Abramowicz J. Changes in the sonographic appearance of the uterus after discontinuation of tamoxifen therapy. J Ultrasound Med 2006;25(4):469–473 PubMed

Case 29

Caspi B, Appelman Z, Rabinerson D, Zalel Y, Tulandi T, Shoham Z. The growth pattern of ovarian dermoid cysts: a prospective study in premenopausal and postmenopausal women. Fertil Steril 1997;68(3):501–505 PubMed

Salem S, Wilson SR. Gynecologic ultrasound. In: Rumack CM, Wilson SR, Charboneau JW, Johnson J, eds. Diagnostic Ultrasound. 3rd ed. St. Louis: Elsevier; 2005:527–587

Case 30

Levine D, Brown DL, Andreotti RF, et al. Management of asymptomatic ovarian and other adnexal cysts imaged at US: Society of Radiologists in Ultrasound Consensus Conference Statement. Radiology 2010;256(3):943–954 PubMed

Twickler DM, Moschos E. Ultrasound and assessment of ovarian cancer risk. AJR Am J Roentgenol 2010;194(2):322–329 PubMed

Case 31

Asch E, Levine D. Variations in appearance of endometriomas. J Ultrasound Med 2007;26(8):993–1002 PubMed

Jain KA. Endometrioma with calcification simulating a dermoid on sonography. J Ultrasound Med 2006;25(9):1237–1241 PubMed

Case 32

Brown DL. A practical approach to the ultrasound characterization of adnexal masses. Ultrasound Q 2007;23(2):87–105 PubMed

Laing FC, Allison SJ. US of the ovary and adnexa: to worry or not to worry? Radiographics 2012;32(6):1621–1639, discussion 1640–1642 PubMed

Levine D, Brown DL, Andreotti RF, et al. Management of asymptomatic ovarian and other adnexal cysts imaged at US: Society of Radiologists in Ultrasound Consensus Conference Statement. Radiology 2010;256(3):943–954 PubMed

Case 33

Salem S. The uterus and adnexa. In: Rumack CM, Wilson SR, Charboneau JW, Johnson J, eds. Diagnostic Ultrasound. 3rd ed. St. Louis: Elsevier; 2005: 545–549

Case 34

Molander P, Paavonen J, Sjöberg J, Savelli L, Cacciatore B. Transvaginal sonography in the diagnosis of acute appendicitis. Ultrasound Obstet Gynecol 2002;20(5):496–501 PubMed

Case 35

Salem S, Wilson SR. Gynecologic ultrasound. In: Rumack CM, Wilson SR, Charboneau JW, Johnson J, eds. Diagnostic Ultrasound. 3rd ed. St. Louis: Elsevier; 2005:527–587

Case 36

Valentin L, Ameye L, Testa A, et al. Ultrasound characteristics of different types of adnexal malignancies. Gynecol Oncol 2006;102(1):41–48 PubMed

Case 37

Lyons EA, Levi CS. The first trimester. In: Rumack CM, Wilson SR, Charboneau JW, Johnson J, eds. Diagnostic Ultrasound. 3rd ed. St. Louis: Elsevier; 2005:1069–1128

Case 38

Doubilet PM, Benson CB. Double sac sign and intradecidual sign in early pregnancy: interobserver reliability and frequency of occurrence. J Ultrasound Med 2013;32(7):1207–1214 PubMed

Laing FC, Brown DL, Price JF, Teeger S, Wong ML. Intradecidual sign: is it effective in diagnosis of an early intrauterine pregnancy? Radiology 1997;204(3):655–660 PubMed

Lane BF, Wong-You-Cheong JJ, Javitt MC, et al; American College of Radiology. ACR appropriateness Criteria® first trimester bleeding. Ultrasound Q 2013;29(2):91–96 PubMed

Case 39

Wilson SR, Withers CE. The liver. In: Rumack CM, Wilson SR, Charboneau JW, Johnson J, eds. Diagnostic Ultrasound. 3rd ed. St. Louis: Elsevier; 2005:77–145

Case 40

Laing FC, Allison SJ. US of the ovary and adnexa: to worry or not to worry? Radiographics 2012;32(6):1621–1639, discussion 1640–1642 PubMed

Levine D, Brown DL, Andreotti RF, et al. Management of asymptomatic ovarian and other adnexal cysts imaged at US: Society of Radiologists in Ultrasound Consensus Conference Statement. Radiology 2010;256(3):943–954 PubMed

Case 41

Thurston W, Wilson SR. The urinary tract. In: Rumack CM, Wilson SR, Charboneau JW, Johnson J, eds. Diagnostic Ultrasound. 3rd ed. St. Louis: Elsevier; 2005:321–393

Case 42

Dogra VS, Gottlieb RH, Oka M, Rubens DJ. Sonography of the scrotum. Radiology 2003;227(1):18–36 PubMed

Woodward PJ, Sohaey R, O'Donoghue MJ, Green DE. From the archives of the AFIP: tumors and tumorlike lesions of the testis: radiologic-pathologic correlation. Radiographics 2002;22(1):189–216 PubMed

Case 43

Vetter K, Kilavuz O, Voigt H.-J. Doppler ultrasound in the diagnosis of fetal anomalies. In: Sohn C, Voigt H.-J., Vetter K, eds. Doppler Ultrasound in Gynecology and Obstetrics. Stuttgart: Thieme Verlag; 2004:111–122

Case 44

Görg C, Cölle J, Görg K, Prinz H, Zugmaier G. Spontaneous rupture of the spleen: ultrasound patterns, diagnosis and follow-up. Br J Radiol 2003;76(910):704–711 PubMed

Case 45

Lake D, Guimaraes M, Ackerman S, et al. Comparative results of Doppler sonography after TIPS using covered and bare stents. AJR Am J Roentgenol 2006;186(4):1138–1143 PubMed

Case 46

Alonso-Gamarra E, Parrón M, Pérez A, Prieto C, Hierro L, López-Santamaría M. Clinical and radiologic manifestations of congenital extrahepatic portosystemic shunts: a comprehensive review. Radiographics 2011;31(3):707–722 PubMed

Remer EM, Motta-Ramirez GA, Henderson JM. Imaging findings in incidental intrahepatic portal venous shunts. AJR Am J Roentgenol 2007;188(2):W162-7 PubMed

Case 47

Salem S. The uterus and adnexa. In: Rumack CM, Wilson SR, Charboneau JW, Johnson J, eds. Diagnostic Ultrasound. 3rd ed. St. Louis: Elsevier; 2005: 545–549

Case 48

Alonso-Gamarra E, Parrón M, Pérez A, Prieto C, Hierro L, López-Santamaría M. Clinical and radiologic manifestations of congenital extrahepatic portosystemic shunts: a comprehensive review. Radiographics 2011;31(3):707–722 PubMed

Remer EM, Motta-Ramirez GA, Henderson JM. Imaging findings in incidental intrahepatic portal venous shunts. AJR Am J Roentgenol 2007;188(2):W162-7 PubMed

Case 49

Salem S. The uterus and adnexa. In: Rumack CM, Wilson SR, Charboneau JW, Johnson J, eds. Diagnostic Ultrasound. 3rd ed. St. Louis: Elsevier; 2005: 545–549

Case 50

Kielar AZ, Shabana W, Vakili M, Rubin J. Prospective evaluation of Doppler sonography to detect the twinkling artifact versus unenhanced computed tomography for identifying urinary tract calculi. J Ultrasound Med 2012;31(10):1619–1625 PubMed

Case 51

Gorman B, Carroll BA. The scrotum. In: Rumack CM, Wilson SR, Charboneau JW, Johnson J, eds. Diagnostic Ultrasound. 3rd ed. St. Louis: Elsevier; 2005:849–888

Case 52

Freire M, Remer EM. Clinical and radiologic features of cystic renal masses. AJR Am J Roentgenol 2009;192(5):1367–1372 PubMed

Case 53

Holloway BJ, Belcher HE, Letourneau JG, Kunberger LE. Scrotal sonography: a valuable tool in the evaluation of complications following inguinal hernia repair. J Clin Ultrasound 1998;26(7):341–344 PubMed

Middleton WD, Kurtz AB, Hertberg BS, eds. Ultrasound: The Requisites. 2nd ed. St. Louis: Mosby; 2003

Case 54

Cho JJ, Strickland M. Lithium-induced microcysts. Ultrasound Q 2012;28(3):179–180 PubMed

Case 55

Singh AK, Nachiappan AC, Verma HA, et al. Postoperative imaging in liver transplantation: what radiologists should know. Radiographics 2010;30(2):339–351 PubMed

Case 56

Barrenetxea G, Barinaga-Rementeria L, Lopez de Larruzea A, Agirregoikoa JA, Mandiola M, Carbonero K. Heterotopic pregnancy: two cases and a comparative review. Fertil Steril 2007;87(2):e9–e15 PubMed

Case 57

Resnik M, Older R, eds. Diagnosis of Genitourinary Disease. 2nd ed. New York: Thieme; 1997

Symeonidou C, Standish R, Sahdev A, Katz RD, Morlese J, Malhotra A. Imaging and histopathologic features of HIV-related renal disease. Radiographics 2008;28(5):1339–1354 PubMed

Case 58

Wood MM, Romine LE, Lee YK, et al. Spectral Doppler signature waveforms in ultrasonography: a review of normal and abnormal waveforms. Ultrasound Q 2010;26(2):83–99 PubMed

Case 59

Bates J, ed. Practical Gynaecological Ultrasound. 2nd ed. New York: Cambridge University Press; 2006

Salem S, Wilson SR. Gynecologic ultrasound. In: Rumack CM, Wilson SR, Charboneau JW, Johnson J, eds. Diagnostic Ultrasound. 3rd ed. St. Louis: Elsevier; 2005:527–587

Case 60

Ginat DT, Bhatt S, Sidhu R, Dogra V. Carotid and vertebral artery Doppler ultrasound waveforms: a pictorial review. Ultrasound Q 2011;27(2):81–85 PubMed

Wood MM, Romine LE, Lee YK, et al. Spectral Doppler signature waveforms in ultrasonography: a review of normal and abnormal waveforms. Ultrasound Q 2010;26(2):83–99 PubMed

Case 61

Baldisserotto M, de Souza JC, Pertence AP, Dora MD. Color Doppler sonography of normal and torsed testicular appendage in children. AJR Am J Roentgenol 2005;184(4):1287–1292

Yang DM, Lim JW, Kim JE, Kim JH, Cho H. Torsed appendix testis: gray scale and color Doppler sonographic findings compared with normal appendix testis. J Ultrasound Med 2005;24(1):87–91 PubMed

Case 62

Andrews EJ Jr, Fleischer AC. Sonography for deep venous thrombosis: current and future applications. Ultrasound Q 2005;21(4):213–225 PubMed

Lockhart ME, Sheldon HI, Robbin ML. Augmentation in lower extremity sonography for the detection of deep venous thrombosis. AJR Am J Roentgenol 2005;184(2):419–422 PubMed

Case 63

Rosenthal SJ, Harrison LA, Baxter KG, Wetzel LH, Cox GG, Batnitzky S. Doppler US of helical flow in the portal vein. Radiographics 1995;15(5):1103–1111 PubMed

Case 64

Bonavita JA, Mayo J, Babb J, Bennett G, Oweity T, Macari M, Yee J. Pattern recognition of benign nodules at ultrasound of the thyroid: Which nodules can be left alone? AJR Am J Roentgenol 2009; 193(1):207–213

Frates MC, Benson CB, Charboneau JW, et al; Society of Radiologists in Ultrasound. Management of thyroid nodules detected at US: Society of Radiologists in Ultrasound consensus conference statement. Radiology 2005;237(3):794–800 PubMed

Moon WJ, Baek JH, Jung SL, et al; Korean Society of Thyroid Radiology (KSThR); Korean Society of Radiology. Ultrasonography and the ultrasound-based management of thyroid nodules: consensus statement and recommendations. Korean J Radiol 2011;12(1):1–14 PubMed

Case 65

Di Salvo DN. Sonographic imaging of maternal complications of pregnancy. J Ultrasound Med 2003;22(1):69–89 PubMed

Durfee SM, Frates MC, Luong A, Benson CB. The sonographic and color Doppler features of retained products of conception. J Ultrasound Med 2005;24(9):1181–1186, quiz 1188–1189 PubMed

Case 66

Yoon JH, Cha SS, Han SS, Lee SJ, Kang MS. Gallbladder adenomyomatosis: imaging findings. Abdom Imaging 2006;31(5):555–563 PubMed

Case 67

Lyons EA, Levi CS. The first trimester. In: Rumack CM, Wilson SR, Charboneau JW, Johnson J, eds. Diagnostic Ultrasound. 3rd ed. St. Louis: Elsevier; 2005:1069–1128

Case 68

Applegate KE, Goske MJ, Pierce G, Murphy D. Situs revisited: imaging of the heterotaxy syndrome. Radiographics 1999;19(4):837–852, discussion 853–854 PubMed

Gayer G, Zissin R, Apter S, Atar E, Portnoy O, Itzchak Y. CT findings in congenital anomalies of the spleen. Br J Radiol 2001;74(884):767–772 PubMed

Case 69

Basaran C, Karcaaltincaba M, Akata D, Karabulut N, Akinci D, Ozmen M, Akhan O. Fat-containing lesions of the liver: cross-sectional imaging findings with emphasis on MRI. AJR Am J Roentgenol 2005;184(4):1103–1110

Prasad SR, Wang H, Rosas H, et al. Fat-containing lesions of the liver: radiologic-pathologic correlation. Radiographics 2005;25(2):321–331 PubMed

Case 70

Huang CC, Ko SF, Huang HY, et al. Epidermal cysts in the superficial soft tissue: sonographic features with an emphasis on the pseudotestis pattern. J Ultrasound Med 2011;30(1):11–17 PubMed

Case 71

Gaitini D, Soudack M. Diagnosing carotid stenosis by Doppler sonography: state of the art. J Ultrasound Med 2005;24(8):1127–1136 PubMed

Rohren EM, Kliewer MA, Carroll BA, Hertzberg BS. A spectral of Doppler waveforms in the carotid and vertebral arteries. AJR Am J Roentgenol 2003;181(6):1695–1704

Case 72

Tchelepi H, Ralls PW. Ultrasound of focal liver masses. Ultrasound Q 2004;20(4):155–169 PubMed

Case 73

Kanterman RY, Darcy MD, Middleton WD, Sterling KM, Teefey SA, Pilgram TK. Doppler sonographic findings associated with transjugular intrahepatic portosystemic shunt malfunction. AJR Am J Roentgenol 1997;168(2):467–472

Case 74

Khati NJ, Hill MC, Kimmel PL. The role of ultrasound in renal insufficiency: the essentials. Ultrasound Q 2005;21(4):227–244 PubMed

Case 75

Bertolotto M, ed. Peyronie's disease. In: Color Doppler Ultrasound of the Penis. New York: Springer-Verlag; 2008:61–69

Case 76

Gallego C, Velasco M, Marcuello P, Tejedor D, De Campo L, Friera A. Congenital and acquired anomalies of the portal venous system. Radiographics 2002;22(1):141–159 PubMed

Case 77

Akbar SA, Jafri SZ, Amendola MA, Madrazo BL, Salem R, Bis KG. Complications of renal transplantation. Radiographics 2005;25(5):1335–1356 PubMed

Case 78

Vikram R, Sandler CM, Ng CS. Imaging and staging of transitional cell carcinoma: part 2, upper urinary tract. AJR Am J Roentgenol 2009;192(6):1488–1493 PubMed

Case 79

Salem S, Wilson SR. Gynecologic ultrasound. In: Rumack CM, Wilson SR, Charboneau JW, Johnson J, eds. Diagnostic Ultrasound. 3rd ed. St. Louis: Elsevier; 2005:527–587

Case 80

Charalel RA, Jeffrey RB, Shin LK. Complicated cholecystitis: the complementary roles of sonography and computed tomography. Ultrasound Q 2011;27(3):161–170 PubMed

Case 81

Sanders R, Winter T, eds. Intrauterine contraceptive devices. In: Clinical Sonography: A Practical Guide. 4th ed. Philadelphia: Lippincott, Williams & Wilkins; 2007:317–340

Case 82

Katabathina VS, Kota G, Dasyam AK, Shanbhogue AK, Prasad SR. Adult renal cystic disease: a genetic, biological, and developmental primer. Radiographics 2010;30(6):1509–1523 PubMed

Khati NJ, Hill MC, Kimmel PL. The role of ultrasound in renal insufficiency: the essentials. Ultrasound Q 2005;21(4):227–244 PubMed

Case 83

Wilson SR, Withers CE. The liver. In: Rumack CM, Wilson SR, Charboneau JW, Johnson J, eds. Diagnostic Ultrasound. 3rd ed. St. Louis: Elsevier; 2005:77–145

Case 84

Katabathina VS, Kota G, Dasyam AK, Shanbhogue AK, Prasad SR. Adult renal cystic disease: a genetic, biological, and developmental primer. Radiographics 2010;30(6):1509–1523 PubMed

Case 85

Cochlin DL, Dubbins PA, Goldberg BB, Halpern EJ, eds. The retroperitoneum and ureters. In: Urogenital Ultrasound: A Text Atlas. Boca Raton, FL: CRC Press; 2006:326–349

De Bruyn R. Pediatric urologic ultrasound. In: Cochlin DL, Dubbins PA, Goldberg BB, Halpern EJ, eds. Urogenital Ultrasound: A Text Atlas. Boca Raton, FL: CRC Press; 2006:361–389

Case 86

Healy KA, Ogan K. Pathophysiology and management of infectious staghorn calculi. Urol Clin North Am 2007;34(3):363–374 PubMed

Case 87

Stravos T. Male genital system. In: Bluth EI, Benson CB, Ralls PW, Siegel MJ, eds. Ultrasound: A Practical Approach to Clinical Problems. 2nd ed. New York: Thieme; 2007:xx–xx

Gorman B, Carroll BA. The scrotum. In: Rumack CM, Wilson SR, Charboneau JW, Johnson J, eds. Diagnostic Ultrasound. 3rd ed. St. Louis: Elsevier; 2005:849–888

Case 88

Caskey C. Ultrasound techniques for evaluating renal masses, renal obstruction, and other upper tract pathology. Ultrasound Q 2000;16(1):23–39

Rha SE, Byun JY, Jung SE, et al. The renal sinus: pathologic spectrum and multimodality imaging approach. Radiographics 2004;24(Suppl 1):S117–S131 PubMed

Case 89

Cokkinos D, Dourakis S, Spyridon P. Ultrasonographic assessment of cirrhosis and portal hypertension. In: Current Medical Imaging and Reviews. 2009:62–70 70.

Case 90

Langer JE, Oliver ER, Lev-Toaff AS, Coleman BG. Imaging of the female pelvis through the life cycle. Radiographics 2012;32(6):1575–1597 PubMed

Case 91

Levy C, Lyons E. Sonography of multifetal pregnancy. In: Rumack CM, Wilson SR, Charboneau JW, Johnson J, eds. Diagnostic Ultrasound. 3rd ed. St. Louis: Elsevier; 2005:1185–1212

Case 92

Corwin MT, Siewert B, Sheiman RG, Kane RA. Incidentally detected gallbladder polyps: is follow-up necessary?—Long-term clinical and US analysis of 346 patients. Radiology 2011;258(1):277–282 PubMed

Kane R. What do I do with gallbladder polyps? Are they significant? Are there any reasonable size criteria that I can use to determine which need follow-up imaging or even surgery? SRU Newsletter [serial online]. July 2013;23(3):7–8

Case 93

Stavros T. Male genital system. In: Bluth EI, Benson CB, Ralls PW, Siegel MJ, eds. Ultrasound: A Practical Approach to Clinical Problems. 2nd ed. New York: Thieme; 2007:135–152

Case 94

Chaudhary V, Bano S. Thyroid ultrasound. Indian J Endocrinol Metab 2013;17(2):219–227 PubMed

Case 95

Sidhu PS. Disease of the testis and epididymis. In: Baxter GM, Sidhu PS, eds. Ultrasound of the Urogenital System. Stuttgart: Thieme; 2009:153–180

Yang DM, Kim SH, Kim HN, et al. Differential diagnosis of focal epididymal lesions with gray scale sonographic, color Doppler sonographic, and clinical features. J Ultrasound Med 2003;22(2):135–142, quiz 143–144 PubMed

Case 96

Dombale VD, et al. Symmetric diffuse lipomatosis of the thyroid gland. J Clin Diagnos Research 2011;5(4):867–868

Gupta R, Arora R, Sharma A, Dinda AK. Diffuse lipomatosis of the thyroid gland: a pathologic curiosity. Indian J Pathol Microbiol 2009;52(2):215–216 PubMed

Case 97

Catalano O, Sandomenico F, Raso MM, Siani A. Low mechanical index contrast-enhanced sonographic findings of pyogenic hepatic abscesses. AJR Am J Roentgenol 2004;182(2):447–450 PubMed

Case 98

McNaughton DA, Abu-Yousef MM. Doppler US of the liver made simple. Radiographics 2011;31(1):161–188 PubMed

Scheinfeld MH, Bilali A, Koenigsberg M. Understanding the spectral Doppler waveform of the hepatic veins in health and disease. Radiographics 2009;29(7):2081–2098 PubMed

Wood MM, Romine LE, Lee YK, et al. Spectral Doppler signature waveforms in ultrasonography: a review of normal and abnormal waveforms. Ultrasound Q 2010;26(2):83–99 PubMed

Case 99

Gillen MA. The spleen. In: McGahan JP, Goldberg BB, eds. Diagnostic Ultrasound. 2nd ed. New York: Informa Healthcare; 2008:801–822

Case 100

Mohaghegh P, Rockall AG. Imaging strategy for early ovarian cancer: characterization of adnexal masses with conventional and advanced imaging techniques. Radiographics 2012;32(6):1751–1773 PubMed

Twickler DM, Moschos E. Ultrasound and assessment of ovarian cancer risk. AJR Am J Roentgenol 2010;194(2):322–329 PubMed

Index

Locators refer to case number. Locators in boldface indicate primary diagnosis.

U

V

W

X